The Anti-ageing Beauty Bible

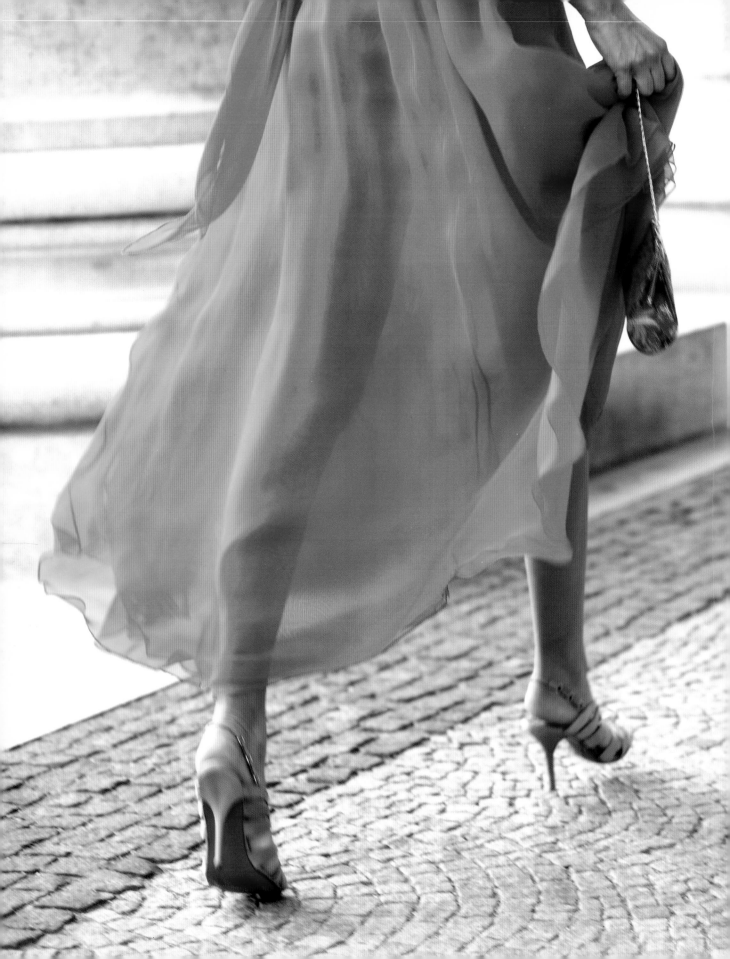

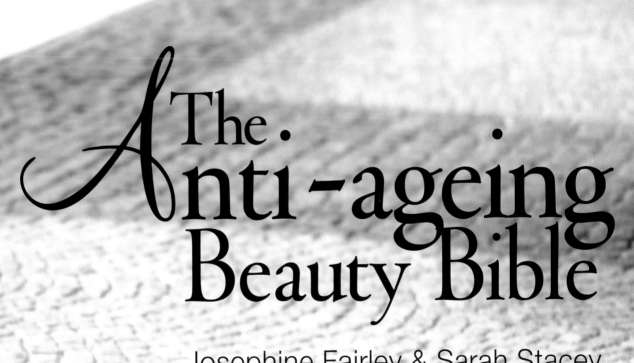

The Anti-ageing Beauty Bible

Josephine Fairley & Sarah Stacey

Illustrations by David Downton

Kyle Books

Contents

It's this simple:

there has never been a better time to age. Every year, billions are poured into research into the creams, the vitamins, the age-spot-zapping lasers (and even magic tummy-flattening pants!), and the light-reflecting make-up innovations which can help us look great for our age, whatever our age

There are fabulous role models out there, too, to give us all hope. Women we know as friends. Women we see in magazines, or on screen, from Helen Mirren (who wouldn't want to look that good in a bikini at any age?), Julianne Moore, Cate Blanchett, Susan Sarandon, Oprah Winfrey, Isabella Rossellini and Sophia Loren. (Even, God bless her, Joan Collins, who just keeps pushing back the threshold for what's considered 'old': first forty, then fifty, sixty, and now – who knows where it'll end…?) We know plenty of women who once would have been written off as 'middle-aged' at forty, who are back-packing, dating, even clubbing (a dance-step too far, for us, but why on earth not…?) up to their eighties.

If you're reading this book, we know one thing: you want to stay looking and feeling your absolute best, for as long as possible. (Without, necessarily, going under the knife or having invasive treatments. Although in *The Anti-Ageing Beauty Bible* we've some advice on that, too – even if personally we'd never help nature along quite so drastically for ourselves.)

The real challenge for so many women is that as the years go by, our confidence wobbles. We can lose our way. We don't look the way we always did, but we haven't worked out how to embrace this new phase. One key thing we've observed as we look around: women can start to 'fade away'. Complexions get paler. Hair colour, ditto. And if we're not careful, we start dressing to match, to reflect the fact we feel a bit low-key, a bit less va-va-voom – in muted shades that eventually make us look like a ghost of our former, younger, more attractive-feeling selves.

But it doesn't have to be like that!!!!! Women really don't have to do a vanishing act. We know, because we've talked to the experts – from globally renowned hair colour wizards to A-list nutritionists, facial massage gurus to experts who know how to keep our brains sharp, too. (Because it's all very well knowing which concealer's going to blitz your under-eye circles, but it really helps if you can remember where you put your make-up bag…! Not to mention the car keys, your glasses, etc.) And if you're bothered by the effects of gravity, we've talked to people who can help everything become that bit more 'pert' again – from faces to thighs, even foot arches!

Crucially, we've tapped into the wisdom of

You're *never* too old to become *younger*

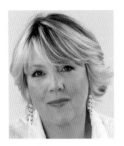
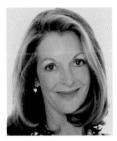

make-up professionals who understand mature faces, because they're facing the challenge of lines and wrinkles or 'sun spots' themselves, every day when they look in the mirror. Because make-up – applied well – can be your quickest way to drop a decade in little more than a flash. In fact, our advice to women who write to us for advice because they're contemplating a facelift is simple: get a makeover first. It is truly, truly, truly miraculous what the right foundation (with primer first), concealer, lipstick and brow pencil can achieve.

But which concealer, which moisturising lipstick, which age-defying foundation? (Not to mention which are the best anti-ageing eye creams, or shine-restoring hair masks, or body firming creams…?) As beauty editors, that's what we're asked all the time, and the signature of our best-selling Beauty Bible series of books has been pointing you in the direction of the products which really, truly perform.

As usual, we recruited 2,400 real women – all aged from 35 to well into their sixties – to put container-loads of anti-ageing products through their paces, over a period of three months or longer. There are super-whizz-bang, high-tech options, and all-natural choices (and our 'daisy rating' – see box right – helps you identify those).

What our testers' incredibly consistent comments and scores (out of ten) confirm is something we've known for a while: that there truly are many, many products out there which can help you look younger. Not as young as your 19-year-old daughter (let alone granddaughter), or the intern in your office. But radiant. Glowing. Not someone who's fading into the distance, but who's right here, right now: enjoying your life, looking and feeling the best you possibly can.

This book is exceedingly close to our own hearts – having a joint age of over 112, as we sat down to put manicured digits to Apple keyboard. But yes, we do constantly get compliments about 'looking good for our age'. Which, frankly, are the compliments that any woman *d'un certain âge* wants to hear.

Through the pages of this book – organised as an A to Z of everything that our friends and readers have told us bothers them about ageing – we are about to help you feel your best. Look your best. And be your best, too. Life is no dress rehearsal and we only get one chance to enjoy this one.

The truth is that when your daily 'self-care' ritual is sorted – from the right skincare to the perfect make-up to haircare to at least a little bit of exercise – then you can do the things you still long to do, explore the passions you yearn to pursue, be the woman you'd really like to be.

Trust us: age really can be a thing of the past.

With love,

Jo Sarah x

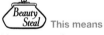
www.beautybible.com Don't forget: you can follow us on Twitter: @Beauty_Bible!

10 important things you need to know about make-up

While perusing 24,000 forms (yes, it nearly killed us) from the ten-women tester panels who trialled literally thousands of products for this latest Beauty Bible (which we believe is the definitive guide to ageing gorgeously), we realised there were some key myths and misconceptions about make-up. And also some key secrets that everyone simply needs to know – because make-up isn't cheap, and you want to get the very best value out of the cosmetics you buy.

So (with apologies to those of you who basically have a degree in make-up and know this stuff already), here goes.

A primer goes over moisturiser, under foundation. Used on their own, primers aren't moisturising enough. And if you're not sure why you need this extra step in your make-up regime, turn to page 89 to find out how primers will help you create the most flawless canvas ever for your foundation – and make it last longer.

Apply eyeshadow and other eye make-up before your base, though. That way, if it 'sheds', it's easy to clean up and won't spoil your foundation.

For eyeshadow, it also helps to own a 'blending brush'. This is quite simply the best way to make sure all the edges of your shadow are seamless. Jemma Kidd recommends dipping the blender brush in a little translucent powder and buffing over eyes to soften. ('The idea is to "sheer down" the colour, not remove it,' she advises.) All brush ranges feature a 'blender' brush, and if you can't identify it – well, that's what sales consultants are for.

The time to apply light-reflecting concealer (or a brightener) is before foundation. If applying under eyes, use the brush/wand to trace a triangle down from the corners of the eye to meet in the middle of the under-eye zone, and then blend with brush or ring finger. On eyelids, start in the inner corner by your nose.

Apply flaw-correcting concealers over foundation. Once you've evened out your skintone, you may not need so much.

Dry, dull-looking skin makes you look much older than you are. Youthful skin isn't powdery and one-dimensional; it's radiant. So we swear by this tip from Laura Mercier to achieve that, fast: 'Use the tiniest bit of a light moisturiser patted around the outer eyes and along the top lip over your make-up. It makes skin look fresh, not dry, and it's a great de-ager as it stops make-up settling into any fine lines.' (You can do this during the day to refresh make-up, too.)

You really don't have to live with dry, cracked lips. But lip balm is only half the answer. Lips respond beautifully to buffing: press a wet flannel on to your lips, then use it to gently rub away flakes and roughness. And then slather on your balm or lip treatment (we've lots of good ones on page 137). Your lip pencil will glide on more smoothly, too: even the creamiest of these can be drying.

There's a quick way to deal with eye-make-up smudges. Don't ask us why make-up seems to flake and speck more now we're older – but it often does seem to, and during a busy day you don't have time to start again. MAC Cleansing Tips are infused with make-up remover, so very handy – but better still, roll a Q-tip in a very little bit of foundation, then roll it back and forth over the eye zone. It removes smudges – but doesn't leave skin 'naked'.

Remember: self-tanner will always look patchy unless you exfoliate and moisturise first. It really is that simple, and not buffing and hydrating skin is the number one reason why we get negative comments from our testers about some fake tans. (OK, this isn't strictly make-up. But we have lots of testers who need to understand this!)

And whatever else you do, get a regular makeover. It's easy to treat make-up like a trusty recipe – finding something that works and clinging to it long after it's stopped doing what it once did for you – so we recommend regular makeovers. These are free (or at the very least, redeemable against purchase). There is no better way to discover what make-up can do to counterbalance the fact that skin has become thinner, thirstier and more transparent, or its tone has altered and faded. A good in-store make-up pro – we particularly recommend the make-up artists at Laura Mercier, Bobbi Brown, Trish McEvoy and on the By Terry counter in Space NK branches – can also help show you tricks to deal with lips that are thinning, eyes that are drooping and a chin or nose that is becoming 'longer'. As the ads say, Just. Do. It. (Please!)

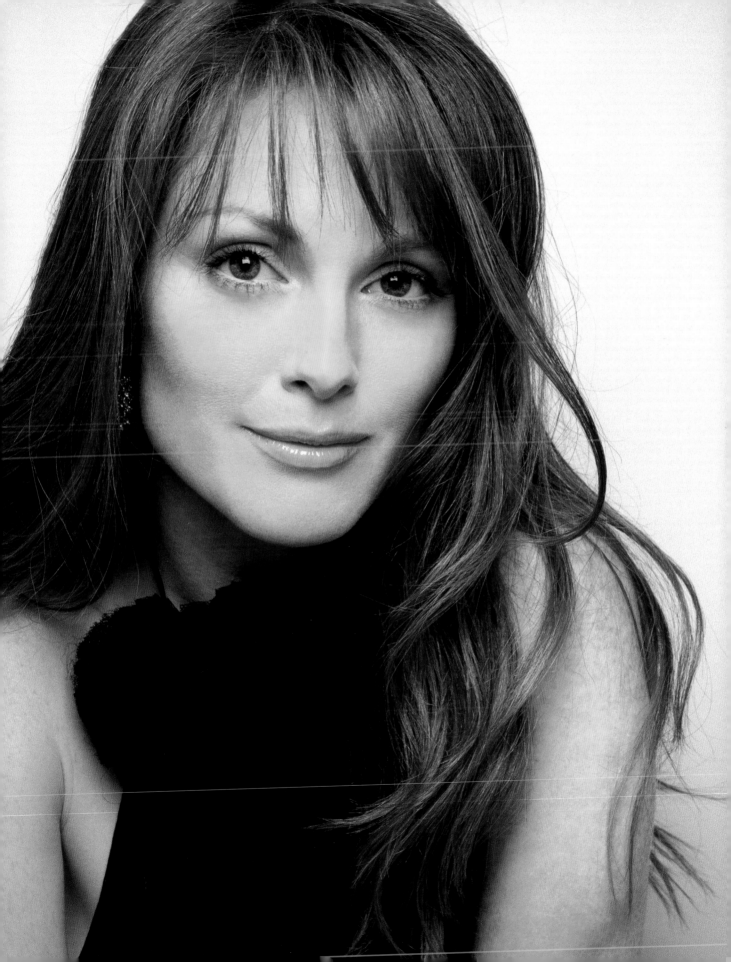

Cosmetics:
your top 10 products

Before you consider a facelift, buy these Make-up Musts

We have four words to say when friends and readers tell us they're considering 'having work done', or even Botox. 'Have a make-up makeover.' Make-up really can work miracles. And showcased here are the ten make-up essentials that we know can melt away the years – blurring lines, delivering radiance and making skin look dewily fresher, smoother and younger. We feel strongly that cosmetic surgery (and even cosmeto-dermatology) should be a last resort. Trust us: by ensuring that your make-up kit features these ten categories of cosmetics, you really can drop a decade – with the wave of a magic (concealer) wand.

1 A make-up primer. With silicones (to smooth the skin) and light-reflective pigments (to 'blur' the appearance of fine lines), a make-up primer also helps solve the problem of make-up that 'disappears' into thin air, which can be a particular problem for drier, mature complexions. (For specific recommendations, see page 89.)

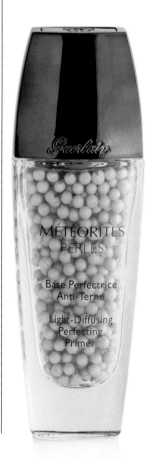

2 A 'line-smoother'. Real magic, these. Again, they feature silicones and sometimes even nylon particles, and can be applied as required to deep grooves and finer lines. (Personally, we favour the type with a teensy nozzle, for targeted application.) They simply 'sit' on the skin's surface, and can be patted into the skin to create a truly velvety surface. Lines? Now you see them. And now, with these, you don't. (Our testers' favourites are on page 95.)

3 An anti-ageing foundation. Many foundations now have age-defying properties. These can work in several ways: through the addition of skin-caring ingredients, plus moisturisers to ensure skin looks 'plumper'. This new generation of 'anti-ageing' foundations also harnesses the power of 'optical pigments'. (Want to know which ones are worth investing in? Turn to page 90 for our testers' experiences.)

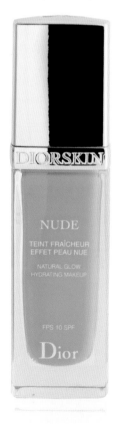

4 A light-reflective concealer. We probably get more anxious queries addressed to www. beautybible.com about dark circles than any other beauty woe. As well as effective lifestyle tips (on page 54), we bring you the low-down on the wand-style concealers which go a long way to disguising the darkest circles, and can lessen the appearance of deep grooves and lines. (For Beauty Bible award-winning concealers, go to page 91.)

5 Cream blusher. Lots of reasons to love this. First, the texture 'melts' into skin, so doesn't look dusty (which is always a risk, as we age). That makes it fairly goof-proof, too. But another reason cream blush should nudge the powder option out of your kit once you hit 35 plus is that it adds another layer of moisturising protection against the elements. (Which versions did our testers rate? Look at page 23.)

6 Lip pencil. Does double-duty, at this phase in life: it not only defines lips (the contours of which can become blurrier with the years), but it helps prevent lipstick from 'travelling' into feathered lines. (For the best, see page 135.)

7 Lip gloss. Recent research showed that the plumpness of lips is a way that we (subconsciously) gauge an individual's age. Lip gloss is the fast-track to a juicier pout: a smoosh on the lower lip makes them look instantly fuller. (But because not all lip glosses are created equal, you'll want to read our panellists' opinions, on page 134.)

8 A bone-coloured cream eyeshadow. You can shade your eyes with a rainbow of colours, but our prescription is always to use a neutral eyeshadow as a base, first. Why? Because it evens out the skintone of the eyelids, which tends to darken and redden as we age, while at the same time creating a velvety-smooth, even base for shadow – whether that's another cream version (turn to page 70 for our testers' favourites), or powder.

9 Brow colour. Because 'not fade away' should be your beauty mantra, at this time in your life – and because defined, groomed brows help give your face much-needed structure. (The most outstanding brow pencils on the market are listed on page 64.)

10 Waterproof mascara. A boon, as we age, because waterproof mascara stays put through hot flushes and survives watery eyes. It's a fact: eyes get touchier and well up more as the years roll by. (It's hard to find a good version – one which neither gives you panda eyes by teatime, nor requires industrial-strength remover – so our testers tried them all on your behalf. See page 73 for those that 'wowed'.)

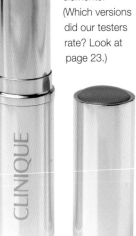

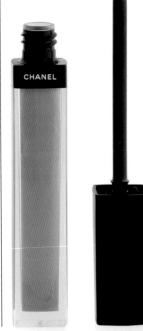

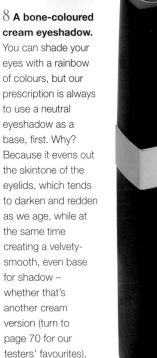

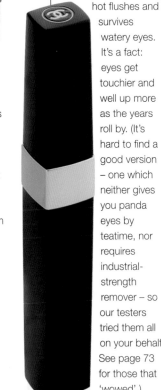

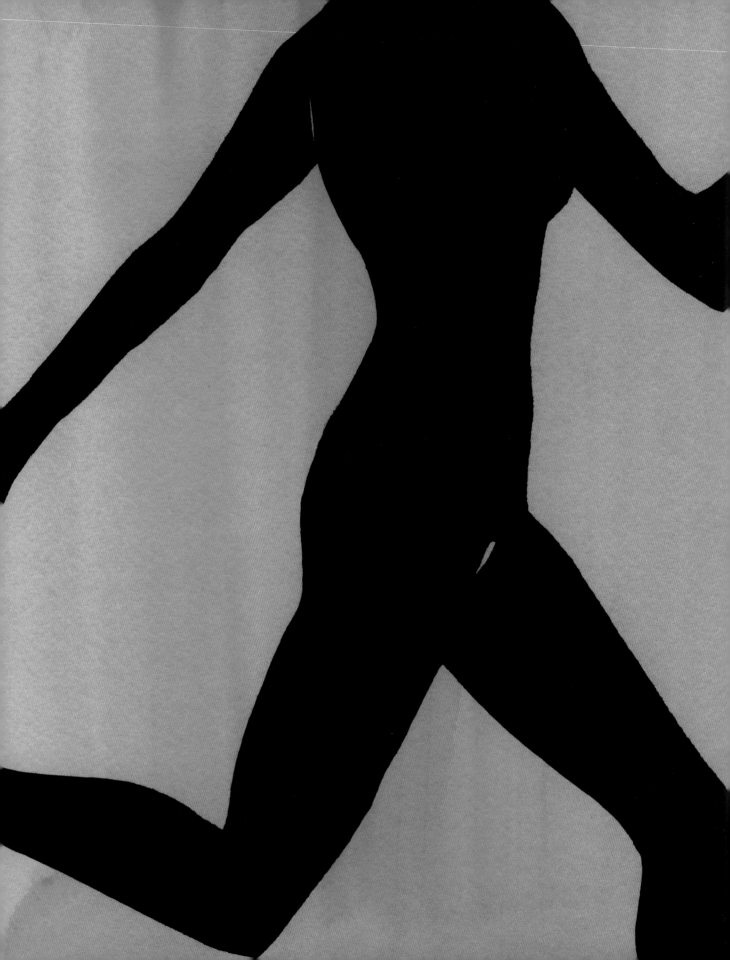

LOVE
the BODY
you're in
...and it will
LOVE YOU
right back

Be more active
(your body will love you for it)

A simple programme of daily exercises will help tone your body – and make you feel happier, too. So counteract the force of gravity by following our 10 easy steps to a firmer, fitter, more confident you…

As the T-shirt slogan goes, 'Gravity sucks'. Because after 35 (if not before), bodies start to head south. At the same time, our bodies get stiffer and less flexible. Some people embark on a major blitz to counteract this – the gym, jogging, Pilates, whatever. But the best strategy to start with is simply to become more active, all the time – then you can add your favourite exercise, as we suggest below. Being more active boosts the rate at which the body burns calories. It firms you up and (done properly) stretches you out. And it also produces feel-good hormones called endorphins so that your mood, as well as your body, feels less saggy.

So if you're standing disconsolately in front of a long mirror in your undies and wondering what on earth you can do to shape up and/or slim down, take heart. Embarking on a simple daily programme of little shifts will really make a difference to your body (and at the same time, to how you feel about showing it – on the beach, to a new lover, or in that Little Black Dress that used to fit but doesn't now). Best of all, you can start in your very own bed. (Although probably better alone, in this instance…)

1 **When you wake up,** lie straight and flat in your bed, take a few slow, deep breaths (in through your nose and very slowly out through your mouth), then lift your arms above your head and point your toes, feeling the stretch right through your body on both sides. Stretch your whole body, then each side, and finish with your whole body again.

2 **While the kettle boils,** tense your buttock muscles ten times for ten seconds each time. The more you practise this, the firmer your bottom will become, so practise whenever you're standing: waiting at the bus stop, stirring a pan, queueing to pay in a shop, etc.

3 **While you brush your teeth** for the recommended three minutes morning and evening, squat down with your back against the wall or door. (It feels weird, but it's a great stretch.)

4 **When you're watching TV,** hide the remote control and when you get up to change channels, do ten squats to tone your upper thighs. As you squat down, with your back straight, push your weight down through your heels so the front of your thighs work harder.

5 **Tone up your arms and bingo wings** by pushing light weights above your head: do ten pushes at a time, as many times a day as you can. No weights? Use cans of baked beans. (We love baked beans – to eat! – especially with a slurp of olive oil and grated Parmesan.)

6 Lose five pounds by improving your posture…

• Stand up straight, as if the crown of your head is suspended from a thread in the ceiling/sky.

• Let your shoulders sink down and back: feel as if your shoulder blades are meeting at the back.

• Do a few shoulder rolls both ways while you are sitting at your desk or on the train.

• Walk like a cat (think model on catwalk…), hips swinging forward with your big toe leading.

7 Walk briskly everywhere you can, swinging your arms (put belongings in a back pack – the kind that fastens across your front is easiest if you carry a lot). Look for hills and climb stairs rather than using the lift. Get in the habit of striding out for at least 15 minutes in the evenings to help you relax. You should aim for 10,000 steps a day – easy to calculate if you have a pedometer.

8 Every time you get up from a chair, consciously pull your belly button in towards your spine to work your tummy muscles. If you are picking up things from the floor, bend sideways while pulling in your tummy to help smooth your love handles.

9 Finally, do exercise you enjoy. Whether it's walking or swimming, dancing or yoga, riding or fencing, if you look forward to it you are far more likely to stick with it and get a feel-good double whammy. Aim for at least 30 minutes, five days a week.

10 Make all of this a habit. It takes 16 to 21 times of repeating an activity for it to become a habit – so in less than a month, all this can become second nature. And by then you should look very luscious in that Little Black Dress.

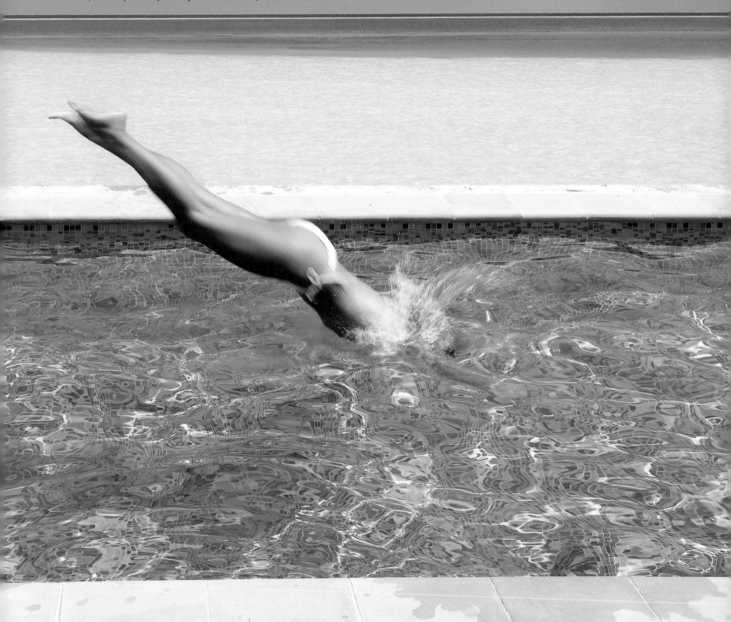

First, find your MIRACLE

We recruited 2,400 women specifically for the all-new trials in this book, and they have confirmed what we've known for years: that there really are creams and serums that magic the years from your face. The challenge is: how on earth do you find out which ones…? Well, there's no need for (expensive) trial and error – because our testers have done the research for you.

For this section of the book, we dispatched over 200 'miracle' products – from high street/supermarket anti-agers right through to the priciest creams on the market. Our ten-women tester panels were under strict instructions: use the treatment on one side of your face, observe and note any immediate improvements, then after two weeks, and finally, at the end of the tube or jar. (NB: many of our testers started out cynical – and were converted.)

OK, so no cream is going to make you look 17 again, waving a wand to magic away every line and wrinkle. But the scores for these 'miracle' treatments featured here are high – and that's despite the fact we ask testers to compare the results with the extravagant promises made on the packaging. So: there really ARE products which, as well as softening and smoothing your complexion, can help plump out deeper lines, make smaller ones disappear, firm skin tissue – and turbo-charge the glow, which has a big impact on how others perceive us. (Age really is in the eye of the beholder…)

We also know that massaging in any skincare product enhances the effect – and indeed some of these products come with instructions. (On page 78 you will find simple guidelines.) For more 'miracles' – in the form of specific night treatments – please see page 156, while miracle serums are on page 172.

Now, just before you dive in… Although, as we've explained, we tested all price ranges for this book, the simple truth is that all the top scoring ones are pretty pricey. However, when we specifically trialled £20-and-under 'miracle' creams for our previous book *Beauty Bible Beauty Steals* (which also comes as an iPhone App, see DIRECTORY), we did get some terrific scores and comments. So in the panel on page 19 you will find a rundown of the winning moderately-priced creams from that book.

Anti-ageing miracle creams: *our award winners*

REVIEWS

L'Occitane Immortelle Divine Cream

 8.98 / 10 A stunning score for this 'divine' combination featuring organic essential oils of the botanicals immortelle and myrtle, from a Provençal-born range which now has a world-wide reach. Silky-textured, it's enriched with 34 per cent plant oils and is formulated to boost cell regeneration and 'increase cellular vitality', which translates to enhanced radiance.

Comments: 'Love the texture and smell, it took a little while to sink in but it was worth the wait; skin instantly looked brighter and much smoother and plumped; after two weeks, fine lines around mouth much less noticeable and skin much more supple, and the improvements continued: my husband said my skin was looking nice and for him to notice is quite remarkable' • 'my skin hasn't looked so good for a long time, so much brighter I look as if I've had a good night's sleep; crêpiness, fine lines, grooves all reduced – a fantastic product and I got lots of positive comments' • 'lovely thick product with fabulous smell, absorbed very well and skin felt so hydrated and really supple; definitely boosts the skin; but do give it five or ten minutes before applying make-up' • 'complexion was more plump, less drawn, less sagging, with really nice bright glow, eyes glowed too and normally ruddy complexion reduced; improvements continued as long as I was using it…'.

Guerlain Orchidée Impériale Exceptional Complete Care Cream

8.88 / 10 You will be seeing Guerlain's name many times in this book, with some truly spectacular results for the Orchidée Impériale range, which (as the name suggests) harnesses a special orchid extract 'to infuse the skin with extraordinary longevity' (!). It falls into the category of a 'supercream', with a slightly heart-stopping price. And, of course, this is blessed with a heavenly Guerlain-esque fragrance.

Comments: '10 marks for this thick cream which was very quickly absorbed and immediately firmed and re-conditioned my skin, fine lines temporarily smoothed and skin nicely plump, very good base for make-up; after the jar was finished, skin appears much brighter, luminous and radiant, incredibly soft, eyes appear slightly lifted, fine lines improved: people have commented on the improvement and asked what's happened' • 'I don't feel embarrassed about going out without make-up now; I wonder if the facial massage improves circulation? Skin feels and looks younger and "lifted"' • 'definite visible improvements, especially smoother and brighter skin, which is younger looking' • 'within 60 seconds, skin has a healthy sheen, over the weeks skin drinks it in with relish – definitely the best moisturiser I have ever used, skin is so much brighter I feel glowing and radiant, soft, smooth and silky – I haven't looked like this since I was in my early twenties – I've even been accused of having a facelift'.

Decléor Excellence de l'Âge Sublime Regenerating Cream

 8.87 / 10 A day cream (Decléor like their customers to use oils at night), this meltingly-smooth cream-textured cream works to enhance firmness, smoothness, hydration, and to even out skintone. As you'd expect from an aromatherapy brand, fragrance is an important part of the pleasure factor, although this is powdery/creamy (with notes of sandalwood, amber and peach) rather than 'botanically-scented'.

Comments: 'I was dubious as this cream looked too rich and thick for my oily combination skin

If you know you have sensitive skin and you want to try a powerful anti-ageing treatment, go carefully. Start by using the product two or three times a week, and build up from there. Alternatively, do a 'patch test' (using the crook of your elbow or the skin just behind the ear), and check for any redness/ irritation/flakiness 24 hours later. If that happens, you may be one of the people who simply can't tolerate some ingredients – and if you do suffer a reaction, it is always worth taking the product back to the counter (although the beauty industry will probably have hit-men trained on us for suggesting this). Sometimes a sympathetic sales consultant feels empowered to give you a refund, confident that you'll be back again in future. (Which you certainly won't be, if they don't.)

but it is amazing, after five weeks skin looks luminous, almost glass-like, firmer, smoother and springy to the touch – rejuvenated' • 'fine lines reduced, deeper grooves too, and crêpiness? There is none! This cream really makes me look better and younger, lots of people have commented' • 'immediate discernable improvements, skin felt softer, less dry, fine lines plumped out and after two weeks, skin looks more youthful, fine lines less visible, skin around eyes and lips less dry and crêpey, overall more radiant and fresh-looking – works wonders on an ageing face' • 'skin looks brighter and love the texture and scent'.

Dermalogica Power Rich Cream

This is Dermalogica's state-of-the-art anti-ageing cream, luxuriously priced (though not as much of a splurge as the Guerlain on page 17). It claims to use a trio of 'pharmaceutical-strength' ingredients, and comes in the format of a 35-day supply of (five) sealed metal tubes, complete with a key (think glamorous sardine tin!), to squeeze out every last skin-regenerating, vitamin-and-antioxidant-powered molecule. One poor score was balanced by the majority who loved this product and marked it very highly indeed.

Comments: 'The first night I applied this I woke up and thought the spa fairies had been at work all night: my skin glowed, had a wonderful aliveness and look of youth and vitality; after two weeks complexion was great despite the harsh weather outside and heating inside – wonderful plump, smooth skin; youth in a tube (the only downside was the rather sweet smell)' • 'wow! What a product, the holy grail of creams, delivered all it promised and more; massive difference between the tested and not tested side: smaller wrinkles faded, pores so much smaller, skintone so much brighter, I LOVE it' • 'skin was much more radiant; initially there was some flakiness after use but after a few days that went, people have commented on how smooth and radiant my skin looks: I would use it every few months as a treatment' • 'the grooves down the sides of my mouth look as if I have been using a filler, they're so plumped up and smoothed out, absolutely fabulous product'.

Melvita Naturalift Anti-Ageing Cream ✿ ✿ ✿

8.67/10

Melvita is a big name in France, now spreading its reach overseas (it's part of the L'Occitane empire). This Ecocert-certified creation blends oligopeptides from hibiscus seed to protect collagen and elastin, argan (for an instant firming action), revitalising chestnut and New Zealand mamaku (derived from a fern), plus potent antioxidants. Subtle but nice scent from rose and geranium.

Comments: 'A friend noticed that my skin looked firmer and my face slimmer; I had seen my skin get brighter and clearer in tone, with less noticeable fine lines, over the time I used it: am very happy with this' • 'my fine lines have improved and that's great, a real visible effect, I enjoyed using the cream because it's very light and yet moisturises very well, also smells delicious and you don't need to use much' • 'as well as skin being brighter, pores finer and less noticeable, and fine lines slightly reduced, this definitely lessened my hyperpigmentation brown patches: I would buy it' • 'no miracles but fine lines and wrinkles plumped out with continued use, and skin soft; did like the lightweight texture and the lovely lemon smell' • 'absolutely wonderful. After finishing the jar, I noted 50 per cent improvement in brightness, 100 per cent in softness and also crêpiness and about 75 per cent reduction in fine lines, plus the two large wrinkles above my eyebrows have reduced in length and depth. I can't believe it! My friends and family have certainly noticed a difference and paid me compliments on looking younger'.

Elemis Cellular Recovery Skin Bliss Capsules ✿

8.5/10

This winner – featuring a programme of single-dose capsules containing facial oils which you open and apply – proves to us that our system works. Elemis actually submitted this twice (an admin error, we think). We sent the product to two different sets of women, six months apart. And the average of their scores was absolutely identical: 8.5/10, from both groups! Use one pink capsule (rose-smelling) in the morning, one green (lavender fragrant) capsule at night, ideally using a facial massage to apply the oil.

Comments: 'Silky, oily texture sank in almost instantly and made skin softer and smoother;

after two weeks, I could see a big difference; handy that you can take just the right number if you go away but make sure they're well-wrapped so they don't puncture and leak' • 'beautiful product with gorgeous smell' • 'definite improvement in softness and brightness, due to the product and the massage, seemed oily to start with but it wasn't; great product overall, lovely smell and I actually looked forward to using them; because of the consistency you are more likely to massage your skin which can only help' • 'by the end of the jar, I knew this is a really clever product, gives radiance and less crêpiness, fine lines less noticeable as well as smoothness and softness'.

NIA 24 Intensive Recovery Complex

NIA 24 is said to be 'the USA's No 1 recommended physician skincare line', taking its name from pro-niacin: a molecule clinically proven to help reverse photo-ageing. (It's so effective at counteracting sun damage that the National Cancer Institute is researching this as a potential skin cancer prevention agent.) A richly-textured cream, NIA 24's winner features tomato complex, peptides, skintone-evening liquorice, with the bonus of light-diffusing ingredients to 'blur' fine lines instantly.

Comments: '10/10: very positive change in my skin from the first use; after two weeks fine lines less pronounced, skin texture very soft, overall glow, my face looks very bright and healthy, less wrinkled and no spots – much fresher and more youthful-looking' • 'sinks in quickly which is a plus, I hate heaviness; definite improvement in softness which I didn't think possible – I keep touching my skin; skin texture slightly improved' • 'really gorgeous fluffy texture and fresh fragrance, sinks in beautifully; skin immediately brighter, very clear and after I finished the jar it's definitely younger-looking, softer and smoother, no dramatic improvements with fine lines and wrinkles but the general glow of wellbeing distracts from them; compliments about looking well and skin looking good' • 'pores look smaller, and seems to have evened out some of my freckles' • 'a facelift in a jar: my skin has never looked better, all my lines have reduced in depth, tone is brighter and more even and jawline more defined: old colleagues who I hadn't seen for ages told me I look fabulous!'.

Beauty Steals

As we explained on page 16, these 'miracle' products did incredibly well in our book *Beauty Bible Beauty Steals*, which is also available as an App for your iPhone (see DIRECTORY). So if you're having a budget-watching time, they're really worth considering.

L'Oréal Derma-Genesis Cellular Youth Nurturing Night Cream

This high-scoring product springs from L'Oréal's labs and reflects their huge commitment to age-defying R&D. Like its sister anti-ageing eye treatment (which also scored highly in *Beauty Bible Beauty Steals*) this contains high levels of skin-plumping hyaluronic acid, plus L'Oréal's patented Pro-Xylane ingredient.

Comments: 'Gorgeous product; lavender-coloured light cream which is quickly absorbed and a real pleasure to use; the first morning my skin was visibly brighter and slightly plumped; after two weeks, fine lines across forehead and round mouth definitely less visible; neck smoothed, and complexion dramatically brightened' • 'really delighted to find such an effective product at a price I could afford'.

Neal's Yard Remedies Frankincense Nourishing Cream

Beauty Bible has trialled this natural product over several years and it has always scored spectacularly with some testers (a few found it too heavy). The rich botanical cream has very high levels of frankincense essential oil, which was used in mummification – so no wonder it's so good at preserving skin. The blend includes oils of wheatgerm, almond and myrrh – renowned for their regenerating and moisturising properties. It can be used under make-up or at night.

Comments: 'I thought it would be too rich for my oily skin but it was miraculous! Skin looked so much younger and plumper and seemed to reduce breakouts: I've never seen such initial dramatic effects which were maintained' • 'the immediate feeling of plumpness has been replaced by a smooth uplift and youthful tightness' • 'I always felt my skin looked colourless and grey until I tested this product'.

Soap & Glory Make Yourself Youthful Rejuvenating Face Serum

A triumph for the amazing Ms Marcia Kilgore with this light, sinks-in-fast serum. It is probably all oily skins need (under fifty), but can be layered under something richer if you're dry-complexioned or post-menopausal. It contains a collagen-stimulating tetrapeptide, a 'superactive stimulating organic oxygenating complex', ginseng, shea butter, sweet orange peel essential oil (which gives the lightest of fragrances) and a 'moisture-trapping complex'.

Comments: 'Glided on the skin wonderfully and sank in quickly; after two weeks a marked improvement to skintone and softness, fine lines slightly less evident, skin had a lovely bright glow' • 'significant improvement in radiance in first 24 hours, skin on neck and chest looked smoother, fine lines a little softer' • 'skin looks younger because more glowing and well hydrated'.

Plump up your cheeks!

If you're looking pale and wan and your cheeks (like the rest of you) are beginning to head south, you can create a brighter, more uplifting appearance in next to no time…

Every woman with a thinnish face knows that when you're tired or under par, you're liable to look a lot less than radiant – peaky, sad and, at worst, like Lady Macbeth's rather haggard first cousin (as Sarah knows all too well…). As the years go by, the upsides of a slender form mean your cheeks tend to drift downwards with the rest of your body. But there are immediate ways to give your cheeks (and thus your whole face) a lift – plus some mid- to long-term strategies which we promise can transform you.

For instant lift, apply a 'pop' of blush to your cheeks (see overleaf for more). And marvel at the mirror…!

Pinch your cheeks. No blusher? Gently pat and pinch your cheeks for a few seconds until they glow rosy pink. Better still, if you have five or ten minutes, do some star-jumps.

Pop on some earrings. Sparkly, shiny or lovely fat pearls, in colours that flatter your skintone – and never, ever dangly. If you can, find ones that wing their way upwards taking your face with them. (Sarah's favourite pair are rather Art Nouveau-ish wings in blue, green and amber-y faceted glass.)

Sweep your hair up. Brush your hair back and up, clip it on top, pop in pretty combs, roll into a pleat… Anything to take the eye of the beholder upwards.

For instant lift, apply a 'pop' of BLUSH to your cheeks, and MARVEL at the mirror!

Try milk! Drinking it, that is – which is a suggestion given to us by Beverly Hills make-up artist Valerie Sarnelle. One of her starry clients (there's a galaxy flashing in and out of her elegant salon) – a *femme d'un certain âge* with divinely plumptious cheeks above her slender form – told Valerie they were due not to cosmetic fillers but milk! We suggest organic full-fat milk from grass-fed moos because it should have more conjugated linoleic acid (CLA), which may help your facial muscles. (Cheeks are the 'meatiest' part of your face, and increasing muscle mass will make them look fuller.) Milk will definitely give you magnesium – great for your mind as it's a natural tranquilliser, and helps with teeth, bones, muscles and sleep, among lots of other things. (We love magnesium!)

Apply skincare products upwards. Whenever you apply skin cream, oil or lotion, always stroke upwards from your chin to your cheekbones, then out to your temples. Facial therapist Suzie Mitchell suggests: 'Put a little facial oil or cream in one palm and rub your hands together, then smooth over the face, neck and bosom. Rather than fingertips, use the big muscle in the cushion at the base of your thumb, always working upwards. Start by fanning out over and round your neck, then work round and up your jaw and cheekbones to the temples, then across and up your forehead to your hairline. Repeat, covering the whole face for five to ten minutes. The oil or cream will be absorbed, skin velvety, and your face look rosy and "lifted".'

Pop some supplements. Consider supplementing with omega-3 essential fatty acids, hyaluronic acid (HA) plus Sun Chlorella. The first two keep skin cells

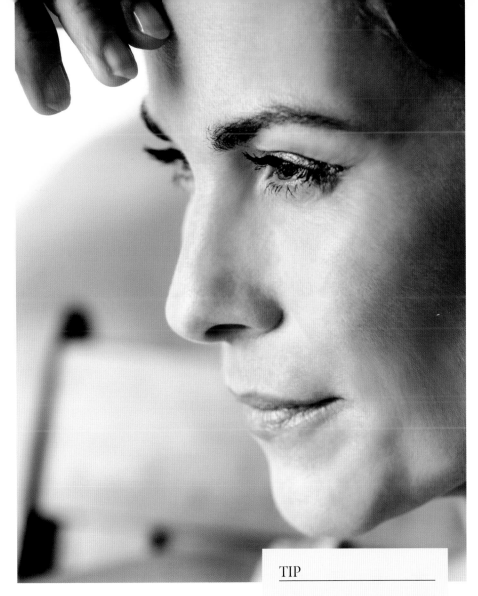

NB: we recommend doing these exercises in private…!

1 Put a finger in your mouth, close your lips round it and suck on your finger for five to ten seconds, as hard as you can while sucking in your cheeks. It's like a child making a fish face. Release, and repeat 15 more times. This will help strengthen your cheek muscles and enhance the circulation and oxygen flow to your face, so your cheeks look more pink and full. It also helps prevent lip lines.

2 Tone your cheeks by placing your fingertips on top of your cheekbones. Now inhale and tilt your chin down towards your collarbone; exhale and push the skin and muscle fibres of the cheekbones upwards. Then open and close your mouth five to ten times, feeling the muscles tightening as you do so. Do this three times a day or as often as you can.

3 Place your index finger and middle finger on each cheek and then slowly rub in a circular motion. This will stimulate the muscles, which will thicken them up and cause them to look fuller. (It also makes your cheeks rosy!)

at optimum lipid (fat) and hydration levels, and we also suggest Sun Chlorella A, a Japanese brand, to keep your gut happy; it really does show on your face, due to the two pairs of stomach meridians which run down the face – one pair down the sides to the chin, one pair from under the eyes to the chin. If your tum's upset, your face gets longer and more gaunt; keep your gut in good shape and you won't believe the difference! Sarah's skin plumped and peachified almost incredibly when she started taking Sun Chlorella, which she anticipates taking for life. (Also see the Supergreens Facelift Diet, page 176.)

Sign up for a course of facial acupuncture. And have regular maintenance sessions (see page 155).

TIP

Supermodel Carmen dell'Orefice recommends doing any inverted (upside down) yoga pose, such as Downward-facing Dog, to bring colour to your face. If you don't practise yoga, simply plant your feet a hip-width apart then try touching your toes. Hang there for a few seconds as the blood pours to your head.

Keep regular appointments with the dentist. Teeth and gums need to be in optimal shape to support your facial bone structure.

And if slimming down rather than plumping up your face is your problem, see our section on facial contouring, on page 44.

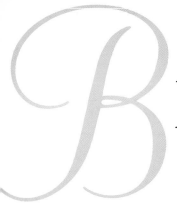

Blush becomingly

A subtle hint of pink blusher applied to the cheeks will bring a youthful glow to your complexion (and we mean subtle – you certainly want to avoid an alarming doll- or clown-like appearance). And it's uplifting too. Here's how to make it work for you…

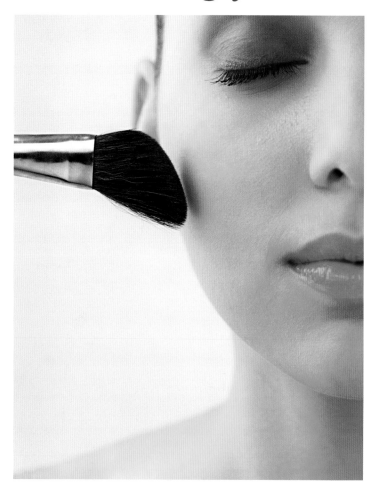

Choose a transparent rose blusher. 'By mid life you are naturally losing that youthful "rosiness",' explains Terry de Gunzburg, 'and you want to recreate that. That doesn't mean turning into a babydoll, but finishing with a hint of blush: a nude rose or a transparent rose, even a pinkish coral, high on the cheeks. Even if you have "couperose" [rosacea/redness], it's very important, but in that case use a beige-y rose. Blusher gives an instant "lifting" effect.'

If you prefer powder blushers, try Chanel Joues Contraste in No 15 Orchid Rose. We're mostly cream blusher girls but less dry skins may be fine with powder. This looks really muddy in the compact but in fact it's a whisper-light soft rose that Mary Greenwell uses on everyone on the planet, with (as we now realise) good reason.

Use the right brushes. Of course cream blushers can be applied with fingers, but we find the best way to apply cream blusher (and to get longer-lasting results) is with a foundation brush; just 'feather' it into the skin with the lightest touch. Jo uses the flip side of her regular foundation brush, but if you do the same, you need to be religious about washing your brushes once a week or the blusher shade starts to 'pinkify' the foundation (to be avoided at all costs). For a powder blusher, apply an angled blusher brush with the short side on top, laid against your

TIP

Cream (or gel) blusher tends to fade on your cheeks, so 'set' it with a touch of translucent powder, and remember to take it with you for touch-ups.

cheekbone, to wrap the colour around without overloading it. Try them out in store to find one with a handle that suits your grip – personally we don't like too-short handles, but they might suit you.

Remember: nobody blushes brown. Because many women with high colour are scared that pink blusher will draw attention to that, they're tempted to use bronzer instead of blusher, so that it won't pick up the redness. Don't go there. Instead, use foundation to tone down that redness and then – as above – a very soft pinky shade on the top.

And never forget that less really is more. You need a whisper of colour not warpaint.

Cream blushers: *our award winners*

Cream (and cream/gel) blushers are much friendlier to mature skins than powder versions. They never look dry and dusty, and are pretty fool-proof (you can use fingers for blending – although see opposite for more secrets of truly seamless application). An increasing number of brands now offer cream blusher formulations, and we trialled almost 20 different versions for this book. We requested suits-all-skintone shades – usually a mid-rose tone. The challenge we then set our testers: identify the brands which deliver a healthy flush that looks subtly, naturally glow-y – but crucially, stays put too.

REVIEWS

Clinique Blushwear Cream Stick

 Silky and oil-free, this water-resistant formula is specifically created to deliver long-wear results. It's non-drying (thanks to plant sterols and lecithin in the creamy blend), and comes in just four versatile shades which are designed to be universally flattering. It swivels up for direct application to cheeks – but ideally, we advise using a brush for blending.

Comments: 'Top marks; very easy to apply stick straight on to skin then blend with fingertips, looked natural, glowing' • 'am buying more and for my friends!' • 'colour looks vivid at first but mellows and lasts for hours' • 'worked well over liquid foundation, but not over mineral powder' • 'great product; much more dewy and healthy looking than powder blush; applied in the morning and still had a glow by evening' • 'don't usually wear blusher as end up looking like Coco the Clown, but was very happy with this'.

Bobbi Brown Pot Rouge for Lip and Cheeks

 You could use this as a cheek tint – as our testers do – but it also does double-duty on lips, too. (Bobbi's memory of her grandmother using lipstick on her cheeks inspired this product.) It's creamy but sheer – with a matt finish – and comes in a pot (as the name suggests), with a twist-off top. Nine shades; our lot got Blushed Rose.

Comments: 'Colour was wonderful, more tan than powder pink, and easy to put on, though needed to learn some tricks for best results, eg, putting on with fingers, warming it slightly on cold days, and applying on freshly moisturised skin or creamy/

AT A GLANCE

Clinique Blushwear Cream Stick

Bobbi Brown Pot Rouge for Lip and Cheeks

Cosmetics à la Carte Bare Blush

Marks & Spencer Lip & Cheek Tint

♡ WE LOVE...

In Jo's kit you'll find Cosmetics à la Carte Bare Blush: a twist-up stick of colour that's a breeze to blend (as prescribed for her by our make-up artist friend Jenny Jordan), which was much-liked by our testers, too. Sarah loves Jemma Kidd Blush Wear Crème Cheek Colour in apricot-y Paw Paw – looks bright orange until you blend it, then abracadabra, it's a natural glow (Jo nearly pinched it on a recent train journey...).

liquid foundation, not over powder' • 'didn't need to reapply all day' • 'dream to apply and blend in, much lighter and more vesatile than a standard cream: hands-down winner for being true to colour, easy to apply, long-lasting and so natural' • 'colour doesn't usually last on me but at mid-afternoon I still had a lovely glow'.

Cosmetics à la Carte Bare Blush

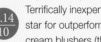 This is Jo's blusher-of-choice (she's on her third swivel-up stick). Cosmetics à la Carte is a London-based brand which has been making cosmetics (and offering terrific make-up lessons) for the past 35 years. (We're big fans.) A signature of the brand is that they'll create 'couture' colours for individual clients, but our testers received an off-the-peg shade: Rose.

Comments: '10/10: went on smoothly, no patches, gave a very even natural coverage, sheer finish that lasts all day' • 'perfect to have in your make-up bag and much more long-lasting than a powder' • 'went on very smoothly with my fingers, and gave glowing natural finish – if not applied too heavily!' • 'offers a nice tint if used sparingly, or richer colour with two layers – very long-lasting' • 'matt but somehow dewy! Also looked wonderful on my lips' • 'love this; long-lasting, sheer silky finish'.

Marks & Spencer Lip & Cheek Tint

 Terrifically inexpensive, this deserves a gold star for outperforming many far pricier cream blushers (though a couple of testers simply couldn't get the hang of it). Flip open the see-through plastic lid of the little compact to find a super-sheer (too much so for some testers), blendable texture which can also – like Bobbi's – be used on lips for a stain-like effect.

Comments: 'Great to use and looked fantastic – sheer finish with touch of shine, but needed touching up at lunchtime' • 'skin looked natural, a little dewy, and glowing: quicker and easier to apply with foundation brush' • 'went on surprisingly smoothly and blended easily, whole effect natural and subtle colour, and surprised how well it performed for both cheeks and lips' • 'hated this at first but when I learned to use it was surprised how much I liked it – too dry for my lips though'.

'When you're *younger*,
you want to be
PERFECT,
but *later* you learn
that perfect
isn't really that
INTERESTING'

Susan Sarandon

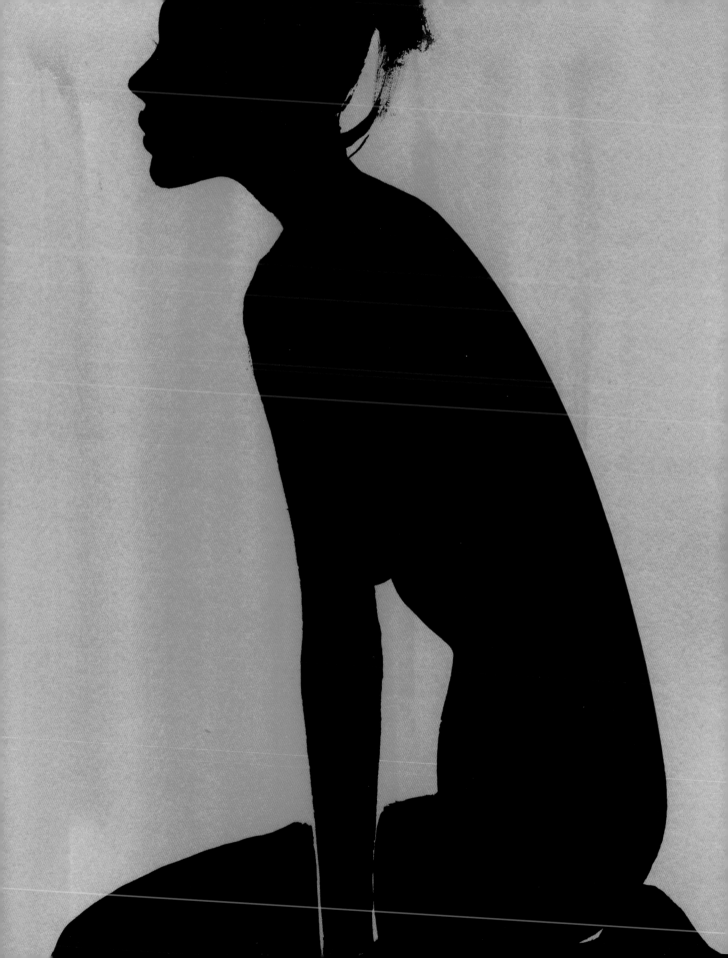

Body: how to look better naked (*truly*)

We have a sneaking admiration for nudists of mature years, who throw caution (and just about everything else) to the wind, and go naked. (And even play badminton or volleyball *au naturel*.) Are we about to do the same? Not for all the tea in Fortnum's...

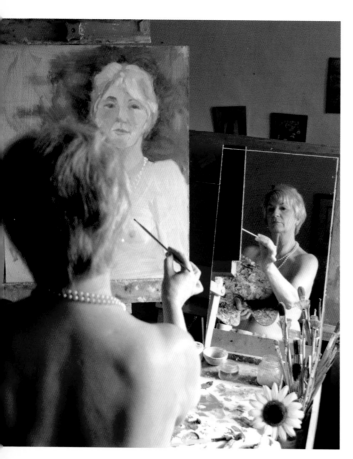

Bodies, like our faces, show signs of gravity and sun damage. And often they're more neglected than our faces: swathed in layers of clothing for much of the year puts crêpey skin, bingo wings and even saggy knees out of sight – and off our beautycare radar. Even when it's roastingly hot, we see many women hiding under kaftans and sarongs feeling self-conscious about a body that's less than Elle Macpherson-esque.

But the naked truth is that nobody is ever going to judge you as harshly as you judge yourself. Just think of that little mental dialogue when you shop for a swimsuit: 'Omigod, look at my backside.' Contrast that to the thoughts running through a man's head when he catches sight of you naked: 'Whoo-hoooo!'

However, there are ways for every woman to feel a bit more 'Whoo-hoooo' about her own body. Overleaf, you can read about creams to slather on which, according to our testers, really can help body skin be more resilient, more velvety, more bare-able (and stroke-able, too). But there's a lot more that you can do to look better naked – which in turn, makes you feel better in your clothes. We just love that French phrase: '*être bien dans sa peau*' – literally 'to be good in your skin' – meaning 'to be content with yourself', which we think is definitely worth aspiring to. So, here are some suggestions that we're confident will make you feel that bit more comfortable in your own skin...

Stand up straight. Good posture not only makes you look an inch or two taller, but magically takes an inch or two off your mid-section, by un-sagging it. We've explained this on page 15, but it's so vital that here it is again! Imagine lifting your rib-cage as if there was a string going up from your breastbone to the ceiling. At the same time, gently pull your shoulder blades back and down. It's pretty easy to remember to do this every time you catch sight of yourself in a mirror, but you want to make more of a habit of it than that. For enhancing posture permanently, nothing beats Pilates (though yoga and the Alexander Technique come pretty close), through which you become much more aware of how you're standing, sitting and moving. And strengthening the core muscles in the tummy (the aim of Pilates) and the obliques creates an invisible 'corset' around the body, flattening your abs with absolutely no need for Playtex or Spanx.

Soften your water… and you'll soften your skin. Hard water is really drying, leaving skin looking and feeling papery. If you aren't sure whether your water is hard or soft, try the soap test: if your soap lathers extremely well and is hard to rinse away, it's soft. If it lathers only moderately and leaves skin rapidly squeaky-clean upon rinsing – or if there's a chalky residue on your shower door or curtain – then it's hard. You can actually buy a gizmo which fits into your shower to help remove the minerals, softening the water you use for washing your body. (See DIRECTORY, or simply Google 'shower water filter'.) The lower-tech alternative for dealing with the effects of hard water is to keep baths and showers short – under five minutes, if possible. Use a mild soap and use it only in areas of skin folds – underarms, neck, feet and, er, 'bits'.

Quit smoking… We can give you a gazillion reasons why you'll be better off not smoking, but in this case it's because the swirl of smoke around your body has an ageing effect on skin, bombarding it with free radicals – which break down collagen and elastin. There's some suggestion that smokers have a more negative body image, and the more a woman smokes, the worse she feels about herself.

…and get moving. On the other hand, the act of exercising actually makes you feel better about your body (never mind the physical improvements), according to a study from the University of Florida.

Get rid of 'goosebumps'. Shy to take that summer cardie off because of your bumpy upper arms? Blitz with a twice-weekly scrub. If that doesn't beat the problem, you may have an inherited skin condition called keratosis pilaris (KP), for which a consultant dermatologist recommends using a product called Dermol 500, with Vaseline Intensive Care Lotion to remoisturise afterwards. In fact, we recommend body-scrubbing to everyone as a preparation for any anti-ageing body lotion/butter/oil: a top-to-toe rub-down with a sugar- or salt-and-oil-based scrub, followed by moisturiser, is an instant skin makeover.

Tackle dry shins. Skin over the shins is particularly prone to dryness and can even develop cracks that look like a dry river-bed. Also, observes beauty therapist extraordinaire Nichola Joss, 'We're generally unaware how much waxing and shaving can dry out the skin.' There's another good reason for keeping shin skin supple: later in life, this is where leg ulcers can develop – hard to shift and unpleasant to live with. Prevention is very definitely better than cure, here. We cannot recommend too highly that you try This Works Skin Deep Dry Leg Oil, which we love because it's absolutely miraculous for easing the itchiness and

TIP

If you're heading for a 'red carpet'-type event, you might want to consider this advice from Kylie Minogue: 'My real skin tip is that I use all-over body make-up, which makes a real difference because you get this even, lovely finish everywhere. When you hit forty, you need a little more help.' Recommended products are Per-fékt Body Perfection Gel, a gel-mousse that slides on to give a natural build-upable coverage and smooth airbrushed glow, and Prtty Peaushun Skin Tight Body Lotion, a natural product with light-reflecting particles devised by Hollywood make-up artist Bethany Karlyn, which helps even out skin tone and enhance muscle tone. MAC does a range of body make-up, including Face and Body Foundation, which is water resistant and available in a wide range of colours.

tautness of dry shins. You could also follow Nichola's advice: 'Use a body oil first because it penetrates deeper into the skin, then double up with cream on top to hold the moisture in.'

Apply a self-tanner. According to all the beauty pros we know, the very fastest way to look slimmer is with a body self-tanner, which helps create the illusion of a slimmer body (a little like the way darker clothes do). Self-tanner can also help conceal the dimpling and puckering from cellulite. If you're self-tan-phobic, we recommend one of the gradual options which can be massaged into the skin in circular movements, just as if you were applying a body lotion: favourites with Beauty Bible testers include Joico Gradual Self-Tanner, St Tropez Everyday Body, Nivea Sunkissed Skin Body Lotion and Palmer's Cocoa Butter Formula Natural Bronze.

Use camouflage. If you're self-conscious about red veins on your feet and legs, you have three options: make-up, sclerotherapy or lasers (see page 203). Sclerotherapy (generally using local injections of saline) has been tried-and-tested over the years and it's a fraction of the price of lasering (for questions to ask before venturing into either of these procedures, see page 46). But for occasional pin-baring, Nichola Joss recommends concealing veins (or other blemishes) with Laura Mercier Secret Camouflage concealer, which works as well on legs as it does on faces: she advises applying with fingers as the warmth helps the make-up 'meld' into skin for a seamless finish. It's pretty budge-proof, too. (And see also our suggestion above about self-tanner: flaws of all kinds are infinitely less visible when the rest of the leg is 'sun-kissed'.)

Gloss up. Polish off your body make-over with a spritz of 'dry' (ie, non-greasy) body oil on shoulders and bosom (we love Soap & Glory Easy Glistening Dry Oil Body Gloss), and a slick of varnish on toes and hands.

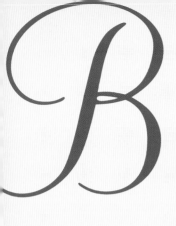

Anti-ageing body treatments: *our award winners*

The women we know are finally waking up to the fact that, yes, skincare should extend below the neck-line. In fact, right down to your toes. Firming, smoothing and moisturising ingredients can deliver rapid results, improving dull, papery, flaky (and even saggy) body skin – and with it dramatically boosting body confidence

AT A GLANCE

Decléor Aroma Sculpt Divine Rejuvenating Cream

Huiles & Baumes Gentle Dry Oil

L'Occitane Milk Concentrate Firming & Smoothing with Almond Milk

Natio Wellness Body Lotion

Yes to Carrots C is Smooth Body Moisturizing Lotion

Guerlain Super Aqua-Body Body Serum

Yes to Carrots C Through the Dry Spell Deliciously Rich Body Butter

Among the dozens of products sent out to our panellists there were creams, butters and oils which made a big difference to the resilience, smoothness and touch-me-softness of arms, legs, bums and tums. (Though if it's cellulite you want to blitz, see page 38.) So which texture – lotion, oil, cream, serum – and fragrance (or not) should you go for? We suggest choosing whatever you'll enjoy most – because as our testers found, that's what inspires regular use. And goodness, how they enjoyed these!

REVIEWS

Decléor Aroma Sculpt Divine Rejuvenating Cream

 A really outstanding score from the well-known aromatherapy-powered brand, with a scrumptious cream featuring a cocktail of essential oils (rose, chamomile, lemongrass, lemon, grapefruit, frankincense, myrrh), plus shiitake mushroom extract, tamanu and macadamia oils. Pearlescent particles deliver a lovely instant radiance, while the cream is designed to have a draining, firming and even a 'lifting' effect, making it ideal (so Decléor promise) for use after weight loss, as well as for general anti-ageing. **Comments:** 'I would give this 12/10 if I could; it's a smooth, silky cream that's firm enough to take a scoop and rub it in; I used to be a bit slapdash but the improvement is so noticeable that I apply every morning: I can now go out bare-legged!' • 'skin no longer flaky, tone has improved, and I got a compliment on how smooth my legs are' •

'fabulous fragrance, my skin feels so much fresher and softer, and looks almost shimmering; compliments from my other half were a nice side effect' • 'I have to confess that I only did the trial on one side of my body for two days: the instant difference in skintone – especially on my legs – made me switch to using it all over'.

Huiles & Baumes Gentle Dry Oil ✿ ✿ ✿

 Ecocert-certified organic goodness from a French all-natural brand, this dry oil spritzes on to the body but sinks in fast, with a blend of coconut, olive, rosehip, borage and evening primrose oils. It's delectably scented with tiaré, grapefruit flower and vanilla, and though not specifically meant to be anti-ageing, that's the test we set it – and it passed with flying colours. **Comments:** 'The first body oil that truly soaks in so you're not left feeling greasy and can get dressed immediately; smells nice but very gentle so won't overpower any perfume; definitely improved skin condition and left it hydrated and comfortable, smoother and a better colour' • 'easy to spray on, skin felt nourished, and after a week was very soft!' • 'much smoother skin immediately, shins really benefited; after a few days, definitely silkier feel and a sexy sheen' • 'loved the subtle chocolate-orangey fragrance, very natural and relaxing'.

L'Occitane Milk Concentrate Firming & Smoothing with Almond Milk

 The 'sister' product to a high-scoring cellulite treatment that features later in this book, this body cream melts easily into skin to nourish with a blend of silicium and almond proteins, which are akin to collagen. It's rich in almond oil, hence the name – but smells clean and fresh, rather than marzipan-y.

Comments: 'Loved this product with its light almond-y smell, felt instant lifting and toning, definitely a treat' • 'absolutely gorgeous smell, luxurious light silky buttery texture, left skin very soft – my husband thought my bare legs were silky pyjama bottoms!' • 'so nice I spent much longer massaging it in after bathing, would buy it again as a treat' • 'skin feels smoother and softly hydrated, loved the fab vintage-inspired tub with silver lid; worked well on sensitive skin and any trouble areas such as chest, tummy and thighs'.

Natio Wellness Body Lotion

 Not quite a 'steal', but a reasonably-priced product from an Aussie brand with a natural focus (Natio is that country's fastest-growing beauty brand, though they've actually been producing cosmetics for 75 years). A non-greasy formula, rich in aloe vera and vitamin E plus potent antioxidant pomegranate.

Comments: 'Very effective body moisturiser, skin is much softer, silkier, smoother and has healthy glow; and yes, younger-looking – smoothed it into recent surgery scars and they are less visible and not so lumpy' • 'skin feels velvety, absorbed quickly so no worries about using before you get dressed and fantastic smell' • 'liked everything about this: and the benefits are lasting with regular use' • 'skin a lot less dry and plumper, very easy to smooth in, and instant results – skin lovely and silky-smooth'.

Yes to Carrots C is Smooth Body Moisturizing Lotion

 YTC (as we know them) are positive superstars in our *Beauty Bible Beauty Steals* book – and here we put those award-winning products through their paces anew, specifically to tackle the problems manifested by ageing body skin. Loaded with carrot juice, sweet potato, melon, pumpkin (for beta-carotene), plus Dead Sea minerals, it's light-textured but rapidly quenches skin.

Comments: 'Skin certainly looked happy and well-hydrated, soft and healthy; this natural product does a great job and is quickly absorbed' • 'really liked the light, fresh smell, and skin felt smooth and moisturised 24/7' • 'lovely to smooth

in, just needed gentle massage, no rubbing and no sticky after-feel so I could get dressed immediately' • 'I do prefer the idea of natural skincare, as I have always tried homoeopathic and flower remedies first rather than prescription drugs' • 'divine smell and rich, creamy texture, could tell instantly this is a super product'.

Guerlain Super Aqua-Body Body Serum

 As you read on through this book you'll see Guerlain's name reappear frequently. This serum is a bit of a legend in body-care circles, a super-luxurious 'soft touch' treatment that delivers long-lasting hydration, boosting skin's resistance to environmental stresses and ageing, and revitalising with cell-renewing Desert Rose Flower Complex. Soft-focus powders deliver an instantly even-toned, luminous finish.

Comments: 'Lovely to use if you had a special function coming up, after a week skin felt very smooth, well-hydrated and silky, drier areas disappeared' • 'skin appears more youthful, radiant and healthy after using this for a few weeks, I feel my skin has had a real treat! It's soft, smooth and supple, has a healthy sheen and feels as if it has more elasticity' • 'loved this product, smell was divine, and skin condition has improved significantly, now very smooth, toned and even. Gorgeous!'.

Yes to Carrots C Through the Dry Spell Deliciously Rich Body Butter

 This features similar ingredients to the lotion, left, which scored just a few fractions of a point higher – but this comes in a rich, luscious butter format. A star of previous books, we retrialled this – and it impressed several of our mature dry-skinned testers, though some others weren't keen on the smell (you do tend to love or hate it) and/or texture.

Comments: 'Fabulous texture, really easy to apply and absorbed almost straight away; loved the smell, really inviting and totally natural; gave lovely sheeny skin that felt soft, after a few days the dry skin on my legs had cleared completely; a patch of dermatitis has also improved. Love this product, it takes the time and effort out of using a body cream' • 'gorgeous fragrance and my skin lapped up the product' • 'sweet, pleasant, natural smell, skin was instantly softened and after three days' use, felt much smoother, silky after a week; I liked that and I like using natural body products which are less harmful to the environment, and to me!'.

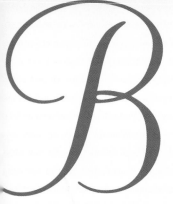

Body scrubs: our award winners

When you want fast body improvements, we say: reach for a scrub. These are pretty darned miraculous for transforming dry and rough skin in about 30 seconds flat. (Especially when the exfoliating particles are suspended in an oil base that delivers a softening, sensual 'slick' on the surface, to nourish as it sinks right in.) What's more, if you then choose to layer another body oil, lotion or cream on to body-scrubbed skin, the ingredients will work their cell-plumping magic more effectively because you've buffed away the dead surface cells first

AT A GLANCE

Ila Beyond Organic Body Scrub for Energising and Detoxifying

REN Moroccan Rose Otto Sugar Body Polish

Balance Me Skin Brightening Spearmint Exfoliating Polish

Dermalogica Exfoliating Body Scrub

Urban Retreat UR Exfoliating Body Scrub

Lulu & Boo Vanilla Sugar Body Scrub

So: our Beauty Bible recruits trialled several dozen body scrubs (there are now so many on the market) – and these were their super-smoothing favourites, with some truly stellar scores. More than half of those also earn at least two daisies for naturalness. (See page 7 for more about our daisy rating.) Most testers preferred natural ingredients and were put off by synthetic chemicals, such as sodium lauryl sulphate and parabens.

REVIEWS

Ila Beyond Organic Body Scrub for Energising and Detoxifying

 Ila's the Sanskrit word for 'earth', and this all-British luxury spa brand – founded by an aromatherapist who set out to fuse holistic wellbeing with beautiful skin – prides itself on being all-natural, too. Hand-blended in the Cotswolds, the scrub's based on Himalayan mineral salts to detoxify and restore energy, with a sense-awakening essential-oil blend of organic rose geranium and juniper. Congrats to Ila for a truly outstanding score (very few products ever exceed an average of 9/10 from our testers).
Comments: '10/10! The skin on my legs looked dull and tight, overall my skin lacked lustre; after using this it shone, smelt fragrant, was smooth and very moisturised – and didn't need any body lotion; after a few uses skintone visibly

improved' • 'I looked like a pork sausage before it's been cooked! But instantly my skin really glowed, with a lovely sheen, and after using twice a week it looks more toned and less pasty' • 'gorgeous smell of rose geranium' • 'luxurious packaging and nice-sized pot, slightly drier than other oil-based scrubs, with nice grainy bits of salt which dissolved in water, now have silky soft thighs and arms' • 'worth the price 'cos it's two treatments in one'.

REN Moroccan Rose Otto Sugar Body Polish ✿✿

9:27/10 Oh, we love it when this happens… Yes, this product has featured previously in *The Green Beauty Bible* – but we sent it out to ten different testers specifically for this book, who awarded the scrub virtually the same impressively high score as when previously trialled. With Paraguayan cane sugar, skin-conditioning olive and almond oils, kola nut and tea extracts – and the heady fragrance of rosa Damascena oil (you lot really are suckers for rose scents), we're elevating this to the Beauty Bible Hall of Fame.
Comments: '10/10! Not really messy, easy to rub in, beautiful rose smell, good texture like soft sugar, washed off quickly leaving nice soft film on body; lovely to use in bath – rose-scented water – or shower. Very luxurious lovely product, and softer skin!' • 'left skin very smooth and moisturised, no need for body cream on my very dry skin; bumpy

skin on upper arms has gone after a month of using regularly' • 'like a spa treatment! Skin more even in tone now, I loved this – the best scrub ever!' • 'moisturising lasts for days, skin silky and much softer and clearer, particularly around my thighs and buttocks, and bumpy arms reduced – fabulous'.

Balance Me Skin Brightening Spearmint Exfoliating Polish

One for the mornings, we'd say, with its zingy, wake-you-up spearminty scent. A (non-runny) blend of natural salt, coconut and sweet almond oils, it buffs and moisturises in one – in common with most of these winning scrubs. Balance Me – created by two British holistic therapists (one a former Lancôme PR) – 'believe in straightforward, natural skincare that works and lasts', of which this is a classic example.

Comments: 'Top marks! Skin on my legs was dry and quite flaky – lizard-like – texture is perfect, and skin felt fabulous, moisturised and smooth with no stickiness or irritation. The best exfoliating polish I have ever used, didn't need a body cream after' • 'stubborn rough patches on knees and feet from kneeling to bathe my toddler are definitely smoother and more moisturised; rinsed away well, leaving no gritty bits; would be great to use before waxing – I shave and found I had fewer ingrown hairs than usual' • 'lovely minty smell, perfect texture, tough enough for dry skin around knees and elbows without being too abrasive; skin felt gorgeous after, really soft and smooth – as good as my expensive brands – a great product'.

Dermalogica Exfoliating Body Scrub

Unlike the other winners, Dermalogica's is a lightly-foaming creamy body scrub (in a shower-friendly, flip-top tube) which polishes, energises and cleanses the body, in one. With antioxidant green tea polyphenols, it's got a revitalising fragrance from oils of lavender, orange, rosemary and sandalwood. Like us, Dermalogica are big on scrubbing as a skin 'prep' for other treatments – and you'd probably need to follow this with a body oil/cream/butter. A couple of testers marked it down for containing sodium lauryl sulphate (the foaming agent).

Comments: 'Very nice aroma, very good texture, not too grainy but thick enough to stay on skin; washed off very easily; left my skin very smooth from first use – and slight improvement in psoriasis on my elbow; really enjoyed it' • 'very easy to use

and good texture' • 'skin felt baby-smooth and glowing instantly, really got the blood circulating; I don't like oil-based products, so this was brilliant for me – though marked down for sand-like particles that needed pushing down the plughole'.

Urban Retreat UR Exfoliating Body Scrub

This creamy body scrub gets its body-buffing power from bamboo and walnut shell particles – which in our opinion makes it more suitable for shower than bath use, as they don't dissolve. Skin-nurturing shea butter nourishes the skin, while a zesty mix of lemon, orange and bergamot is specifically blended to enliven the senses. A truly massive tub, BTW!

Comments: 'Really great for improving skin condition, and fantastic for removing fake tan, also worked well before applying fake tan to exfoliate and moisturise' • 'pleasant refreshing citrus orange smell, mixed with tea!' • 'my slightly scaly skin felt genuinely soft and silky, not oily, no need for extra moisturiser; the single best exfoliator I've ever used' • 'thick creamy consistency, went on easily and evenly – though granules in bottom of bath needed showering away' • 'lovely big tub, easy-to-get-to product and to grip with wet hands' • 'love the fruity smell' • 'texture really creamy and buttery – would probably buy'.

Lulu & Boo Vanilla Sugar Body Scrub

We first discovered this teensy Brit brand while judging the Soil Association Beauty Awards, and Lulu & Boo are certainly punching above their weight with a victory over dozens of better-known beauty names. Moisturising ingredients in the sugar scrub include coconut butter, almond and jojoba oils, but the product's real signature is the good-enough-to-eat essential-oil fragrance of vanilla, orange and cardamom.

Comments: 'Immediate gorgeous-to-the-touch skin; thick, satisfying texture; felt and smelt luxurious, and loved the smell – would buy it' • 'skin felt very moisturised, softer and smoother, no body cream needed' • 'very nice, oily enough to moisturise but didn't feel sticky on skin or make bath slippery; loved the vanilla scent on my skin and in the bathroom' • 'would recommend this after a holiday as it kept my skin glowing and smooth for much longer, but don't get water in the jar!' • 'one of my favourite products: loved everything about it – all blemishes and spots gone after a few weeks, and left with lovely smooth skin'.

♡ WE LOVE...

Well, first of all we'll tell you what we personally don't love: those body scrubs based on crushed nuts and seeds, which drift to the bottom of the bathwater and make you feel like you're sitting in a tub of grit. (Not such an issue if you shower, but we're mermaids.) REN Moroccan Rose Otto Sugar Body Polish (which scored so well with our testers), ESPA Detoxifying Salt Scrub and Les Soins aux Fleurs de Bach Body Scrub (with its amazingly effective 'Anti-Stress' fragrance) all have a place on Jo's bath-side, while Sarah's shower features Essential Care Organic Coconut Candy Scrub (literally good enough to eat), Wild Organics Marshmallow Butter Sugar Scrub, and – a double-duty skin whammy – Yes to Carrots Pampering Hand & Nail Spa, which works all over!

We must, still must, improve our busts...

And we CAN! Starting now, with the right bra – because choosing the right 'underneath' (as fashion guru Amanda Platt calls your bra), is as crucial to looking great as what you put on top

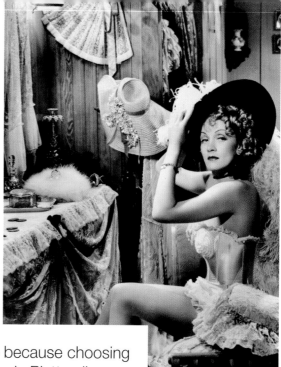

When you can't rely on youthful perkiness, you need a better bra to give you uplift. Undies have become increasingly important in our lives. To put it plainly, at this stage in life you need a bra that's not only pretty but does its job impeccably (and don't forget equally well-fitting knickers). We'd always urge you, if possible, to go to an expert: the difference it can make is staggering. And it's not just a question of looking good: your bra can affect your health.

Think of your bra as a suspension bridge.
You may never have linked your bosom and engineering, but according to chiropractor Tim Hutchful, it really is like a suspension bridge! 'You need a well-engineered bra so your shoulders don't end up doing all the work. Bras that don't fit affect the shoulders and chest and usually cause pain as you get older.' Poorly-fitting bras can lead to all sorts of physical problems, including head-, neck-, shoulder-, and/or back-aches (back pain is common among large-breasted women). Too tight a bra can even restrict your breathing.

Most importantly, wear the right size.
Amazingly, about 80 per cent of women are wearing the wrong-size brassiere. In one

study, most women with shoulder pain found it lifted completely when they removed their bra. (Though the researchers didn't try kitting them out in the right-size bra to see what happened then…) Add to this the fact that our bosoms lose firmness with age and you can see why it's vital to confront the bra issue if you want your *poitrine* to look alluring and feel comfy. Be aware too that, however carefully you handwash them (and never tumble dry), bras lose their oomph as they get older, so depending on how often they're worn you should replace them every six months. (If necessary please shuffle your budget – it's really worth it.)

Become a savvier bra-shopper. There are more types of bra than we've had hot dinners (well, nearly) but whether you choose wired (or not), padded or plain, demi-cup or full, black lace, crimson satin or classic white cotton, there is basic advice that's common to all styles. Plus, for energetic exercisers, you can now find a range of sports bras that is specially designed to keep your bosom stable rather than bouncing with every movement (think of the way a ponytail bobs up and down as you run, play tennis, even do yoga). So…

● First and most importantly, says June Kenton,

BRAS AFTER BREAST SURGERY

June Kenton of Rigby & Peller, who has had a mastectomy herself, is passionate about the concerns of women who've had this surgery. 'Getting a prosthesis and bra after mastectomy is often treated in the same way as getting a pair of crutches, but it should be about fashion, not a medical appliance,' she says. The key is to find a bra which fits the other breast perfectly before choosing a prosthesis. 'Get bras to fit your "good" side then fit the prosthesis so it matches,' she advises. (Find more advice at www.rigbyandpeller. com, and other specialist mastectomy lingerie suppliers.)

owner of Rigby & Peller (the legendary lingerie emporium in London), 'Be really grown-up and have a proper expert fitting. Try on lots. Move around, sit down, stand up, lift your arms – make the bra work for you. Then choose the style which performs best.'

● The two crucial measurements are cup size and band size (the bit at the bottom) – so make sure the fitter measures those each time. The perfect position for your breasts is midway between your shoulder and your elbow. The most common problem is wearing a bra too small in the cup and too big in the band at the back. Most women wear their bra bands too high (see next point), so their measurements are wrong. Often the key is to get a deeper cup and a smaller band. This usually eliminates the dreaded 'back sausages' too.

● The band should sit evenly around the chest, ie, the back shouldn't be higher or lower than the front. It shouldn't ride up but stay parallel to the floor.

● Breasts should be supported primarily by the band around the rib-cage, not the straps.

● Breasts shouldn't bulge over the top or sides of the cup, even with a low-cut style such as a balconette.

● The nipple should be in the centre of the cup.

● The cup should fit smoothly, and not wrinkle, be loose, or cut in at the top so you get a bulge (called 'double-cupping' in the trade).

● The centre piece of the bra should lie flat against the chest.

● If it's underwired, the wires should go under the bust contour and follow it snugly – not cut in or rub.

● Straps should not dig in or slip off the shoulder. Choose straps that are comfortable and make you feel supported. Generally that means wider straps – but they don't need to look bulky.

● A well-fitting bra shouldn't leave marks on your skin – and that means the straps too.

BOOST YOUR BUST... AND BANISH BINGO WINGS!

There are very simple actions that will help firm your bosom – and arms too. Fitness trainer Andy Wadsworth suggests the following for bust uplift, followed by a couple for debagging the dreaded bingo wings! But most important of all for the bustline, he says, is your posture: stand tall, keep your shoulders down and wide, lift your chest. Don't round your shoulders or slouch.

1 **Palm push: standing or sitting, extend your arms in front of you at chest height, elbows bent as if you are hugging a tree (or a person…). Now push your palms together with force. Hold for ten seconds. Repeat ten times. Do this as often as you can. Watchpoint: keep your shoulders relaxed, pushing your shoulder blades down and together.**

2 **Floor press-up: do full press-ups on the floor if you are strong (and used to this type of exertion); if not, keep your knees to feet (you're on tiptoes) on the floor and press-up the rest of your body. Once you can do 20 knee press-ups, try doing a full press-up. Aim to build up to three sets of ten press-ups.**

3 **Wall press-away: stand facing a wall, then extend your arms at chest height a bit wider than a shoulder-width apart, so your hands touch the wall. Bend your arms and let your body fall towards the wall, then push away by straightening your arms. Aim for three x ten repetitions.**

4 **Chest press: lie on the floor (or bench or fitness ball), with a weight in each hand (either a 2kg weight or a full bottle of water). Raise your arms up in the air above your chest. Aim for three x ten repetitions.**

5 **Butterfly: standing with feet a hip-width apart and with a weight (as above for Chest press exercise) in each hand, start with hands at about 45 degrees to the floor; then lift the weights up in an arc to meet in front of your chest. Aim for three x ten repetitions.**

FOR BINGO WINGS...

6 **Tricep dip: sitting on a chair or the edge of the bath, with your feet under your knees a hip-width apart, grasp the sides of the chair or bath while you lift your bottom from the seat and let it drop down and forward; keep your elbows behind you rather than out to the side. Straighten your arms to come up. Move down and up without pausing for three sets of ten, building up to 20.**

7 **Overhead triceps press: put your hands behind your neck with a weight in each (as in exercise 4), then push them up above your head in a straight line. Go up and down smoothly without pausing for three x ten repetitions.**

PS **Any activity that uses your arm and chest muscles will help tone and firm: Jo swims and does yoga, Sarah brushes big horses, mucks out stables – and finds that scrubbing the bath with both arms is an amazing workout for arms and tummy!**

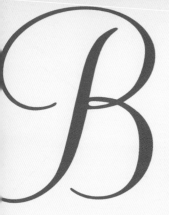

Bust treatments: *our award winners*

You've found the perfect-fitting bra to give maximum support – now lavish your bust with treats that not only leave the skin feeling soft and smooth but, amazingly, claim to make your breasts feel firmer and more pert... So you can reveal your décolletage with confidence

AT A GLANCE

Palmer's Cocoa Butter Formula Bust Firming Massage Cream

Liz Earle Superskin Bust Treatment

Caudalie Firming Concentrate

Clarins Bust Beauty Firming Lotion

Motherhood, gravity, going bra-less when you were a carefree twentysomething – they all take their toll on the bust area. Add to that the effects of gravity over the decades and none of us is as pert as we once were – although good underwear, fitted properly, can be nothing less than a miracle-worker (see page 32 for more). Frenchwomen swear by the perkifying effects of cold water (once upon a time, Clarins even made a device that blitzed boobs with icy water – and rather effective it was, too), but nowadays there are more treatments than ever which allege that they'll firm and uplift breasts, not simply leave the skin soft and silky. (Any body lotion would achieve velvetiness in the boob zone, frankly.) So do these targeted bust treatments achieve the near-impossible and deliver real uplift? To find out, we dispatched well over a dozen to our teams, and got this feedback – which included an overall victory for a real Beauty Steal! NB: they were instructed to use the product for four weeks on one breast alone and note any difference.

REVIEWS

Palmer's Cocoa Butter Formula Bust Firming Massage Cream

7.98/10

Congratulations to this super-affordable brand for notching up a totally stellar score in a challenging category! Palmer's cocoa butter-based products have done well with our testers before; this time round, the team of ten was impressed by this non-sticky, quick-drying, gel-like formula, designed not just to firm and smooth the bust and décolletage, but also for firming and toning use after pregnancy and weight loss.

Comments: 'I loved it!!! So did my husband – thank you Palmer's!!! My boobs were quite plump and firm but after the kids they did decline. I was staggered after the first application on the "test" boob: skin looked young again, plump and smooth with a little glow' • '10/10: bust shape and tone felt and looked smoother and firmer, lived up to its promises in every way' • 'dries in about five minutes so I could put on my bra without feeling sticky' • 'immediately skin looked more soft and toned and bust lines less pronounced; liked the chocolate-y smell!'.

Liz Earle Superskin Bust Treatment

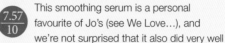
7.57/10

This smoothing serum is a personal favourite of Jo's (see We Love...), and we're not surprised that it also did very well in our trials. Lightweight and cooling, it sinks in fast and is packed with the botanical ingredients you'd expect from the 'naturally active' brand: omega-3 and omega-6 essential fatty acids, antioxidants, quince and green tea extracts, white lupin, plus an ingredient extracted from Kigelia africana (aka the 'sausage tree'!), sourced from a community-based sustainable forestry project in Malawi. Some testers applied it to their necks too, and loved the double whammy.

Comments: 'Skin felt moisturised, softer and firmer; natural herby smell soon went, and skin dried very quickly, not sticky at all' • 'felt like I'd had a mini bust-lift, skin looked luminous and softer; results were excellent though I wasn't fond of the brownish colour' • 'definite improvement in décolletage area, although not in that small area between my breasts; had lost elasticity due to pregnancy and age, and definitely has improved a little; love the smell' • 'bust and neck much softer and less crêpey, and fine lines less noticeable' • 'I

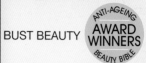

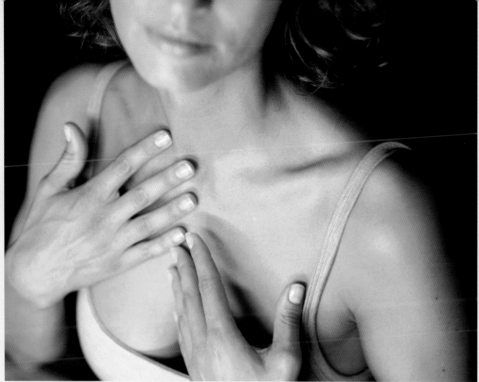

am cursed with a very large chest and there was never a chance it was going to make a huge difference, but it improved my skin, felt gorgeous and smelt divine!'.

Caudalie Firming Concentrate

7.5/10 As with all Caudalie products (which are inspired by the owners' family vineyard in Bordeaux), this 100 per cent natural lightweight oil features vine-derived ingredients – here, grapeseed oil. They recommend it's used not just on the bosom, but to firm the arms and stomach, and what we love about it is the delicious blend of aromatherapeutic oils: sweet mint, peppermint, douglas fir and lemon.

Comments: 'Skin felt soft, moisturised and also more firm and toned, immediately; liked the light, natural fragrance a lot. After two weeks, bust more toned and felt firmer – and it definitely improved the crêpey skin on the underside of my upper arms (put it there too)!' • 'really liked the fresh citrussy smell, skin was softer and smooth, and I really got into the routine of application – no miracle cure for pert boobs but maybe a bit firmer' • 'improved texture and firmness of décolletage, skin looked smoother and more evenly toned' • 'my partner didn't know I used this, and spontaneously commented on the lift and appearance of my breasts – was absolutely amazed it worked, though not sure who'd want their breasts to smell of chewing gum…' • '10/10: skin felt immediately firmer and softer, and I adore the minty fresh smell; bust feels firmer and more

lifted and stretch marks less visible. Have bought some more supplies. I feel more confident and can't live without it'.

Clarins Bust Beauty Firming Lotion

7.05/10 Once upon a time, Clarins had the bust-treatment category virtually to themselves (they've been caring for bosoms for 30 years!). This classic treatment still holds its own today: an oil-free gel with a 'filmogenic texture', to tighten, firm and smooth the skin. Key botanicals are oat sugars, vitamin E, moisturising katafray bark, plus vu sua – a South Vietnamese superfruit. Most testers really rated this though a couple were distinctly underwhelmed.

Comments: 'When it had dried completely after ten minutes, skin felt very silky; skin felt definitely plumper and somewhat firmer after four weeks, and a marked reduction in the look of stretch marks. Boobs weren't any perkier but that might improve over a longer period' • 'after four weeks, skin looked and felt firmer and smoother and a definite difference between the breast I'd applied it to and the other one; I wasn't expecting a radical change but was pleased to see there was a difference; did what it promised, leaving skin velvety soft and smooth' • 'skin looked immediately more youthful, firmer and smoother, but no improvement in tone and tightness; surprised there were no guidelines on how many times to apply, etc' • 'lovely product: after a few weeks, skin is smoother, feels more even and bust feels a bit tauter, in a good way'.

♡ WE LOVE...

We don't really 'do' bust treatments. But Jo does slather Liz Earle Superskin Bust Treatment on her décolletage, for suppleness. (It is a Grade A neck treatment, too – see page 153 for more about that.)

Give cellulite the brush-off

Tone those thighs and de-dimple that derrière. (Because there's a lot you can do to smooth out cellulite)

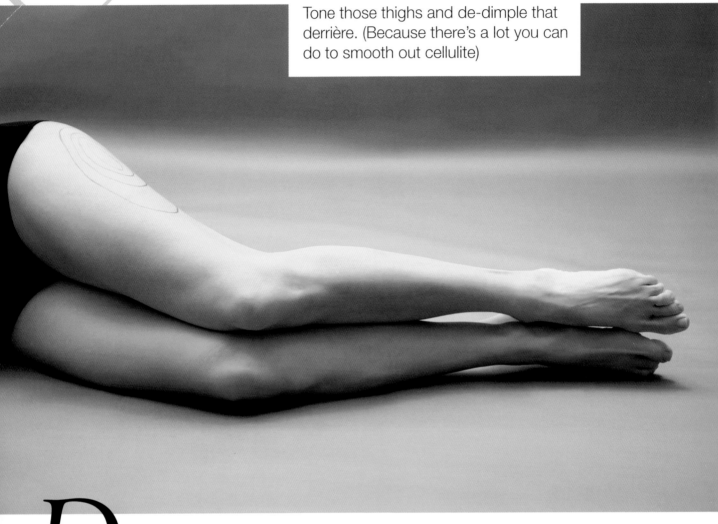

Dimples may be appealing on babies (and handsome men), but on your thighs and backside? Not so charming. So the bottom line on cellulite – hallelujah – is that there's much that can be done to improve it (and thus, in turn, your body confidence). You may never conquer the problem completely – but a combination of nutrition, body-brushing, exercise and localised massage can make a visible difference…

Scrub off the dead skin cells. As well as dry-skin body-brushing (see right), do use a scrub on your backside, thighs and

hips, because any cellulite product you apply to the area is going to penetrate better if it doesn't have to make it through dead skin cells. Targeted body exfoliation also brings about incredibly rapid improvements in skin texture: in our experience it can take less than a week of daily blitzing to combat 'goosebumps' in the cellulite zone and thereby transform skin smoothness.

Body-brush the bumps bye-bye. The skin is a vital (and often overlooked) organ of elimination and nothing is better at stimulating localised circulation than daily brushing. It wakes up a sluggish lymphatic system – and many women have told us it works astonishingly well to improve digestion and aches and pains as side benefits.

First, find your brush: most diligent body-brushers choose a brush with a strap that slips over your hand, and has a removable long handle to get at your back, etc. (Sarah finds her favourite Origins Raffe brush which has a short-ish handle reaches everywhere.) The brush shouldn't be scratchy: if it makes little white scratch marks when you brush the back of your hand with it, it's too hard.

We recommend total body-brushing rather than targeted brushing of the affected area, because you get the all-over lymph drainage and circulation-boosting benefits – here's the how-to:

● Body-brush dry skin, not damp or wet, and never areas that are bruised or irritated, or your breasts.
● Begin by standing in a comfortable position. Place one foot on a higher surface, such as the edge of the bath or a bed.
● Start by brushing the soles of the feet from toes to heel. Move on to the top of the foot and then upwards, with smooth, long strokes – always in the direction of the heart.
● Give extra attention to the skin between the knees and the waist, going over the cellulite area several times. Don't ignore the lymph nodes in the groin. Upwards, upwards, upwards.
● Next, move on to the top half of the body: palms of hands, backs of hands, sweeping towards the armpits (plenty more lymph glands there). Now do your shoulders and back – you'll probably need your long-handle brush here.
● Continue the sweeping movements on the front of your torso, going a little more lightly as the skin can be very sensitive here. (But miss out your breasts and nipples.)
● Brushing should be firm and vigorous, but shouldn't hurt. A rosy glow is fine; red or irritated skin isn't.
● Three to five minutes is ideal. Realistically, two minutes is OK. But the key is: do it daily, and if you can only manage even one solitary minute every morning, that's infinitely better than a once-a-week longer blitz.

Give your fat a mini-massage. Dermatologist Dr Elizabeth Tanzi explains: 'Fat doesn't have a lot of blood flow, so kneading the skin helps increase circulation – and in turn, lessens the appearance of lumps.' Massage with your knuckles, moving up the fronts of your thighs, across your rear and then up the back of your thighs. (If this requires a little contortionism, so be it.) Alternatively, book regular massages with a deep tissue masseur

or practitioner of manual lymphatic drainage (MLD): these can help both to improve circulation and to drain away any excess fluid, which can exacerbate the appearance of cellulite.

Take exercise! As usual, more is better…it works. And you might want to try FitFlops, the footwear range with the inbuilt gym in the sole, for its proven leg-toning benefits.

Eat more veggies and high-fibre foods. They'll help in the war on dimples (and benefit your whole body): loads of veggies and salads (green leaves, onions and garlic); fruit (especially deep reds and purples – so make the most of berries and dark grapes); some wholegrains (brown rice, oats, and anything sprouted); olive oil and herbs. Also go for good-quality protein: oily fish and shellfish, eggs, poultry, tofu and natural live yoghurt. When you're out and about, choose a freshly-squeezed veggie juice or berry smoothie over tea and coffee, and take snack-packs of seeds and nuts (especially Brazil nuts and almonds). Basically, let 'fresh' be your watchword.

And it's about what you don't eat, too. Avoid processed and preserved foods, sugar, refined salt, 'fungal' foods (which means mushrooms, vinegar, blue cheese). Some people find that giving up gluten helps, too, and we also suggest you avoid caffeine and alcohol as much as is realistic. (NB: we do appreciate you're not a nun.)

Take goji. Dermatologist Dr Howard Murad (who's written an entire book on the subject) calls goji 'the cellulite assassinator' (it comes as berries and also juice). We've long espoused an inside-out as well as an outside-in approach to cellulite, and pharmacist Shabir Daya has put together a Cellulite Busting Kit (see DIRECTORY), incorporating the latest guidelines to help minimise the look of cellulite. This includes a food state multi-nutrient, vitamin B50, omega-3 essential fatty acids, glucosamine sulphate and goji berry juice.

And give yourself a break. We know women get incredibly angst-y about cellulite, but we would encourage you to relax a bit about the problem. Cellulite is never as apparent to others as it seems to our own so-critical selves (we've never yet met a man who even quite knew what cellulite was, let alone complained about it on a woman) – and other people see the 'big picture' (your sense of humour/great cooking skills/ your laugh). And if all else fails – well, that's why sarongs were invented.

> FAT doesn't have a lot of blood flow, so *kneading* the skin helps INCREASE circulation

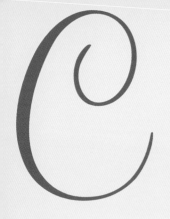

Cellulite treatments: our award winners

It's a fact that even if you've been mercifully dimple-free until mid-life, the breakdown of collagen and elastin which leads to lines and wrinkles in the face can become all-too-apparent on the hips, derrière and (especially) thighs – in the form of cellulite. Certainly, diet plays a role, as does exercise, and we always advise body-brushing which is our own secret weapon. And now there's an abundance of cellulite-blitzing products. Do they really work? Our research with younger readers showed that yes, some definitely do. But we wanted to know – can they rise to the challenge of a more mature body? Almost three dozen cellulite products later – each dispatched to ten testers who 'fessed up to *peau d'orange* – here's the bottom line. (And we were astonished…)

AT A GLANCE

Thalgo Crème Thalgomince

Adonia LegTone Serum

Green People Triple Action Cellulite Lotion

L'Occitane Amande Refining and Contouring Gel

REVIEWS

Thalgo Crème Thalgomince

 Thalassotherapy spa brand Thalgo actually prescribe this for massage twice daily, so that key ingredients – horse chestnut, caffeine complex, plus a plant extract they call 'Adipo-reset' (!) – are able to get to work round-the-clock. It's rich and creamy, enveloping skin 'like a slimming patch', Thalgo tell us, and though it's designed to complement two specific salon cellulite treatments Thalgo offer, our testers trialled it as a stand-alone product, observing impressive results. Several gave it nine or ten marks out of ten.

Comments: 'Lovely light but rich cream, which sunk in immediately; I used it on one leg which was instantly smoother and softer, and after six weeks cellulite definitely less noticeable, orange peel almost gone, firmer, and smoother than it has been for years; lost half an inch around my thigh – loved it' • 'very luxurious product with wonderful aroma, really feel good and my cellulite was a little improved' • 'after six weeks, skin looks and feels smoother and firmer – really loved using this treatment' • 'cellulite markedly reduced, thighs much less uneven and lumpy; when you pinch the skin, the orange-peel effect is much less obvious, plus thighs look and feel much firmer and tighter: expensive but I will be buying more – I love this and recommend it unreservedly' • 'silvery stretch marks and orange peel were much improved'.

Adonia LegTone Serum

We find it a l-i-t-t-l-e hard to swallow that this US serum can 'reduce cellulite by 47 per cent in nine minutes', as their blurb trumpets – but the product is certainly heralded as 'the nine-minute butt lift'…! The 'secret' ingredient is a combination of 'a Greek plant stem cell culture', plus 23 organic oils 'from an Aegean eco-system which have been micro-filtered in a special process to magnify the effect and potency of the Greek Stem Cell Culture'. We'll go by what our testers tell us... (PS: the ingredient list on this product has the smallest typesize of any we've ever seen, and that's saying something!)

Comments: 'Pleasant lotion that sinks in after three minutes then you have to reapply; good clear instructions; skin immediately feels slightly tighter, and incredibly soft and supple; by about three weeks, cellulite is definitely less noticeable, so soft and smooth that I want to stroke it; skin is firmer too' • 'bit of a pain to apply twice but smoothed my skin beautifully, my boyfriend said my thighs, etc looked younger; cellulite looked less – I love my new, much firmer upper legs, they look like they've lost five years – I'm telling all my friends about this product, it's like an iron for your thighs' • 'smooths out unsightly bumps and uneven skintone, so you can throw away the maxi and wear the mini!!!'.

Green People Triple Action Cellulite Lotion ❀ ❀ ❀

7.55/10 This certified organic lotion blends spicy ginger and black pepper essential oils (to pep up circulation), detoxing juniper oil and green tea, pomegranate oil for elasticity, omega-rich rosehip oil, plus bayberries – which are effective at tackling fat deposits. They recommend using it in tandem with body-brushing (twice daily), but our testers didn't do the brushing thing – and nevertheless, made these comments.

Comments: 'Skin felt smoother and firmer after using regularly' • 'liked this silky, fragrant product which was easily absorbed, and gave slight improvement in texture, skintone and firmness, used in tandem with diet, lots of water and exercise' • 'easy-to-follow instructions, had to smooth the cream into skin in circular motion – not the easiest but I did master it; skin is soft and I like this product so will continue to use it' • 'skin is a bit smoother, tighter and firmer but I have been body-brushing and working out a lot so not certain how much down to the cream except smoothness' • 'cellulite is less noticeable and there is general tightness on upper thigh which is my worst spot' • appearance is improved, and skin smoother and firmer'.

L'Occitane Amande Refining and Contouring Gel ❀

7.44/10 A 'contouring gel-cream' with a patented complex of almond proteins, silicium, immortelle flower (a key anti-ageing botanical for L'Occitane), peppermint and

♡ WE LOVE...

Jo was cellulite-free until she hit 50. Then, she observes: 'I suddenly understood what all those "resort wear" sarongs were created for...' She regularly uses a cellulite brush discovered in Germany with copper bristles, and is now devoted to the Decléor Aromessence Slim Effect Draining Contouring Serum and Baume Slim Effect Draining Massage Balm: 'Both the balm and the oil are divine, and 100 per cent natural.' Sarah's dimples are relatively shallow – possibly due to riding and walking for miles every weekend – but she scrubs thighs regularly, applies body lotion most nights and skin-brushes as often as she remembers.

TIP

Double up your daily application of product morning and night. You may get through more, but the active ingredients will have twice the opportunity to tighten and drain. If you just apply once, do it before bedtime: loose night clothes are less likely to rub the product off again than tight daytime clothing.

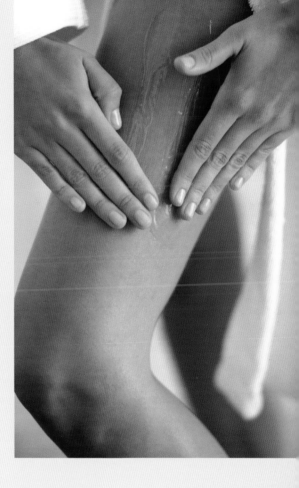

palmarosa. These are complemented by a quinoa extract, caffeine and lemon oil. We like the dispenser: the type which simply twists to release the product, and twists to close again.

Comments: 'Gooey gel cream which sank in very quickly, very easy-to-follow massage instructions, and after all these weeks there is a tremendous difference between the treated cheek and thigh – and I did nothing else! Much smoother, more even tone, slightly firmer; I loved this product and will definitely buy' • 'cellulite slightly reduced, skin smoother and firmer, measurement of thigh less! Very almondy smell' • 'the treated thigh looks very slightly better which surprises me' • 'skin less dimply and contours smoother, very soft texture and a lot more toned – I have been dieting and exercising too'.

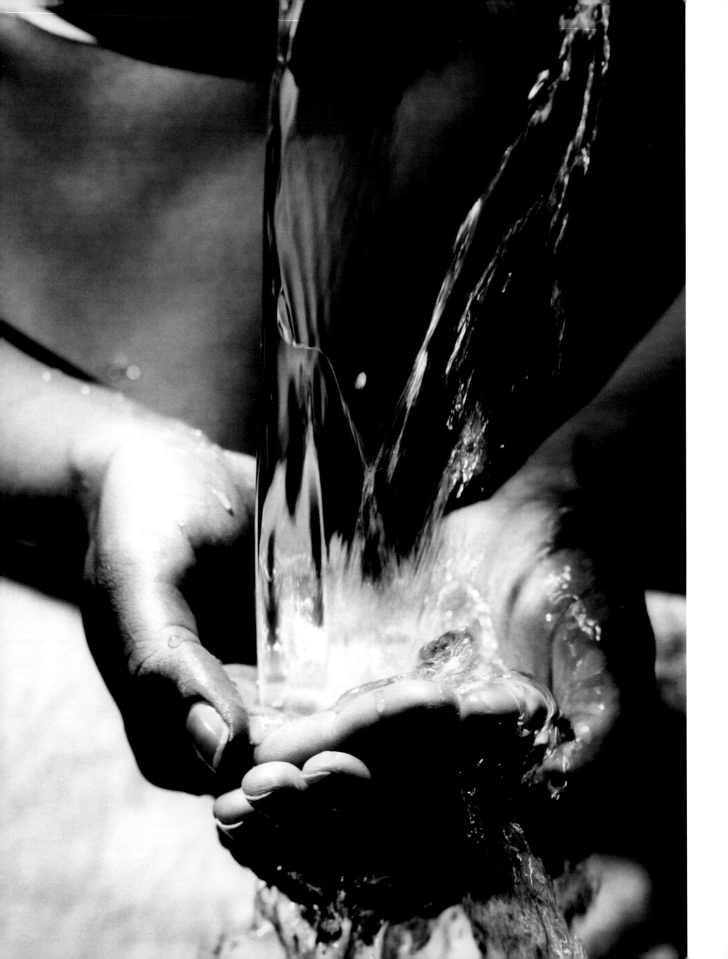

Turbo-charge your cleansing regime

We are the Queens of Clean – always have been – but we know many, many women who are so bored by cleansing they skimp (and even occasionally skip) this important part of the anti-ageing ritual. You can spend hundreds of pounds on an anti-ageing cream (if you really must…) but it's money down the drain if you aren't cleansing properly

The reason is simple: unless you've got rid of the daily build-up of dead skin cells, your anti-ager is just going to sit there. Doing not very much at all. Quite expensively…

Cleansing in this specific way – as espoused originally by Eve Lom and then Liz Earle and now many, many happy and fresh-faced followers – is, in our experience, the most effective way to swoosh away the day and 'prep' skin for everything that comes next.

Step 1 Massage your cleanser into dry skin – balm, lotion, cream, whatever your preference. (Ideally at this stage in life you will have progressed from foaming cleansers, which in general are too drying for mature complexions. And if you're still using soap and water? Stop. Right. Now.)

Step 2 When we say massage, we mean massage. Ideally, use a pressure-point massage, making firm, small circular movements starting at chin-level and working up the cheeks to the eye zone, then shifting along the jaw-bone towards the ears (a distance of around 1.5cm), mid-cheek, cheekbones. And then the same on your forehead. Sweep your fingers more gently around the eyes in a circular but outwards direction. But – important BUT – if you can't be bothered to follow that precise prescription, just general firm massage of your face using circular movements will work wonders for melting make-up, improving circulation and decongesting the skin. You can do this for as long as you like. We recently talked to a Frenchwoman who explained that in France, it's not unusual to spend ten minutes on cleansing. We award ourselves Brownie points if we manage two, but really, the longer you knead your face with your fingertips the more it will reward you for it.

Step 3 Take a hot, wet cloth – a muslin cloth, or a flannel (Sarah prefers that). Press on to the face to remove the first load of cleanser and debris. Rinse under hot water (warm-to-hot water if you are prone to broken veins), then be a bit more vigorous as you swipe away more of the cleanser. (NB: never rub at areas where you have those aforementioned vein problems.) Repeat, until you feel you've swooshed away all remaining cleanser.

Step 4 Rinse the cloth again and wrap a corner of the flannel or cleansing cloth over the tip of your index finger. Rub at areas where skin and make-up build up – particularly in the crease around the nose, the cleft of the chin, and the sides of your face. If you do this, you may never need to use a specific exfoliator. (We rarely do.)

Step 5 As a final step, try swishing the flannel/cloth in cool water and press it on your face. (Jo does this while imagining the day and all its stresses are trickling away down the plug-hole. It isn't compulsory, but she finds it a relaxing technique…)

And overleaf, see the run-down of specifically anti-ageing cleansers. But we say: they'll all work best if you use this technique.

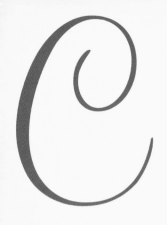

Cleansers: *our award winners*

A good cleanser is in itself a wonderful weapon against ageing. Unless you get the gunk off your face at night thoroughly, you're wasting your money on age-defying moisturisers and serums – because they simply sit on cellular debris and the day's make-up, with no chance of performing miracles. Now, though, there's a new category of cleansers which claim, in themselves, to offer anti-ageing benefits

We've been a bit cynical about that, frankly: a cleanser is meant to be swiped or sluiced away, so how can it do anything more than cleanse and maybe brighten…? This book, however, gave us the opportunity to put several dozen 'anti-ageing' cleansers through their paces, to find out whether you really can cleanse the years away – and these scores would suggest the answer is a resounding 'yes'.

REVIEWS

Elemis Pro-Radiance Cream Cleanser

 Elemis suggest massaging this richly-nourishing, antioxidant-powered cleanser directly into skin, or – if you like a lather – to mix with warm water first. Active 'anti-ageing' ingredients include moringa seed peptides, 'super berry' açai and burdock, while shea butter moisturises, in addition to melting make-up. (Yes, even eye make-up.) It comes with a cotton facial mitt, to be used with warm water for optimum cleansing.

Comments: 'I really love this product – I thought my face was clean when I first used it but when I removed this cleanser with the cloth provided, I was shocked at the make-up that had remained on my face; it also left my skin moisturised' • 'a fabulous cleanser, thick but easily spread, removed all traces of make-up, even eyes and a waterproof lip stain' • 'this cleans effectively, doesn't dry skin, and leaves it looking brighter' • 'I looked forward to the ritual of using it, and skin felt so soft and velvety after that it makes you feel uplifted and good about yourself'.

Dr Brandt Lineless Foaming Cleanser

 We know – because you're always asking for recommendations – that many of you don't feel properly clean without a bit of foam from your cleanser. A real beauty innovation – from Dr Fredric Brandt, one of the US's leading skin cosmeto-dermatologists – this has a 'self-foaming action', yet doesn't strip skin of moisture. Botanical elements include circulation-boosting tangerine leaf oil, apple fruit extract (for firmness), green and white tea (antioxidants), plus grapeseed extract to protect collagen and elastin.

Comments: '10+! Loved its deep-cleansing properties – all my life I've been troubled with clogged pores, but now my skin has never been clearer; I just wouldn't want to be without it, left skin feeling fabulous, superclean and very soft' • 'easy to use, smooth, creamy consistency, skin has benefited' • 'loved the balm-like texture and pump action' • 'liked the fresh smell, skin was improved – looked fresher and possibly firmer'.

Rodial Glamtox Cleanser

 8.75/10 This luxe cleanser, formerly known as the A-List Cleanser (as in the 'red carpet of facial cleansing'…), contains skin-lightening amino acids to target pigmentation and uneven skintone. We're told it has many celebrity fans – but we're more interested in these real-life comments from our somewhat more down-to-earth, un-famous testers.

Comments: 'Pleasure to use this smooth creamy gel balm, with gorgeous smell, removed all traces of make-up including waterproof mascara, the loveliest cleanser I have ever used!' • 'lovely silky, non-sticky texture like honey, left my skin feeling soft and moisturised, even and smooth – but price might make it sit in the "treat" category' • 'felt warm on skin, when washed off skin felt very fresh and clean, not at all dry' • 'removed all traces of make-up, no need for toner' • 'seemed to help the spots I get on my chin at certain times of the month; they disappeared and didn't come back'.

MV Organic Skincare Gentle Cream Cleanser ❋ ❋

 8.57/10 Although this pump-action cleanser doesn't specifically promise anti-ageing benefits, our aged-35+ testers were so impressed by the radiance-boosting results it delivered, we felt we should include it. MV Organic Skincare is an Aussie brand formulated with many certified organic ingredients (although the final product isn't independently certified). One of our fellow beauty editors has raved: 'It's no exaggeration to say that the longer you use this range, the less make-up you'll have to wear.' It's suggested you remove the creamy, make-up-dissolving aromatic formula with a hot compress to decongest skin.

Comments: 'So loved this product: rich, not greasy, not runny, just lovely! Like putting a lemon syllabub on skin – delicious! Removed all make-up and skin felt great' • 'worked really well, smelt lovely, easy to use, great!' • 'nice and rich for my dry skin; makes my face feel really clean and moisturised' • 'love the rose and chamomile smell, fantastic cleanser which calmed and soothed my skin and left no tightness, everything an all-in-one cleanser should be; looked forward to using it' •

'perfect texture once hands are damp – if dry it's too hard to spread' • 'comes with fabulous large, thick muslin cloth'.

Natura Bissé The Cure All-in-One Cleanser

 8.33/10 According to the blurb, this 'provides a soft, glowing and plump appearance from the very first application' – but don't worry: Natura Bissé are only talking about your skin, once you've used this gentle, creamy cleanser. It's been formulated to boost radiance as well as all the usual cleansing benefits (make-up/grime removal), while preserving the skin's moisture levels.

Comments: 'Absolutely love this thick, luxurious and silky product; glides on effortlessly; I've never used a cleanser that removes my make-up so efficiently, and skin felt extremely moisturised, lush and plumped after' • 'lotion melted into a sort of oily consistency, which made it very easy to apply; took off all make-up though mascara needed a bit more effort and time; my mature skin felt very soft after and it was a pleasure to use!' • 'definitely the best cleanser I've ever found, skin felt wonderful after, beautifully moisturised, looks visibly better and feels fabulous'.

Inlight Organic Face Cleanser ❋ ❋ ❋

 8.22/10 Formulated by doctor and homeopath Dr Mariano Spiezia, this 100 per cent organic balm is formulated to suit all skin types, including the most sensitive, and those with acne and rosacea. It's based on moisturising and nourishing coconut oil, astringent green tea, antibacterial and purifying clove bud and rosemary essential oils, plus ginger to stimulate and tone; they reassure that any tiny white granules of condensed shea butter will melt on application.

Comments: 'Only need a pea-size, easy to smooth over face, one of the best balm cleansers I've used' • 'easy to use, nice to apply, loved the texture and wonderful results, took all my make-up off and skin felt amazing, clean, hydrated and soft' • 'I was very sceptical but this soon warmed up and was gorgeous on my skin; cleansed and brightened, left it soft and smooth, and make-up went on really well after' • 'texture is like softly-set butter, quite slippy and oily – perfect if you use fairly heavy make-up – left delicious nourished feeling'.

Learn to contour and sculpt your face

Over the years faces lose definition, with saggier and more padded cheekbones and jawlines. Here, make-up expert Mary Greenwell shares the secrets to creating a more sculpted, slimmer look

A little extra weight as we age can be flattering to the face. There's an old saying: 'After a certain age, you have to choose between your face and your a**e', and it's true. A little fat on the face plumps out the lines from within (as you'll know if you've seen, say, a fiftysomething friend lose a lot of weight – and watched what happens to the depth of her wrinkles).

However, the flipside is that as faces fill out they lose definition. Cheekbones and jawlines get more padded, pouchier and saggier. Even beauties like Grace Kelly and Catherine Deneuve look heavier-jawed, with less gloriously-winged cheekbones. Here, international make-up pro Mary Greenwell – who's made up many a gorgeous older face in her three-decade career – gives us the secret of 'contouring', for a slimmer-looking, more sculpted face. (And it's not the conventional wisdom.)

Always even out your skintone with primer and foundation first. Contouring on to bare skin, even if moisturised, could look dingy. Prepping properly gives the best effect plus staying power.

Use a fawn-y eyeshadow or a mineral powder. The traditional wisdom is that you should use bronzer for contouring but both Mary Greenwell and Terry Barber, director of make-up artistry at MAC (whose products Mary recommends for contouring) say, simply, don't! 'Look at the colour of the shadow under your chin,' says Mary. 'It's fawn. To mimic that, you need something with no red in it, and zero sparkle or shimmer.' Terry recommends MAC's new-generation powder called Mineralize Skinfinish Natural, in a shade a couple of notches deeper than your skintone. It's 'satiny matt to give a moisturised finish', and will add definition without creating dull 'theatre' shadows. Terry advises a two-step approach: 'Add a hint of bright, fresh rose or apricot quite high on your cheekbones, then sweep the deeper colour in from your temples, under the lower half of your cheekbones.'

Use a blusher brush to apply the shadow (an angled one is good). 'Think "shade" here. Sweep the brush across the eyeshadow and tap the handle on a hard surface to remove any excess. To refine the jawline, sweep the brush along the underside of the jaw from edge to edge,' says Mary.

Don't forget right underneath the jaw. 'If you look at someone's chin and jaw, you'll notice that a real shadow goes all the way back to the angle at which the underneath of the chin meets the neck. So should the contouring. Apply lightly, and then add more until the jaw is more defined.'

Give yourself cheekbones, too. 'The principle is the same for under your cheekbones as under your jaw: same product, same brush. Start at the hairline by your ears, and sweep the shadow under the cheekbone. For a truly natural effect, you can apply a whisper of blusher (or blusher and bronzer) to your cheeks, as you normally would, on top of the contour powder.'

Spend an evening practising at home in front of the mirror. Ideally, use a 'triptych' mirror or angle a couple of mirrors so that you can see yourself from the side. If you long for a slimmer-looking face, contouring is an art worth mastering.

If you long for a slimmer-looking face, contouring is an art worth mastering

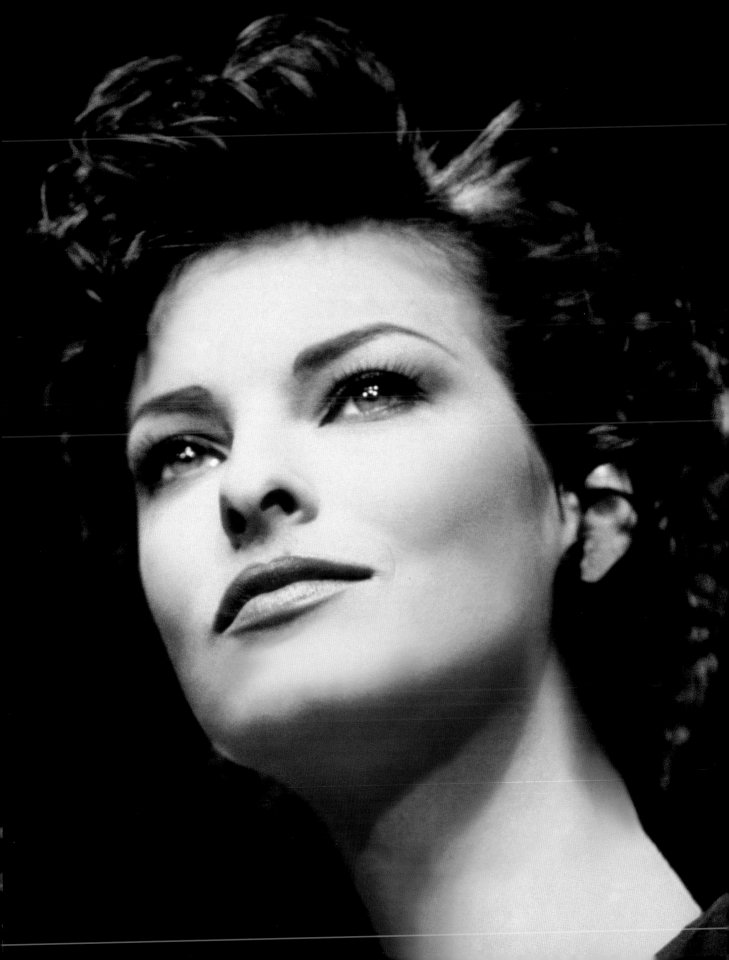

Before you sign up for cosmetic fillers, read this!

If you're considering filler injections, laser treatment, a peel, Botox or even a facelift, it's essential to get as much information as you can first. Cosmetic surgery expert Wendy Lewis tells you all the questions you need to ask to help you get the best possible result

Whenever we want the lowdown on cosmetic procedures and clinical treatments, we turn to Wendy Lewis – aka The Knife Coach, who runs the truly independent Global Aesthetics Consultancy in the UK, Europe and America (as well as writing books, which we list at the back of this one). There is nothing Wendy doesn't know about who's the best, what's new – and the questions that every single woman should ask, not just before undergoing major surgery, but even having what may seem like a minor procedure such as Botox.

As Wendy says, there are – amazingly – people who sign up for fillers, Botox, lasers, peels and even full-blown facelifts without giving the issue much more thought than if they were shopping for a new face cream.

We can't tell you whether you should have a filler injection, or whether you really need a facelift. We believe this is very much a matter of personal choice (though ours is not to). But it is vital to know the right questions to ask before you take the plunge – to optimise your chances of a successful treatment and a good outcome.

Get real. Although some of the most popular procedures are non-surgical, none of them are non-medical. They should be performed in a clinical environment under good lighting and under the direction of a qualified and medically-trained professional. For example, wrinkle-relaxing and filling injections should only be done by a medical aesthetics practitioner, which in the UK includes doctors, nurses and dentists.

Have an initial consultation. Make an appointment with one or preferably two healthcare practitioners. Insist on having adequate time with the individual who will actually be carrying out the procedure – not an assistant or sales person. Your relationship with the person who will be doing your treatment is most important, and he/she is not interchangeable.

Ask serious questions (see box right).

Ask for detailed printed information on every procedure you are considering. Every doctor should have his own materials, pre- and post-treatment instructions, or at least brochures from companies whose products he/she is using, and there should be more consumer information on the websites of all of these brands. However, be aware that no honest or responsible practitioner can guarantee a specific result – we are all individuals and everyone responds differently.

Ask to see photographs of other patients. You should be able to look at real photos of clients who have undergone the procedure/ technique carried out by this specific practitioner. This is most important: there have been instances where one doctor may be showing patients another doctor's results, or labelling the filler company's 'before-and-after' photos as his own work. The caveat: be aware that you can expect to see only photos of the best-case scenario and judge from there – no one will show their worst results. It is impossible to predict the

TIP

Before treatment, Wendy recommends:

● **Avoid aspirin products (Nurofen, ibuprofen), blood thinners or vitamin E for one to two weeks before treatment to prevent increased bleeding and bruising.**
● **Don't have a treatment on an empty stomach – you may get dizzy or faint.**
● **Ice packs before and after can help with pain and swelling.**
● **Bring concealer with you to cover up bruises or needle marks.**

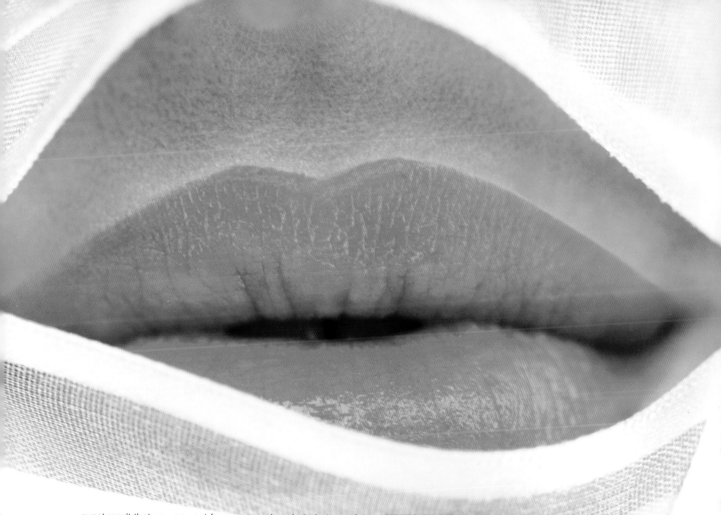

exact result that you may get from a procedure, but photographs offer a good guideline for what is reasonable to expect.

Check out the practitioner's qualifications, experience and training. Find out what professional organisations he/she is a member of and visit their websites for confirmation if needed. Check online to see if the practitioner has had any legal cases brought against them, and what the outcome was.

Tap into your intuition. How do you get along with the person who is going to be wielding the needle? You should feel you can trust him/her with your face and/or body. If you don't get a good vibe, move on. There are many practitioners and clinics to choose from.

Have a good look round. Is the clinic clean and orderly? Does he/she employ professional assistants and nurses? Ask to see inside the room where the procedure will take place, and satisfy yourself that it's the proper clinical setting necessary for a medical treatment. Also look at the other patients in the waiting room – do you like the way they look? And do you like how the staff and even the doctor look? If not, run a mile!

See DIRECTORY for organisations where you can research your practitioner and/or clinic.

WENDY'S VITAL QUESTIONS TO ASK

● What is the medical name of the treatment the practitioner is recommending?
● How long has it been on the market?
● How long has the practitioner been using it?
● What is the name of the manufacturer and where are they located?
● What clinical studies have been done?
● What is the source of the filler material – is it natural, animal or synthetic?
● What are the possible side effects?
● Could I be allergic to it?
● What does a reaction look like and how long does it last?
● What can be done if I have a reaction?
● How many treatments will I

need and how often will I need to come back?
● How much will each treatment cost?
● If I don't like it, what can be done?
● Can I still have other treatments (fillers, wrinkle relaxers, lasers, peels) later?
● Is this the best laser technology/filler/injection to accomplish my goals?
● What are the alternatives?
● Does it have a CE mark (ie, comply with European Health and Safety legislation)?
● Is it approved by the US Food and Drug Administration (FDA) and UK Medicines and Healthcare products Regulatory Agency (MHRA)?
● Is it licensed for cosmetic use?

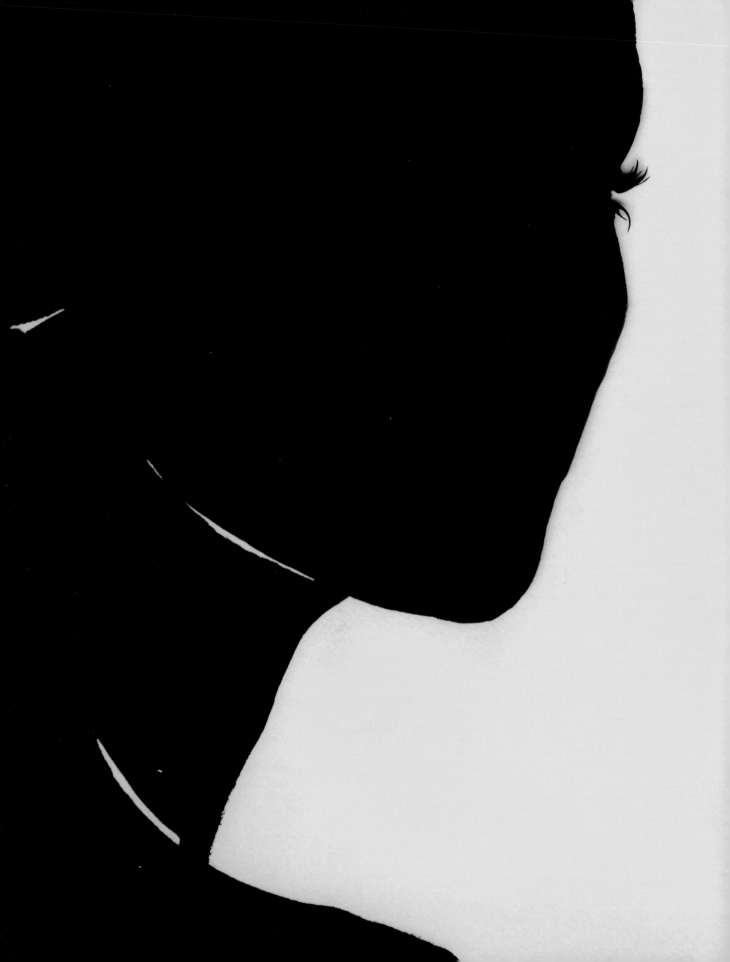

'I NEVER want
to lie about my age.
The actresses I *admire*
are all women who
have not fought
growing older, but
EMBRACED it –
like Sophia Loren or
Audrey Hepburn'

Penélope Cruz

Keep your eyes on the prize

For eyes, read 'angst'. They can be top of many a woman's list of beauty woes, as the years roll by. Think: puffy bags. Think: dark circles. Think: 'laugh lines' (that's the nice way to describe them). And then there's the challenge of applying eye make-up when a) skin's just not as smooth as it was, and b) you can barely see what you're doing anyway…

But leaving vanity aside (temporarily!), what should be absolutely paramount is eye health. Beauty may be in the eye of the beholder, but the bottom line is that we all want to go on beholding everything. So before we give you a rundown of products over the next few pages which will help with the beauty challenges, and share some fabulous make-up tips, here's how to optimise eye health – and help prevent eye-lines at the same time.

Don't frown! Forgive us for stating the obvious but how do you think frown lines get there…? Exactly. But looking after your eyes isn't just about a smooth forehead: taking very good care of eye health in general is absolutely vital as we get older. So…

Wear big sunglasses. Choose glasses which are UVA/B protective. And slap on a broad-brimmed sunhat, not just for the sake of your skin and hair but also, very importantly, for your eyes. Just look at the way people screw up their eyes and face in bright sunlight… Even in not-so-bright conditions, wind is a damage-doer too – and sunglasses provide great protection from dust, specks of dirt and the eye-drying effect of a mistral. Remember, they're also instant glam!

Take reading glasses everywhere and *wear* them. Sarah recently looked at a photo of herself trying to decipher a Christmas cracker joke and nearly choked as she saw the two deep lines scored down her forehead. Motto: must take specs – in chic case, possibly hanging round neck – with you at all times. (Jo keeps a pair in every room of the house, which is also very much appreciated by presbyopic friends.) If you are caught out and about without them, get someone to read to you – the menu, the programme, whatever. (One super-elegant friend takes a lorgnette out and about…!)

Have regular eye tests. The right specs help you read, work at a computer screen, drive safely and prevent frown lines and headaches. Testing can also pick up any other conditions such as glaucoma, which damages the optic nerve and may cause blindness if untreated. Every two years is a minimum when you're over forty, and every year if you have glaucoma in the

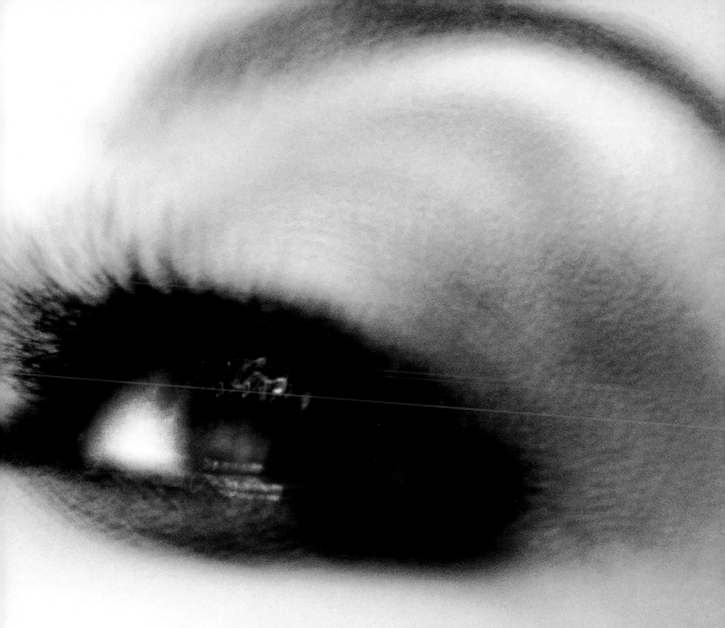

family. NB: women over sixty in the UK can claim free eye tests and will usually get a discount on spectacles. (Remember to get at least one pair of prescription sunglasses, too.)

Attend to dry eyes. OK, it's age again! Like our skin, eyes get drier as we get older, especially if you work at a screen and/or in an office with aircon. If your eyes are itchy, sore, red, stick together on waking and, more seriously, you have any blurred vision, consult your family doctor or talk to your optician. Hopefully, it will just be a case of applying drops once or twice a day. (Sarah swears by Viscotears, a thin gel/ointment you can apply any time – but beware it can blur your sight for a few moments.)

Invest in a good, strong reading light. According to consultant ophthalmologist Professor Charles Clark, 'This can improve vision enormously, slow the deterioration of sight – and reduce frowning!' Obviously, this isn't just for reading but for any close-up fine work, such as tapestry (which Sarah does – very slowly – in the dark winter evenings; Jo knits!). We like the range of lamps from www.seriousreaders.com, which have options for everything.

Consider a supplement. The 'Age-Related Eye Disease Study', sponsored by the US National Eye Institute, reported that two nutrients – called lutein and zeaxanthin, which are both found in healthy retinas – may help your vision and protect your eyes from the age-related condition called macular degeneration. A product called Brite Eyes Formula by LifeTime Vitamins is based on bilberry and eyebright, which contain these nutrients, plus a range of other helpful ingredients. Fish oil, which contains omega-3 essential fatty acid, may also help vision. But you should still eat lots of green, red and orange vegetables and fruit (full of lutein and zeaxanthin) plus at least two portions of oily fish weekly, if you're not vegetarian.

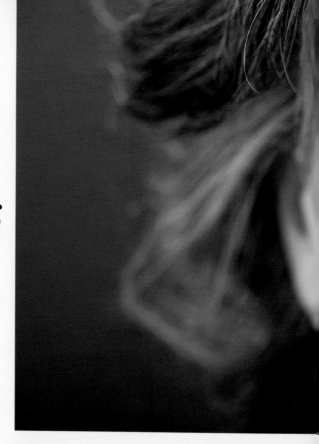

Anti-ageing eye creams: *our award winners*

Because eyes are so expressive – conveying joy, or sadness, or anger – the skin around them wrinkles faster than anywhere else on the face. The skin beneath the eyes also contains less collagen and elastin than the rest of the face. And as a triple whammy, this fragile skin is fine as eggshell – only one quarter as thick as that on the soles of your feet. (Precisely because it's so thin, moisture evaporates very easily)

But – hallelujah – we do know, from years of trials on real women, that there are plenty of products out there to make a difference to those expression lines. For *The Anti-Ageing Beauty Bible*, we sent out over 100 creams that we've never trialled before to our panellists, requesting them to use the treatments on one eye only. There were some truly spectacular performances by some of the winning products – so read on.

REVIEWS

AT A GLANCE

Barefoot Botanicals Rosa Fina Intensive Eye Serum

Murad Intensive Wrinkle Reducer for Eyes

Medik8 Pretox Eyelift

Celgenics Eye Essential

Barefoot Botanicals Rosa Fina Intensive Eye Serum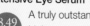

8.49/10 A truly outstanding score for this high-potency serum-style treatment product, which – despite featuring argan and rosa mosqueta (rosehip seed) oils – sinks in fast, according to delighted testers. Other key botanicals in this all-natural winner include frankincense, antioxidant vitamins A, C and E plus vitamin B5. The bonus: witch hazel promises instantly firming benefits.

Comments: 'Divine smell, I liked this product very much; went on very easily, sank straight in, and I did notice a difference in crêpiness which in turn seemed to make eyes brighter. Would definitely buy' • 'the best eye cream I've tried so far; pleasant to use, didn't give me spots and lumps, fantastically hydrating, and made the skin look a little brighter and more radiant' • 'sank in very easily and could apply make-up straight after; skin looked much more hydrated around eyes and certainly had an effect on fine lines which looked smoother because skin plumper; had a positive effect on puffiness and seemed to calm skin around eye socket; dark circles did diminish slightly' • 'really light, silky product; lines much, much fainter after six weeks; wrinkles less deep, skin much smoother; really loved it!' • 'made my eyes look younger and the eye area more perky' • 'lines have significantly reduced and people commented I look "fresh"'.

Murad Intensive Wrinkle Reducer for Eyes

8.43/10 Dr Howard Murad's was one of the pioneering dermatologist brands in the skincare world, founded in 1989, and this features a breakthrough ingredient derived from the superfruit durian, alongside powerful antioxidants including goji berry, plus anti-inflammatories and moisture-boosting hydrators. Fantastic reviews, with the only negative comment about 'over-packaging'.

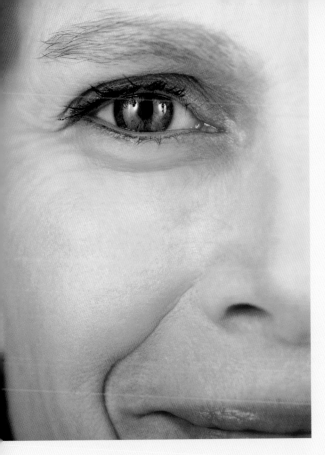

longer-term benefits. Again a few negative comments about over-packaging.

Comments: 'Skin felt instantly tighter, and once gel had dried in, it made eye area look fresher and brighter' • 'my 70-year-old mother really liked this, though she said it sank in slowly, but it did improve fine lines and wrinkles slightly; made eyes look much brighter, reduced puffiness and my father commented on how much better she looked' • 'sinks in very easily and skin felt moisturised and smooth; concealer went on better than usual, lines improved after six weeks, and eye area brighter. Loved it and will buy more' • 'very cooling and refreshing' • 'skin felt moisturised and plumper immediately; under-eye make-up usually gathers in the fine lines but after this it smoothed on fine; after six weeks, plumped skin, lines and wrinkles much less noticeable, reduces crêpiness significantly but if you put too much on it peels off unattractively' • 'quite an effect on dark circles, too'.

Celgenics Eye Essential

8.17/10 OK, suspend your disbelief (for those of you not into crystals or 'healing energies'), because the bottom line is that this eye treatment scored unbelievably well with our panellists – beating dozens of other contenders – and that's what really counts. Products are handmade in small batches, feature organic vegetable oils and natural spring water (plus witch hazel and eyebright in Eye Essential), and come in airless pumps (eliminating the need for preservatives). Celgenics creations also 'carry the vibrational energy of healing, love and peace'. (And personally, we love that.) This eye treat is meant to help with tired eyes from computer use too.

Comments: 'Fine lines did disappear, so much that I had to use on both eyes after four weeks as the difference was so obvious, reduced dark circles to barely noticeable, eyes looked brighter, more awake and alive, ten years younger' • 'make-up went on really well after 10–15 minutes, fine lines improved and much softer, wrinkles more diffused and not as harsh-looking; tested eye slightly brighter, and softness helps to create "lift", smooths eyelids' • 'liked the modern packaging, which delivered a specific amount of very light, well-absorbed cream; foundation easily applied over it; lovely to use' • 'puffiness reduced – one of the most powerful effects, tightening feeling on application, and dark circles much improved although I've been really tired; good long-lasting hydration'.

Comments: '10/10: fabulously hydrating, improved wrinkles, lines, puffiness, dark circles and crêpiness, made eyes look brighter and seemed to "lift" the area; my partner said the "test" eye looked better' • 'needed to be firmly pressed into skin, not massaged; absorbed well once I got the hang of it' • 'fine lines improved, deep lines less deep and defined, eye area looks younger, eyes much, much brighter and tired bags almost gone. I can see a real difference in the left eye. One of the best products I have used in a long time!' • 'rather overpackaged but finer lines definitely improved and skin more elastic and smoother, wrinkles less prominent, crêpiness of eyelids improved and disappeared after four weeks, puffiness definitely down, dark circles not gone completely but am hopeful. Several people said I look well'.

Medik8 Pretox Eyelift

8.28/10 Medik8 is a British cosmeceutical brand, set up to create effective anti-ageing ingredients and formulations suitable for even the most sensitive skins. The sci-fi sounding ingredients in this 'serum-y, cream-y gel' are too numerous to list (think: Dermaxyl and Eyeliss, etc), but together they target fine lines and wrinkles, dark shadows and puffiness, delivering a fast fix – plus

Lighten those dark circles

Fact: we get more anxious questions about under-eye circles to www.beautybible.com than almost any other subject (except eye bags and crow's feet). In a survey by Clinique of 13,000 users, about 53 per cent cited dark circles and puffiness as their number one concern. So here's how to make shadows, well, a shadow of their former selves

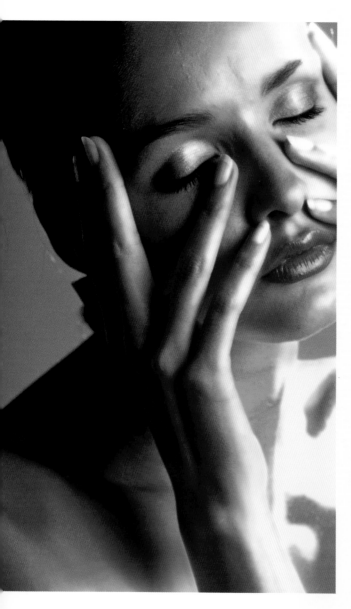

Conceal, conceal, conceal. Overleaf, you'll see the top light-reflective concealers, in our testers' considered opinions. If there's a shade choice, pick a yellow-based concealer if your dark circles have a purple or blue cast; go with a peachy colour if they are browner in tone. Meanwhile, women with darker skintones may find that light-reflective concealers just don't work for them – so you'll want to know that Guerlain Precious Light and the legendary YSL Touche Eclat come in darker shade options. And Bobbi Brown actually created her Corrector concealer specifically for dark circles, with the darkest shade being Very Deep Bisque.

Try Traditional Chinese Medicine. In TCM (as it's known in the holistic realm), dark circles can be linked to an imbalance in kidney energy – which can be helped by acupuncture. With TCM, as with all complementary therapies, seek out someone who is qualified and registered (see DIRECTORY for more details).

Drink plenty of water. For some women, dark circles can be a sign of dehydration. Another good reason to sip those eight glasses a day.

Consider using a cream targeted at 'sun spots'. For some women, dark circles can be linked to hyperpigmentation (see box opposite), in which case it may be worth trying one of the age-spot-lightening creams which performed best in our trials (see page 190). Don't apply so close to the eye that there's a risk of the product 'travelling' into the eye itself, as these can contain potent ingredients that might sting.

Try a D-I-Y Ayurvedic eye mask. Ayurvedic beauty expert Monisha Bharadwaj swears by a recipe for tackling dark circles handed down by her family. 'Crush five mint leaves in a little water with a pestle and mortar. Strain the juice and add to one teaspoon of almond oil and half a teaspoon of honey. Stir until completely mixed and apply a tiny amount under the eyes before going to bed.' Works wonders, she swears.

Clear your nasal passages. As nasal congestion is a common cause (see box right), clearing the respiratory tract may help. If it could be an allergy, try a supplement such as Aller-DMG, and also a barrier product (balm, cream or spray) in your nose which helps to prevent allergens being inhaled. A steam 'head bath' (also brilliant for your complexion) clears nasal passages a treat: fill a bowl with very hot water, add a few drops of essential oil such as eucalyptus, peppermint, rosemary, cover your head with a towel and steam gently for five minutes.

Try an antihistamine. If you think your underlying problem could be an allergy to an airborne substance (as in hayfever, or an allergy to something in a fragrance or cosmetic), an antihistamine could be a simple solution.

Eat dark-circle-busting foods. Certain antioxidant-rich foods may help to strengthen capillaries: edible eye TLC comes in the form of blueberries, cranberries, bilberries, blackcurrants, onions, peas and beans, as well as green and black tea.

Follow the dark circles blog! Believe it or not, there is an entire community on the net, written by dark-circle sufferers and focusing on women's experiences with many of the creams and non-surgical treatments on the market targeting this beauty challenge – www. mydarkcirclesblog.com is pretty commercial (and US-based), but it will at least reassure you that you are far from alone.

WHAT CAUSES DARK CIRCLES?

There are multiple causes for dark circles (medically called periorbital hyperchromia), according to medical research.

Genes They can be genetic, affecting any skin colour and type, but Asian and Afro-Caribbean races and southern Italians are particularly prone to them.

Hyperpigmentation The browner type of dark circles, rather than the bluish-hued type, could be the results of post-inflammatory hyperpigmentation due to sun damage or hormonal fluctuations, notes dermatologist Dr Nicholas Perricone.

Older, thinner skin As we age, we become more prone to permanent dark circles – simply because, as skin thins, the blood vessels in the under-eye zone show up more. Airborne allergens cause blood to pool in the vessels under the skin, worsening the appearance of any dilated blood vessels.

Nasal congestion Famously, they're linked with lack of sleep, but consider this insight from beauty guru Liz Earle: 'The most common cause of dark circles is nasal congestion. When your nose is bunged up, veins that usually drain from your eyes into your nose become dilated and darker.' Ask yourself if you tend to get them with hayfever during the summer, or ongoing colds in the winter. Equally something in your beauty regime could be the culprit (we have often found the finger pointed at a new mascara or eye cream, which may also cause puffiness).

Stress Dr Perricone also blames stress: 'When your body is in fight or flight mode, your brain, like every other organ, leaches every single molecule of oxygen it can from the blood, so a darker, more deoxygenated blood flows through your veins. This dark blood is most visible in the transparent skin under our eyes, and is what causes the appearance of these discoloured veins.' (The skin under the eyes is the thinnest on the body.)

Drugs Some drugs, including the contraceptive pill and HRT, can darken the eye area by dilating blood vessels.

Smoking Women who smoke – which affects micro-circulation long before it leads to heart and lung problems – can be prone to dark circles, too.

'I choose *NOT* to hang on to this **ideal** of looking 20 years old but **understand** that I have a wealth of EXPERIENCE to share. I make the *best* of what I have, but I don't long for who I *used* to be' Elle Macpherson

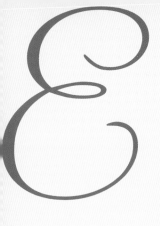

Concealers for dark circles: *our award winners*

At our age, a woman needs a (small) wardrobe of concealers. Here, you'll find the best candidates for disguising dark circles under eyes, which also work well on pigmentation

AT A GLANCE

YSL Touche Eclat

Guerlain Precious Light Rejuvenating Illuminator

La Prairie Light Fantastic Cellular Concealing Treatment

Bobbi Brown Creamy Concealer

TIP

Don't only apply light-reflecting concealer under the eye: a couple of dots at the inner corners of your eye, near your tear ducts and on the bridge of the nose, instantly makes eyes look fresher.

Three out of our top four are light-reflecting so they also blur lines – stroke them in grooves and wrinkles too, to see the effect of the 'optical pigments'. Light-reflective concealers can also be used to highlight the brow bone, or accentuate a pout, when stroked along the top lip; they can do double-duty as an eyeshadow base, too. Of the many, many choices now out there, our testers help you by narrowing it down to these top picks. (And for concealers to hide those other flaws, such as veins and redness, turn to page 91. For products to help puffiness, see page 60.)

REVIEWS

YSL Touche Eclat

 We make no apologies for the fact that this classic concealer has appeared in previous books – because we sent it out to be trialled all over again for *The Anti-Ageing Beauty Bible*, and Touche Eclat (aka Radiant Touch) romped home in first place with a fah-bu-lous score, just as it did before… Created by Terry de Gunzburg (who now has her own By Terry range) in 1992, it was the first of its type. And its legions of fans still think that this pump-action, pen-style concealer – with its built-in brush and light-reflective, line-blurring formula – is unrivalled. Our testers were assigned No 1 (Luminous Radiance), which has slightly peachy-pink hints. (NB: women with darker skins might like to know that at some duty frees and a handful of spiffy department stores, you can find a deeper shade of Touche

Eclat – No 3 – though it beats us why it's not universally available.) A Hall of Fame product, if ever there was one.

Comments: 'Perfect for dark circles – the best product in my opinion! Didn't cover completely but blended them in and made them less noticeable' • 'looked very natural; I always carry one in my make-up bag' • be careful not to overdo or it can look too pale' • 'blended in well over a moisturiser or cream foundation but not as good over a mineral base; great cover-up job on thread veins round my nose and sun spots under eyes; ideal quick fix before morning school run' • '10+++ for this brilliant camouflage for dark circles, also great for lines on my forehead' • 'my magic wand – I thought it was all hype, but how wrong I was! It's easy to use, gives an amazing effect – so many comments about how well I look!!!'.

Guerlain Precious Light Rejuvenating Illuminator

 Like Touche Eclat, this comes in a sexy gold wand, with a brush at the tip to sweep on a formula enriched with Gold Radiance Pigments and Precious Rejuvenating Complex. Which means that… Precious Light claims to offer skincare benefits as well as the instant cosmetic boost. Myrrh – known for its invigorating and rejuvenating powers – is a key ingredient. In three shades – our testers had the lightest, 01.

Comments: 'Fantastic at covering up quite dark circles under eyes, also small scars; a pigmentation mark on my forehead became invisible' • 'very easy to apply, blended well; brightened up dark

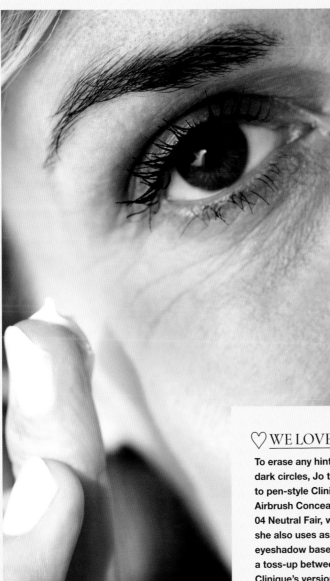

La Prairie Light Fantastic Cellular Concealing Treatment

 8.11/10

The winning contender from this Swiss luxury skincare brand also promises longer-term benefits, as well as a quick dark-shadow-fix, with ingredients such as horse chestnut (to target dark circles), soothing Roman chamomile and arnica, plus papaya extract to target wrinkles, and LP's signature Exclusive Cellular Complex. It comes with the luxurious price-tag you'd expect of a La Prairie creation, but a refill (it's available in three shades) comes with the cylindrical silver-coloured container. It did divide testers, some of whom really rated it – while others were less impressed.

Comments: 'Very easy to dab in, covered and improved dark circles, worked well on small brown age spot by eye; certainly improved look of eyes without looking too made-up' • 'lightened and brightened eye area immediately, but would have preferred something more nourishing like my usual Touche Eclat' • 'not a miracle worker but I looked fresher and well-rested, can use under or over foundation to give a natural-looking foundation' • 'I like the luminosity it brings to the eye area, as if I've had a jolly good night's sleep'.

Bobbi Brown Creamy Concealer

 8.10/10

'Good concealer is the secret of the universe,' maintains our friend Bobbi Brown – and we rather agree. This isn't actually a light-reflecting product but relies on her favourite yellow pigment to camouflage dark circles (and blemishes of all kinds). It also boasts skin-conditioning ingredients like vitamin A. We especially like the fact that this comes in 14 shades (we trialled Beige), including some really dark options for Asian/black skins, which are so often overlooked in the shade-creation process.

Comments: 'Top marks, fits the bill perfectly, am really pleased' • 'very easy to apply with fingertips or concealer brush, I used powder to set it; did a reasonably good job of covering my terrible dark circles, needed a lot of moisturiser underneath (which is fine)' • 'fantastic at taking the darkness away, excellent on pigmentation – lasted well and looked very natural' • 'quite creamy, and moisturising, and covered well – dark circles, thread veins, scars and pigmentation – but accentuated wrinkles'.

♡ WE LOVE...

To erase any hint of dark circles, Jo turns to pen-style Clinique Airbrush Concealer in 04 Neutral Fair, which she also uses as an eyeshadow base. (It's a toss-up between Clinique's version and Dior Skinflash, which is more obviously light-reflective, and – she finds – better after dark.) Sarah gives thanks daily for Trish McEvoy's Correct and Brighten twist pen for shadows and darkness; it wouldn't cover very dark circles but is fab for brightening the eye area; swipe under eyes and over inside half of lids.

circles, small scars looked less obvious; good coverage' • 'a must for your make-up bag' • 'very clever at reflecting light away from my face – great product' • 'very effective on my very pale skin; when I get tired it looks so obvious and this created a good complexion' • 'smooth consistency and didn't cake when built up thinly; made eyes look younger, also covered freckles and hyperpigmentation' • 'I used a lot on my dark circles but it didn't cake or crack, despite an evening of laughter and smiling'.

Unpack those eye bags

Maybe you get them just sometimes. (We all do.) Maybe they're the bane of your life. (As for many of our readers.) The simple truth is: none of us likes excess under-eye baggage and, as we age, skin loses elasticity, so the eye area can be more prone to swelling. Here are the best fixes we know…

Sleep with an extra pillow. If you can get in the habit of sleeping on your back (not everyone can – and remember it is the sleep position most linked with s-n-o-r-i-n-g), then this extra elevation can help to prevent fluid from building up in the eye area overnight. (Most puffy-prone women find the problem's worst before lunch – good reason never to be photographed until the afternoon…)

Check out eye products containing caffeine. In our experience (and anecdotally that of our testers), some products containing caffeine as an ingredient can be especially helpful for smoothing away puffiness.

Or give your eyes a drink of tea. Since caffeine has proven useful for banishing dark circles, a low-tech solution is two tea bags (black, caffeinated, rich in natural tannins), kept in the freezer rather than the fridge and placed on the eyes to constrict blood vessels and drain fluid.

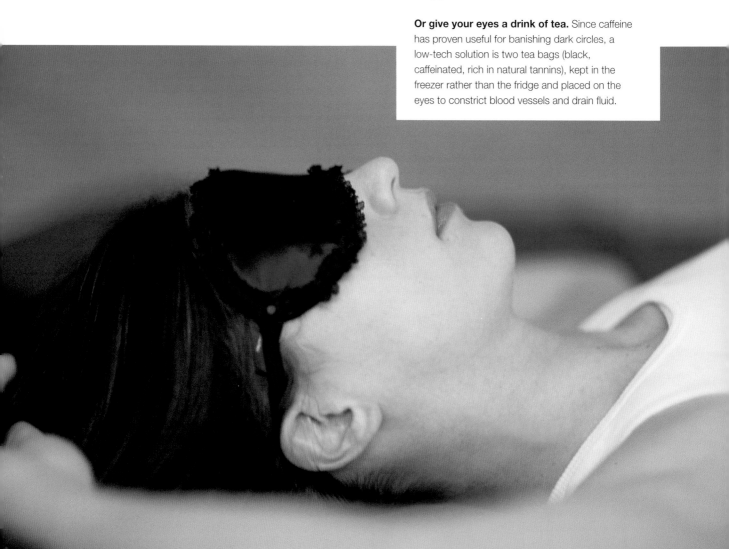

Try a roller-ball. It makes perfect sense to us that something which has a physical action can literally smooth away puffiness – and sure enough, metal roller-balls can prove amazingly effective. You literally roll them around the puffy area in a circular/outward motion, to disperse fluid. As a low-tech version, real silver/silver-plated teaspoons kept in the fridge can be used to 'tap' away fluid. Jo uses a little silver-tipped applicator – like a baby drum baton – that she got with a Crème de la Mer eye product, for the same task: 'miraculous', is her verdict. It's an expensive way to get your hands on one of the most brilliant eye de-puffers of all time… so failing that, go the teaspoon route.

Have a chilled, gel-filled mask on standby in the fridge. There are quite a few on the market, although we prefer the type that don't have eye-holes, as they offer more even pressure (and cooling action) on the whole eye area. (The Body Shop's Aqua Eye Mask is excellent, or see DIRECTORY for other sources.) Lie prone, place mask on eyes for 10–15 minutes and let the cool gel work its soothing magic.

Eliminate your eye cream itself from the list of culprits. Sometimes a product which is designed to deal with lines and wrinkles can very annoyingly trigger puffiness. If you think there's any chance at all that your puffy eyes are product-related, stop using the potential culprit for five days and note any difference. If it's the cream, you'll know because you'll see an improvement. If it's not, your puffiness will be unchanged. Be aware that eye gels are less likely to 'travel' into the eyes themselves than creams; only gels or serums can be applied on the lids themselves, as there's a risk with any oil-based product of getting into the eye – and puffiness, as well as redness, is your body's sign of rebellion.

Reduce salt intake and drink less alcohol. Oh, we're a couple of killjoys, but if you're serious about this, cut down on salt and alcoholic drinks, both of which are notoriously linked with fluid retention. Ditto any foods containing MSG; you can ask in

WHAT CAUSES PUFFINESS?

As with dark circles, there's a long list of potential culprits and it can help to try to 'unpick' your personal trigger/s, so that you can take the lifestyle steps needed to minimise the problem. First (darn it): heredity – your genes may simply incorporate the DNA that leads to thicker fat pads under the eyes, in which case there may not be much you can do to tackle the problem. There is surgery available for fat-removal under the eyes, but if performed too early in life (or if too much fat is removed), this can lead to a really hollow look later on (not a good look). Second is water retention – which is linked with diet, sleeping habits, alcohol and even hormonal roller-coastering. Third, allergies can be responsible if you're allergic to pollen, pesticides, latex, certain foods, including grains and additives including MSG, cosmetics or fragrance. These can all trigger puffiness. And even the most smooth-eyed among us can get all pouchy with a cold.

Chinese restaurants for this ingredient to be left out, but it features in a lot of ingredient lists on processed foods, often by different names such as glutamic acid, vegetable protein extract, hydrolysed vegetable protein/HVP, sodium caseinate or even yeast extract. The safest way to avoid it is always to eat fresh, unprocessed foods. Foods which have a diuretic (water-banishing) effect include celery, cucumber, watermelon, radishes and parsley.

Do plenty of cardiovascular exercise. It revs up your circulation, which helps to eliminate excess water through sweating. In our experience, everything just 'flows' better when we've exercised – and a brisk 30-minute walk can work wonders for unpacking that eye baggage. A workout followed by a sauna or steam bath can flush out puffies almost miraculously.

Make like Linda Evangelista. Readers of our earlier books may be familiar with this trick, but it sure as hell is worth repeating: stroke an ice cube over the skin, working in an outwards direction. If you're prone to broken veins, wrap it in clingfilm first. Jo watched Ms Evangelista do this on a photoshoot and it was right up there with the miracle of the loaves and the fishes in terms of transformations. (Sarah has been known to order a bowl of ice simply to stroke round her super-sensitive, prone-to-puffies eyes.)

ℰTreats for tired & puffy eyes: *our award winners*

There are two eye issues that we get more emails about to www.beautybible.com than almost anything else (except skin problems). First, dark circles (which we help you to conceal on page 56). Second, under-eye puffiness. Even if you've never had tired-looking eyes in your youth, the mid-years can be a time of excess eye baggage and shadows. Since bright, sparkling eyes make you look instantly rejuvenated, we're delighted to bring you the results of this trial – which proves that there are effective treatments to tackle these Big Beauty Challenges. Yes, in the blink of an eye…

AT A GLANCE

Estée Lauder Stress Relief Eye Mask

Repêchage Cell Renewal Eye Rescue Pads

Lavera Faces My Age Cooling Eye Roll-on

Urban Retreat UR The Eye Cream

TIP

'I keep a bottle of witch hazel lotion in the fridge for when I wake up a bit puffy around the eyes. Soak two cotton pads in it, place them on your eyes and lie down for a few minutes. It really takes away the tiredness.' – Mary Greenwell

REVIEWS

Estée Lauder Stress Relief Eye Mask

 8/10 These see-thru gauze pads come in sachets (two pads per single-use sachet), to be pressed on to the under-eye zone while you relax for ten minutes and allow ingredients such as vitamin A palmitate, hyaluronic acid (for a moisture boost), aloe vera, cucumber, allantoin and bisabolol to soothe, hydrate and reduce redness.
Comments: 'A bit of a hero product this: puffy eyes from a cold visibly reduced, and my life-long dark circles much improved; also I am a big investor in eye creams and concealers and both work much better if I have used the mask before; when eyes are tired, tight and sore, the effects are very soothing, cooling and moisturising' • 'my sensitive eyes look brighter, fresher and more hydrated, made me awake again after a very hard day – brilliant when you want to go out after a long day' • 'love the cooling sensation, and made the dehydrated skin around my eyes look more plumped and moisturised – does what it says and is worth the money'.

Repêchage Cell Renewal Eye Rescue Pads

 7.98/10 These are pads, too (from a Manhattan spa brand): circular cotton versions, infused with moisturising seaweed elements and no less than four types of antioxidant tea to reduce puffiness and tone the area. Again, ten minutes should do the trick.
Comments: 'Eyes felt clear and bright and skin smooth and moisturised; the packaging for these pads says these are a vacation for the eyes and it really is the case' • 'because I felt so refreshed I needed less concealer around my eyes, and didn't pile on so much make-up; would absolutely buy' • 'really liked these pads which I kept in the fridge for extra de-puffing; using them in the morning after a late night was bliss!' • 'reduced puffiness and eyes did look brighter and renewed – very relaxing and great for a little pamper session'.

Lavera Faces My Age Cooling Eye Roll-on ✿✿

 7.56/10 For wannabe-natural beauties out there, a NaTrue-certified formulation which glides on to skin via a metal roller-ball (which delivers a lovely instantly-cooling sensation). Soothing botanicals include white tea to boost micro-circulation, vitamins, minerals, aloe vera and salicylic acid, a red and brown algae extract plus nurturing karanja oil (known to help prevent formation of new pigmentation marks), and beachberry to target existing age spots. A couple of testers marked it right down for packaging issues but loved the actual product.
Comments: 'Putting this on after a long day was wonderful, very refreshing; my husband loved it too – and you can't get higher praise than that;

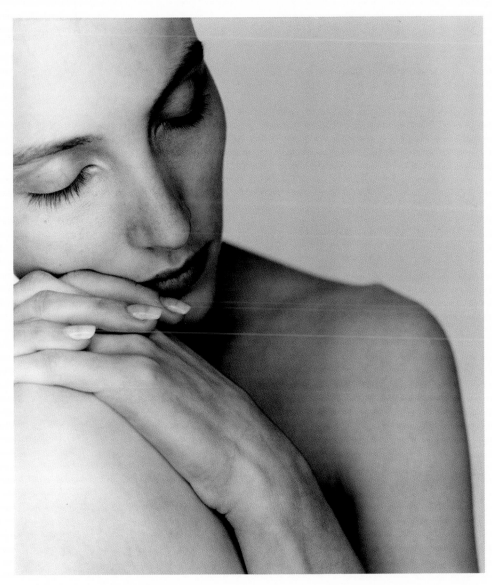

♡ WE LOVE...

Jo has plenty of beauty woes, but puffy eyes and shadows aren't really among them. However, when her eyes feel computer-weary, she reaches for eyeSlices: cooling gel pads infused with soothing botanicals, perfectly shaped to the eye zone, which makes them feel instantly rested. (No need to keep them in the fridge, either: they're quite cooling enough when stashed handily in the bedside drawer.) Sarah does have puffy eyes – but no dark circles – and reaches for the ice cubes first thing in the morning, then strokes on Origins No Puffery Cooling Mask, which works best of anything she's found so far and, vitally, doesn't irritate her supersensitive eyes. A little squirt of Bach Rescue Remedy on and around her (closed) eyes is fab for reducing tired, sore itchiness.

fantastically – and surprisingly – reviving' • 'lovely cooling effect that reduced puffiness and eyes were very refreshed' • 'eye area was clearer, less puffy and incredibly refreshed – felt fantastic' • 'roller-ball is very easy to use, and the light gel soaks in easily, gives a moisturising and firming effect as well as brightening and refreshing; very impressive little product that I would buy'.

Urban Retreat UR The Eye Cream

7.55/10

From the brand originally created for Harrods' spiffy Urban Retreat salon on the Fifth Floor (by their in-house experts), a lightweight soothing cream to target dark circles and puffiness, packed with aloe vera, rosehip oil, cucumber, chamomile and eyebright.

Comments: 'Eyes clearer and brighter, very refreshed, soothed and comforted; quite good at reducing puffiness' • 'looked like I'd had a full eight hours sleep when I definitely hadn't' • 'very good at reducing puffiness, and was pleasantly surprised how quickly' • 'I've had quite a few late nights due to work but my colleagues don't believe me as I have no bags under my eyes' • 'a little miracle; a tiny bit goes a long way and the effects are brilliant; combated tired eyes, dry lids, dark circles, puffiness – and left skin around eyes really soft and moisturised. Love this!'.

Don't let your eyebrows fade away...

Brows disappear – f-a-d-i-n-g away – if we're not careful. They may just get more sparse or go grey. Whichever, your face will quite simply lose definition – brows are the architecture of the face – if you don't either tint them (your hair colourist may be able to do this, albeit somewhat sneakily), or colour them in

TIP

Lots of clients ask expert Jenny Jordan about cutting unruly brows. She advises investing in a cheap pair of hairdressing scissors for this task. Brush brows upwards first, using a little soap on the brush to make them stick up. (It works a bit like a wax.) Then trim with the scissors – but not too close: brow hairs will fall downwards naturally and if you don't leave a bit, you may create 'huge' holes, she warns. Our advice: proceed with caution, but it can be done.

Brush on a mid-taupe/grey-ish powder shadow to colour your brows. This is most flattering for almost all brows, at this stage, to define them. Too dark and you risk that Cruella look. (Alternatively, use a pencil with a soft chalky texture – read about those which our testers got on with, overleaf.)

Extend the brow outwards, not downwards. Of course you need to follow the natural line of your brow, but by now many of us have lost the 'ends' of our brows (just plain vanished into the ether we guess) and if you need to recreate them with make-up, make sure the line wings out towards your temples, rather than down towards your cheeks. (Also see 'Plot your brow line', right.)

Brush your brows to groom them. By now, for many of us, brow hairs are literally all over the place – it sometimes seems as if they're all making a bid for freedom in different directions. A brow brush – or make-up genius Terry de Gunzburg recommends an old mascara wand that's been thoroughly washed – does the job beautifully. Brush them, apply colour, brush gently again. It makes for a much more natural effect. Legendary Hollywood make-up artist Valerie Sarnelle finishes off with her own Valerie Brow Tamer to keep them in place all day. London's brow goddess Jenny Jordan favours Tweezerman Browmousse, a gel which 'sets hairs in place without them getting crispy'.

And brush them again, if you use face powder. If you powder your face after you do your brows, you need to brush them one more time or (as expert Mary Greenwell notes), 'they can look dusty and dirty. And "clean" brows are really important at this time in life'.

Or you could try a stencil. This creates a stronger brow look than many women are used to. And we admit: when Valerie did our brows we had fits at first – they were so much more prominent than we were used to. But she's not known as 'the brow queen' for nothing, and the reactions from onlookers were so positive, we grew to love (slightly trepidatiously) the routine for special occasions. (In LA this means everyday…!) Valerie's range is simply called Valerie Beverly Hills, and her trademark Star Stencil Kit includes a foolproof stencil system for brow perfection. You choose the shape that's most flattering for you (from a wide range), then literally fill it in with a Brow Queen Pencil. Valerie teams 'significant' brows with a sheer wash of eyeshadow and lots of mascara, or even false eyelashes for a 'gorgeous, wide-awake look'.

Balance your brows with your eye make-up. More on your eyes means subtler brows; less eye make-up means you can play up your brows (as per Valerie's advice, above).

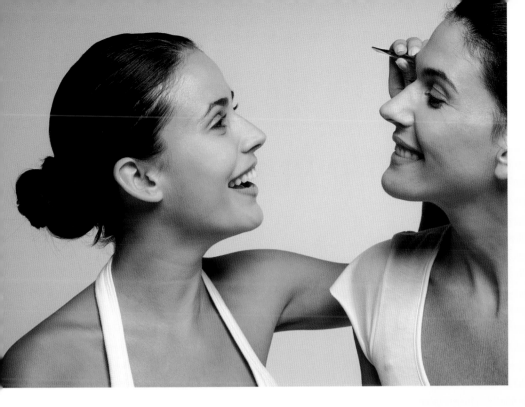

Generally

● Always tweeze in bright daylight, with a hand-held magnifying mirror, facing a window.

● Make sure the brow area is clean and grease-free.

● Use sharp, slant-edged tweezers which grip each hair from the root. Pointy tweezers are difficult to use on yourself.

THE EYEBROW FACELIFT

There's no doubt that 'clean and tidy' brows are essential to a glossy, groomed look. If you have thick brows (lucky you!), then getting them professionally shaped – at least to start off with – can be very helpful, and makes for easier home maintenance. Even if your brows have become sparse, a professional can often improve the shape. (Sarah's were mostly blown off in a gas oven explosion years ago, not helped by over-plucking before that, and they used to skyrocket up at the arch, giving her a rather shocked look. Manhattan expert Eliza Petrescu overcame the problem by carefully plucking hairs above the brows to 'flatten' the arch somewhat, which also worked to create the illusion of widening her thinnish face.)

There's tweezing, waxing, threading, depilatories – a bunch of professional ways of shaping and tidying your brows. Whichever you choose, do talk through what's going to happen and the results you can expect with the practitioner first: it's a bit like a haircut – you can sit like a rabbit in the headlights while your brows are exterminated, which happened to Sarah with threading... (Though Jo swears by it.)

At home, we think plucking – with good slanted tweezers – is by far the easiest way to tend brow shape. We have these tips from Jenny Jordan, whose Eyebrow and Make-up Clinic in London is a mecca for those in search of perfect brows. 'If you want to see the difference that brows make to a face, try putting plasters across your brows. Without them, your face has no shape,' says Jenny. 'As you get older, your brows can literally hitch up and hold your face in place. In the past few years, a new, straighter, upwards-slanting shape has emerged which is as good as a facelift.'

A word of warning: avoid over-plucking. If your brows are scanty, neglect them for a bit; applying olive oil or Vaseline every night may encourage them to grow (OK, that's a folk tale but a lot of people swear by it).

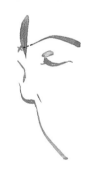

Plot your brow line

● The line slants gently up, starting at a point above the inner corner of your eyes, but with brows never more than an inch apart over your nose.

● It goes out to a wide-angled bend (rather than the old-fashioned extreme arch), above the point where the white begins at the outer rim of your eyeball.

● Then let the line straighten up, winging towards your temples. To find the outer edge, lay a slim pencil (or a slender-handled make-up brush) up from your nostril, past the outer corner of your eye – where it crosses your brow is the natural finishing point.

● The line should be neither fat nor slim, gently tapering to the outer edge – but do avoid the dated 'tadpole' shape.

● Swipe your tweezed brows with a cotton bud dipped in pure tea tree oil, which is a natural antiseptic.

● To fill in the line, Jenny likes to brush on taupe powder so it smudges into the line, and then fixes it with brow gel.

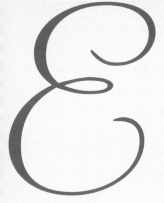

Brow pencils: *our award winners*

Life isn't fair. Just as hairs start randomly sprouting elsewhere on the face (see page 146 for how to tackle that), brows become finer, lighter – and can fade away drastically. Some go grey. Others just get fairer. Or sparser. But a well-defined brow – even if you have to 'fake' it – is near miraculous for helping to accentuate your features and give the face 'structure'.

Although brow powders are now available on the beauty counters, we were interested to find that none of those we dispatched did well enough to be included in our winning line-up. Testers definitely preferred these pencils... NB: do try different shades, and remember that a lighter, softer shade than your natural brows can often work best.

REVIEWS

MAC Eye Brows

 Probably the slimmest and most streamlined pencil on the market anywhere, this is self-propelling and self-sharpening. (Which means you're never at risk of harming skin with a wooden pencil stub. And yes, we know it happens!) It's super-easy to create fine, feathery strokes, and the initially waxy texture transforms to a budge-proof finish. Six shades to choose from (more than most brow colour options), spanning fair to dark; our ten testers received Lingering, a light taupe.
Comments: 'Very easy to apply, went on smoothly and beautifully, the fine tip is perfect for precise feather strokes and you really can't go wrong with the colour; slight waxiness helped hold brows in place; looked very natural – as if I had no make-up on' • 'the perfect brow pencil, beats all the others hands down – although I have very dark brows, the light brown looked really natural on me, and blended in easily' • 'was amazed how much difference this made to my appearance – very easy to apply, I'm not used to using these but found it a doddle!'.

Rituals Natural Eyebrow Pencil

 A built-in brush on the cap, a highlighter at the opposite end to the brow pencil: this is an all-in-one grooming and 'lifting' pencil. (Add a touch of the lighter shade under the brow, and pow! Eyes look more open.) It's got a pretty hard texture (which ensures the colour stays put), and initially has a super-sharp point that we suggest you blunt ever-so-slightly on the back of your hand before feathering on to the brow-zone. Three shades; ours was Hazel.
Comments: 'Very easy and smooth to apply, perfect length pencil to hold lightly and follow arch, super-easy to blend with a small brush' • 'very long-lasting and natural-looking; very easy to sharpen with my own sharpener' • 'hard pencil – but it didn't drag – so I could draw in fine lines for brows and they didn't go smudgy; the best pencil I've used' • 'liked the comb, and the light end for under brows' • 'very impressed with this – the best I have tried; I'm a victim of over-plucking and this gave me exactly the definition I was looking for – only marked down as no sharpener' • 'amazingly natural, even better than my Chanel brow pencil! Brilliant, will absolutely buy'.

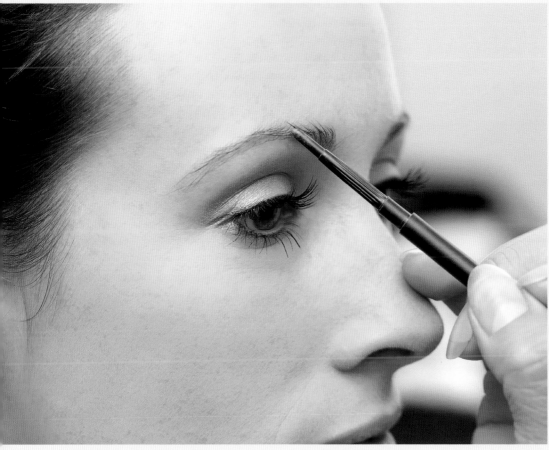

♡ WE LOVE...

Brow pencils are an essential part of our make-up arsenal: without them, Jo says her eyes 'vanish'. Having read our testers' comments Jo is a new and evangelical convert to the MAC award winner featured here; other long-term favourites include **Dior Sourcils Poudre Powder Eyebrow Pencil with Brush** (which gives the effect of a powder shadow, stroked on in pencil format) and the waxier **Jemma Kidd I-conic Eyes Brow Pencil**, in 01 Honey Blonde, perfect for anyone with fair hair (it not only comes with a brush but also a built-in pair of tweezers in the lid). Sarah is another brow pencil devotee – as a victim of over-plucking plus an exploding gas oven! Her all-time favourite is **Arch de Triumph Brow Shaper by Soap & Glory**, a double-ended pencil with foolproof soft taupe one end and pink highlighter the other. Plus it comes with three pop-out brow stencils, should you feel like playing...

Benefit Instant Brow Pencil

 7.41/10 Available in three shades, a more soft-textured pencil which transforms from a creamier texture to long-wear powder, and can then be smoothed with a brow-brush built right in to the other end of the pencil itself. Benefit pride themselves on brow expertise; they've over 500 brow bars in 22 countries and if you're looking to have yours shaped for the first time, these bars aren't a bad place to start.

Comments: 'Nice soft pencil and good brush; needs sharpening regularly for precise application; liked the fun packaging and the simple instructions' • 'went on very smoothly, no effort at all; smooth consistency with fine powdery/waxy look; very easy to blend' • 'lasted all day without touching up' • 'easy to use and subtle effect' • 'almost frighteningly easy to apply! Needs a very light touch but I liked the quite pronounced finish' • 'good waxy texture and once you've mastered the touch it is very effective'.

Une Eye Brow Pencil ✲

 7.4/10 Une is an exciting new brand (a sister to Bourjois) offering an incredibly wide range of stylish make-up options for the wannabe-more-natural beauty. Featuring certified organic beeswax and jojoba oil, this smooth-textured pencil comes in six shades – we had B01, the fairest.

Comments: 'Quite waxy (but wouldn't melt in warm weather) and very easy to apply, no drag, just use gentle strokes for an even look; good shade and blended in fine' • 'hard to get excited about a brow pencil but this is fine and I'd certainly buy' • 'good product and easy to apply' • 'very easy to make precise natural-looking lines, didn't need retouching all evening; I don't usually use an eyebrow pencil but this could persuade me' • '10/10: quite waxy so went on well without dragging, easy to sharpen and didn't keep breaking like some pencils do, soft but not kohl-like finish which settled in well with my blonde/mousey colouring'.

Your eyes are changing

…and so should your eye-make-up technique

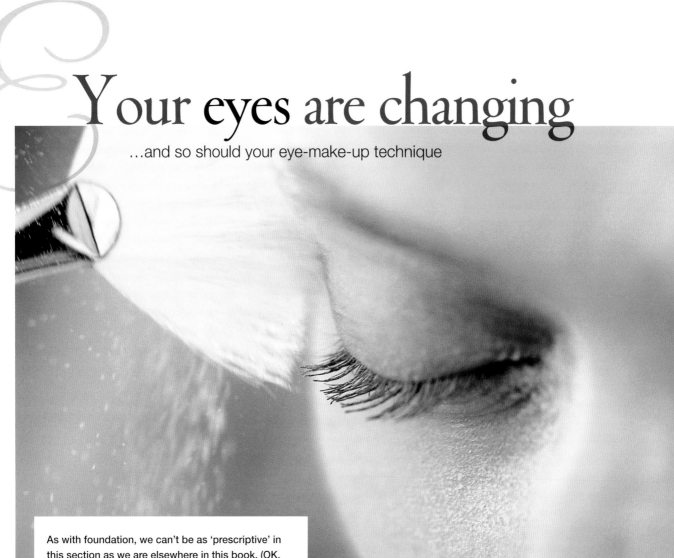

As with foundation, we can't be as 'prescriptive' in this section as we are elsewhere in this book. (OK. Bossy!) That's because eyes present very different challenges. But here are your options, depending on your particular eye make-up 'challenges'. As make-up artist Terry de Gunzburg explains, 'The eyes become smaller and less "defined" as we age – but you can't just add lots of shadow, because the texture of the skin has changed and too much shadow, or the wrong texture (especially shimmer or pearlised products), can draw attention to wrinkly or saggy areas.'

'Of course, you can draw attention to your eyes,' says make-up guru Barbara Daly, 'but in a different way. Aim for a clean, defined look – smoky if you wish, but never that messy, come-to-bed-look of our youth…'

Try applying an eye base under your eye make-up. Then try again, without an eye base. See which looks better on you. Mary Greenwell believes that eye bases can make your eyes look over-done and over-made-up, but some women feel very self-conscious about the redness of their lids and like an eye base (aka eye primer) to smooth out the skintone before shadow. As an alternative, Mary suggests: 'Try going with the colouration. I love seeing a real eyelid. Apply eye cream and allow it to sink in, so your shadow has something to "cling" to; then put a bit of smudgy brown shadow on the lid – soft, warm, even mossy brown – and leave it at that, with light liner at the base of the lashes, and mascara. That may be enough.'

Eliminate dark circles under eyes with a light-reflecting concealer. Apply the concealer in the hollows under your eyes to brighten the area. (Our recommendations for the best products are on page 56.) A great tip given to us by expert Trish McEvoy for correctors and for brighteners is to stroke the product on as a triangle of lines, one under your eye, then the two sides sloping down to meet at a point on your eye-socket bone: then pat in lightly with a finger to cover the area.

A word on puffiness. If you tend to puffiness under your eyes, which Sarah does (often due to various ingredients in cosmetics or foods, also hay fever), first stroke an ice cube round your eye area for a few minutes then try a specific product such as Origins No Puffery (which we think is 'genius'!), or one of the other treats for tired and puffy eyes, on page 60. And don't draw too much attention to your under-eyes; a little mascara winged out to your temples, a fine line under the outer third of each eye and a spot of brightener (as above), under your eyes, high on your cheeks and also on the browbone draws attention away from the puffies.

And some secrets for hooded eyes. If your eyelids are actually drooping over your eyes, the only truly corrective option is surgery. But for less pronounced cases, use a highlighter/luminiser under your brow to 'lift' the eye, a very soft wash of taupe on the upper lid to mute it, mascara to define upper and lower lashes, plus fine eyeliner pushed into the lash-line along the lower lashes to draw the attention downwards.

Define the shape of your eyes differently. 'Using a dark shadow to create the "crease" in the socket, as you might have done when you were 20, just won't work,' says Terry de Gunzburg. She advises this approach to open up your eyes: over the lid try a sheer wash of matt eyeshadow, in a neutral shade (eg, mid-taupe – a sort of mushroomy-pink tone, but nothing muddy), then focus on eyeliner and mascara to frame the eyes. Try a sharpened eyeliner pencil or liquid product with an inbuilt fine brush – in grey, deep brown, aubergine or navy – pushed well into the lashes. (If you like, and have time, 'set' liner with a similar shade of powder eyeshadow on top. We often don't bother…)

Top with two coats of mascara. Apply the second coat before the first has dried to avoid clumping. We think soft dark brown can be more flattering for many women – though Trish McEvoy is a firm believer in black 'to enhance definition', for virtually everyone. (Jo goes for black, always.) Waterproof mascara avoids panda eyes, especially during hot flushes. (For more about eyeliners recommended by our testers, see page 68.)

If your 'socket crease' is unlined and droop-free, use a taupe-y grey or even a pale purple shade to accentuate the socket. We rather like a tip from our smooth-lidded singer friend Lulu, who applies powder shadow to the socket of her eye holding the mirror a good two feet (60cm or so) away, so she can gauge the effect from the distance most people see you from. (But then blend so the edges are seamless using a blender brush, holding the mirror up close.)

Add a touch of highlighter on the browbone. This is universally flattering (except possibly for those who have very high eyebrows, in which case it can make them look loftier). Dot on a touch of ivory or bone-coloured shadow, and if (but only if) the skin is smooth, it can be very subtly shimmering.

If you wear stronger shadow and eyeliner, play down your brows. Terry explains that it's all a question of balance. 'If you're wearing quite a bit of eye make-up, and you add a strong brow, you'll look like you've put on way too much make-up. But if you wear a sheer wash of shadow, and fine eyeliner, you can afford to add a bit more brow definition.' (See page 62 for more brow wisdom.)

There is truly no substitute for analysing the different effects yourself, in a mirror. With a discerning friend if available. Eye make-up is an issue where we can't be psychic and make up your mind for you about what looks best: you're going to have to experiment (do give yourself plenty of time for this), based on the advice above. And, of course, you can go and get free make-up consultations in-store from most brands, which might give you valuable tips and info (even if it's to show you what you don't like).

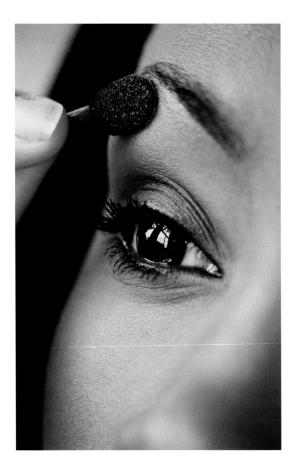

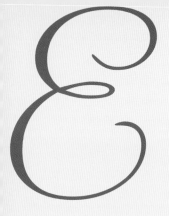

Eyeliners: our award winners

Mascara is only half the answer for lashes, which invariably become sparser over the years. An eye-defining eyeliner also works extremely effectively to create the illusion of thicker, longer lashes. There are many options: pencil, gel, liquid, cream – and they all make a big difference to 'eye-oomph'. We recommend you experiment with different textures till you find the formulation that works best for you – and if you've never trialled a gel or cream liner, do give them a go. Check out our testers' favourites. (NB: maybe it's the shaky-hand thing, but the liquid liners with a fine brush didn't go down well at all)

AT A GLANCE

Bourjois Effet Smoky Pencil

Sue Devitt Eye Intensifier Pencil

Estée Lauder Double Wear Stay-in-Place Eye Pencil

Bobbi Brown Long Wear Gel Eyeliner

REVIEWS

Bourjois Effet Smoky Pencil

8.61/10 An excellent score for this very affordable pencil, which comes in a range of smokily dark shades – and we sent a selection to our testers, including Dark Purple, Deep Green and Smoked Brown. (We try always to send out identical products but sometimes brands don't play ball!) A creamier pencil for someone who wants a sultry, maybe even smudged effect from their eye definer: it has an impressively high-quality built-in brush at one end, for blending.
Comments: 'Top marks: pencil goes on perfectly, very easy to apply precisely; smooth texture without being too soft, smudges easily but controllably; after a week of wearing I'm addicted' • 'you can create different effects by layers and smudging, for day or evening' • 'comes with a brush on the other end which is ideal for softening and smudging (much better than a sponge)' • 'cheaper than my usual Clinique pencil and just as good for my very sensitive eyes' • 'didn't drag at all, and went exactly where I wanted it' • 'I *love* the pointy brush, so you can soften the line precisely as you want it and make it look natural; product wore well all day'.

Sue Devitt Eye Intensifier Pencil

8.04/10 This stubby, velvety-textured pencil is one of Jo's faves, because it delivers quite intense effects very speedily. Like the

Bourjois entry, this is one for the Bardot-esque smoky-eye look. But there's a useful 50 seconds to play in before the colour sets: we tried Bangalore and there's a choice of 12 shades. NB: some testers were put off by the lack of a sharpener as the size can be hard to find. And some loved the chunkiness, while others didn't.
Comments: 'So easy to apply I didn't even use a mirror; soft creamish texture; excellent sponge tip for smudging but once applied didn't smudge unintentionally – fantastic!' • 'haven't used an eye pencil before but will definitely use this now' • 'dream of a product, and very soft – glides on like silk, most amazing texture of any I've used' • 'amazingly easy to apply, no skill needed, although it's fat and chunky is better than its slimmer sisters' • 'I use lots of eye pencils from all brands, but this is the best ever, blends like a dream and has real staying power' • 'couldn't draw a very fine line but gives a good smudgy look – an instant eye make-up when you can't be bothered to do the whole eye thing!' • 'lovely colour that went with everything – nice soft mossy green with a touch of metallic bronze'.

Estée Lauder Double Wear Stay-in-Place Eye Pencil

8/10 As the name implies, this double-ended pencil (colour one end, blender/smudger the other) comes from a capsule Lauder

ANTI-AGEING AWARD WINNERS BEAUTY BIBLE

collection created to deliver specifically long-wear results. Easy-to-blend and soft (almost 'cushiony' in texture), it features silicone technology to deliver stay-true colour for up to 12 hours. We normally ask for black or dark neutrals, but on this occasion our testers enjoyed the subtly shimmering Bronze shade, one of seven jewel-rich tones. A slightly mixed bunch of reviews with some marking down as difficult to smudge – others finding it easier.

Comments: 'Anyone should find it easy to apply precisely, and also very smudgeable – and it stayed like that until I took it off, how refreshing!' • 'reasonably smooth to apply, particularly on bottom lid; needed to be sharpened regularly; loved the nice deep bronze colour, and could get good sharp effect or smudgy, smoky look – easy to use in the main' • 'very useful and versatile, and lasted well' • 'creamy, easy to apply and sticks to your skin until you remove it' • 'what a dream, perfect consistency for an eye pencil, went on smoothly and evenly, and precisely, as long as I kept it sharp' • 'rare to find such an easily applied and long-lasting liner'.

Bobbi Brown Long Wear Gel Eyeliner

7.83/10

One of the first gel eyeliners on the market, it's a beauty classic, created to withstand heat, humidity, even rain. As you get to know this product – which glides on smoothly – you'll learn it can be layered easily, for extra intensity. Packaged in a chic little 'inkwell'-style bottle, our testers tried Caviar Ink, which is a deep black brown. It comes in ten shades, some of them shimmering. Generally, we think you're better off with matt blacks or browns, but experiment (book a makeover and see if different colours suit you). Some testers marked it down for being fiddly and needing practice to apply, though they liked the results. Others found it simple! NB: it doesn't come with its own brush so you need to acquire one.

Comments: '10/10: perfect for a novice, really easy to do a smooth line, and good for me as a contact-lens wearer; needed a separate brush; lovely creamy, smooth texture which lasted well with no smudging or flaking; really opened up my eyes – they looked brighter too' • 'top marks: amazingly easy to apply – no skill required, and I'd given up on liquid eyeliners' • 'this is now my desert island product, it survived two weeks in a very humid Florida, including a torrential rainstorm with no umbrella' • 'I was very nervous about trying this and thought the colour would be too dark but it made my lashes look a lot thicker, and it's long-lasting if you apply a base or powder shadow first'.

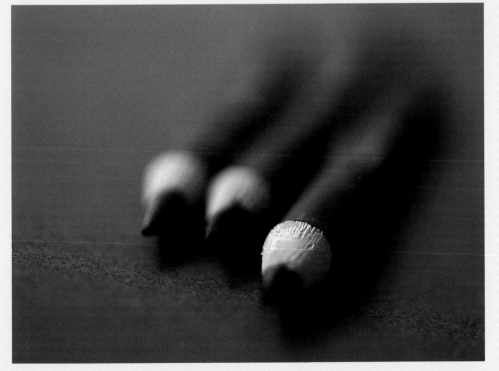

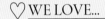

♡ WE LOVE...

Jo is a sucker for a smoky eye pencil, in particular the ultra-chunky Valerie Beverly Hills Smudgey Pharaoh Pencil (Black), and Sue Devitt Eye Intensifier Pencil. (These are both fat pencils, so invest in a 'matching' sharpener.) But she often layers a gel eyeliner over the top, to enhance the staying power of these soft pencils: Bobbi Brown Long Wear Gel Eyeliner, Clinique Brush-On Cream Liner for day, or New CID Cosmetics i-gel (she likes Granite, Graphite and Carbon, a trio of deep grey/blacks). Sarah's eyes just don't look good smoky, so she bucks the pencil trend and loves YSL's liquid Easy Liner.

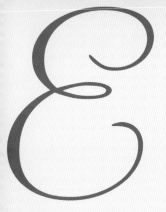

Cream eyeshadows: *our award winners*

Cream shadows are easiest to blend on more 'mature' eyelids – and in a pale neutral can also become a fabulous base for other shades. They're also a lazy, 'everyday' option for a fast make-up effect if you swipe on a taupe-y neutral shade. The right formulation is a must, though – because you want to avoid 'creasing'. With that in mind, we dispatched a couple of dozen cream shadow options to our testers, asking for feedback on smoothness, ease of application and endurance. (As always, we asked for neutral shades that would suit all of you…)

REVIEWS

Clinique Quick Eyes Cream Shadow

 Despite its lightweight texture, this super-high-scoring cream shadow offers heavy-duty performance benefits: long wear (up to ten hours), water-resistance, transfer-resistance – and it's creaseproof with a glide-on formula that sets to a soft, powdery finish. Dot the eyelids using the applicator and blend with fingertips, Clinique recommend; you can also build the shadow, for greater depth. Of the nine shades (many of which are pretty shimmery), our testers were sent Lucky Penny. Like the entire Clinique range, it's fragrance-free and hypoallergenic.

Comments: '10/10! Very simple and effective to use with the sponge applicator; smooth, creamy texture, half way between matt and discreet shimmer; by the end of a long day it was as fresh and uncreased as when I set off, excellent!' • 'loved the soft sheen, enough to illuminate eye area but subtle for daytime; lovely silky consistency; lived up to the claim of staying in place for ten hours!' • 'gave lovely pearly sweep of fabulous neutral shade which really suited my fair skin, blonde hair and brown eyes' • 'loved everything about this! I used to be just a mascara and lip gloss girl but this is now part of my daily routine' • 'recommended to anyone who's a bit scared of getting eyeshadow "right"; it's really easy and very forgiving!'.

Bobbi Brown Long-Wear Cream Shadow

 'At last, a cream eyeshadow that stays on and doesn't crease', promises the Bobbi Brown blurb – and as our testers' comments go to show, this pretty much lives up to that. In a cute small pot (you dip with fingers or use a synthetic brush), it offers a 'breathable polymer technology' (which delivers the long wear and makes it crease resistant), and it's also recommended 'for oily eyelids'. Bobbi is of course known for her super-wearable shades – and there are 20 to choose from, mostly matt but some with a slight shimmer. Our testers trialled Cement, which they found good for daytime on its own, or as a base for evening colours. NB: as some testers pointed out, the little pot is not the most portable.

Comments: '10/10 for the easiest to apply eyeshadow I've ever used, either with brush or finger; the smoothest most velvety texture, matt finish but not flat; have binned all my other eyeshadows and bought several more of these' • 'made the slightly crêpey skin on my eyelids looks as smooth as a teenager's again' • 'long, long, long, long-lasting! Stayed put with great finish and same colour – work means my make-up can be on for 16 hours, this was still fresh at the end' • 'seemed to fill all imperfections; made eyeliner apply easier and last longer on top of it; wish I'd discovered this before' • 'loved the creamy texture

AT A GLANCE

Clinique Quick Eyes Cream Shadow

Bobbi Brown Long-Wear Cream Shadow

Benefit Creaseless Cream Shadow/Liner

Shu Uemura Cream Eye Shadow

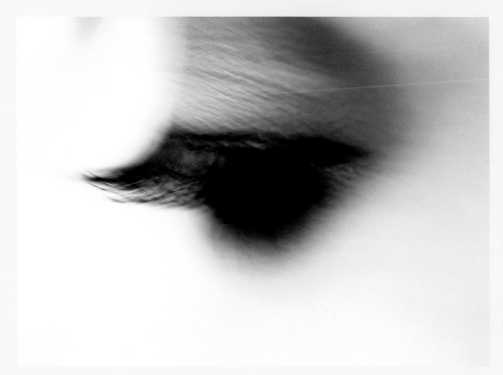

which was easy to apply, and the colour, and it lasted! But found the opening of the pot too small for fingers once the contents went down a bit, so you need a brush' • 'gave soft wash of colour that you could build up, didn't cake at all, just a smooth veil of colour'.

Benefit Creaseless Cream Shadow/Liner

 8.25/10

Crease-proof, smudge-proof, offering 'buildable' colour with a choice of 12 shades. Our testers tried Flatter Me, a creamy metallic rose gold colour, with quite a lot of shimmer (some felt too much) but a smooth, flattering finish, they commented. No applicator is provided, so you may need a brush. Benefit may sometimes seem like a young range but pros love their make-up 'Fix-Its' (and so do we).

Comments: 'Can I give this 11 out of ten? Easy peasy to apply, and so simple to layer up if you want to, use both fingers and brush; shimmery but subtle finish, a sheen rather than shadow – yes, oh yes, I would buy, I loved this and so did the other women in my family (had to lock it away) – it gave me so much pleasure!' • 'very easy to use with a brush, spread easily to give a wash of colour and could be built up into stronger coverage; so you could have it subtle or dramatic' • 'lasted about four hours' • 'felt like a creamy powder, if that makes sense! Quite smooth to use, and easy to

blend in and didn't cake' • 'packaging is adorable – glass container, with a large lid in a pretty little box, makes applying it feel like a ritual'.

Shu Uemura Cream Eye Shadow

 7.6/10

Loved by make-up artists the world over, Shu Uemura are known for their bold shades – but search hard, and you'll find some wonderful, more neutral tones within the Shu range, including the Taupe our testers trialled. Again, the shadow's creators promise that it won't fade, crease – and that this comfortable 'stretch' formula is even waterproof.

Comments: 'Great product; never used cream before but I really liked it for a natural daytime look; lovely and kind to small lines and creases' • 'silky finish that glided on, really smooth and crease-resistant, blended beautifully and stayed put all day and into the night' • 'finish improved when I set it with a little powder, which prolonged it too' • 'best applied with a brush and once I'd achieved an even colour it looked great; slight shimmer which looked best in the evening for me, lasted a lot longer than my usual powder shadow, and the overall finished effect was more dramatic' • 'stayed put brilliantly, lasted all night without any signs of disappearing (out late so didn't take off make-up, naughty I know!)' • 'lasted well in a hot climate'.

♡ WE LOVE…

Oooh, lots in Jo's case, most particularly her Ellis Faas Creamy Eyes pen-style shadow in neutral brown E105 (a taupe-y brown) which can be used very subtly or (unlike some) reapplied for a much more intense smokiness. She also likes the award-winning Bobbi Brown Long-Wear Cream Shadow you can read about, left, in Ash – a medium brown – and Bone (as an eyelid base/ brow highlighter) but adds: 'The jar opening's a little fiddly, so this is best used with a synthetic shadow brush, not fingers. It lives up to its long-wear promise, though.' Sarah hardly wears eyeshadow but always applies a brightener on lids to lift the area before applying a teeny bit of foundation, then eyeliner and mascara. Then for parties she smudges on a bit of taupe-y powder, such as the fantastically good-value Bourjois Ombre Stretch in Brun.

Mascaras: our award winners

Lashes get thinner and sparser over time, so mascara is even more essential to help define the eyes and structure the face. However, there's no such thing as a one-type-fits-all mascara – so here are the top recommendations with details of what they do. On this page, the non-waterproof versions – see opposite for the brands to get you through rain and weepy films!

AT A GLANCE

Non-waterproof

Estée Lauder TurboLash All Effects Motion Mascara

YSL Luxurious Mascara for False Lash Effect

Clinique High Impact Mascara

Lancôme Hypnôse Drama Instant Full Body Volume Mascara

Waterproof

Chanel Inimitable Waterproof Mascara

No7 Extreme Length Waterproof Mascara

Guerlain Le 2 de Guerlain Waterproof Mascara

L'Oréal Telescopic Waterproof Mascara

TIP

Do replace your mascara every three months for best results and to avoid 'bug' build-up.

NON-WATERPROOF MASCARAS

Estée Lauder TurboLash All Effects Motion Mascara

 $\frac{8.89}{10}$ Suddenly, there's a new category of mascara: vibrating mascaras, which imitate the effect of wiggling the brush from root to tip, for extra curl and coverage. A gimmick? Not according to our testers, who gave TurboLash a really excellent mark. The long, slim brush makes it easy to access all lashes – and a bonus is that once the battery in the LashSonic brush has breathed its last, you know it's time for a fresh mascara. Jo has found that it's the only mascara she's ever used which can be reapplied after a day at the office, as the vibrations break up clumps. (NB: a little D-I-Y is required to install the battery!) The best all-rounder, it's good for sparse, fine lashes.

Comments: 'I laughed when I saw this! What next? But it's just a gentle whirring, then it's magic! You put the wand against your lashes and it starts to coat, separate, curl, lengthen – golly!' • 'lovely! I was very sceptical but this is excellent, making lashes longer and thicker with two coats; but had to decode instructions for battery first!' • 'no clumping, good separation of lashes, fantastic lengthening and thickening effect – looked like false eyelashes!' • 'lashes looked longer, thicker, curlier – not natural but not overly heavy looking'.

YSL Luxurious Mascara for False Lash Effect

 $\frac{8.7}{10}$ A bit of a legend in beauty circles, this: we know lots of beauties who swear by the va-va-voom results False Lash Effect delivers, and this was backed up by our testers. The formulation includes beeswax, carnauba and candelilla waxes plus pro-vitamin B5 for lash-conditioning, nylon micro-particles to boost lash diameter – and the brush is generously fat. Good for volumising. (Also in a waterproof version.)

Comments: '10/10 for the lustrous finish and lengthening plus natural curl; loved the wand' • 'no clumping, excellent glossy, lustrous finish, very good at thickening, excellent lengthening; a new-found gem for evenings' • 'looked realistic but in an exaggerated way! Just what I want in a mascara, one coat was plenty' • 'fat brush was very good for top lashes, a little harder to angle on lower ones, lashes looked longer, thicker and curled nicely – and not false' • 'fantastic lash-lengthening, looked glossy and loved that it was "extra-black"' • 'I love YSL for perfumes, and I felt the same expertise created this mascara'.

Clinique High Impact Mascara

 $\frac{8.42}{10}$ We love Clinique's precision: this, they say, gives 'up to a 26-degree curl'. We know from experience there's plenty of 'playtime' while you're applying, but the high-impact brush delivers results with just a few sweeps. This too has lash-conditioning waxes in the blend. (Particularly good for extra length and curl.)

Comments: 'Excellent at body and definition, which was very flattering; easy to use, very good at lengthening and thickening; lashes looked natural and curled upwards' • 'wand design made it easy to access lashes' • 'I have contact lenses and wear mascara every day, so it's an important product for me – this is excellent and not too expensive, easy to remove, too' • 'good for defining my very fine lashes, made them a little thicker and curlier, very natural – like I had better eyelashes! I would buy'.

Lancôme Hypnôse Drama Instant Full Body Volume Mascara

7.62/10 This looks wonky when you take the wand out of the tube – but it's specifically curled like an 'S' to follow the lid-shape, allowing for easy access to even the shortest lashes. A smooth, non-sticky formula promises easy glide through lashes for dramatic, volumised results. The original Hypnôse mascara became the world's best-seller after its 2004 launch. (Good for volume, testers say.)

Comments: 'Excellent, did a great job at lengthening lashes with lots of volume; matt but not dull finish, just needed one coat; I like the wand design' • 'smudged a few times on application but didn't flake through the day – excellent staying power' • 'very noticeable how much longer my lashes appeared; definitely in the glossy and lustrous camp, the best mascara I have ever tried'.

WATERPROOF MASCARAS

As we age, eyes become more sensitive to light, and often to allergens. The result? Eye-wateriness. Our panellists put 24 waterproof mascaras through their paces in daily life (as well as the shower and pool). Here are their enduring (!) favourites. Those promising curl and length did better than volumising ones. Be warned: you need specialist waterproof eye-make-up remover!

Chanel Inimitable Waterproof Mascara

8.12/10 The revolutionary rubber wand (technical-speak: 'soft elastomer') grips lashes beautifully, enabling a real curling action, plus definition and separation. (Great for sparser lashes, we've observed.) In this waterproof formula there's a touch of beeswax, to condition lashes. But, as testers observed, you need a really effective remover to get it off when you want to.

Comments: 'Fab product, really great performing mascara, which made lashes longer, thicker, more curly and separated, with glossy lustrous finish – and no mascara to be seen on my face in weepy movie or shower' • 'didn't budge through rain and weepy movie, though smudged slightly in shower and swimming pool; didn't flake or crumble; lengthening effect very good' • 'especially good on bottom lashes, made them significantly thicker without glooping together, very pretty: my eyes really stand out – cut onions with no problem'.

No7 Extreme Length Waterproof Mascara

7.44/10 This also features a flexible, good-grip rubber wand for clump-free application – we have a hunch these will eventually replace bristle brushes in all mascaras. Most testers felt it was a good basic product.

Comments: 'Looked like my lashes but better, needed two coats, didn't flake, crumble or smudge, and is very waterproof – really stays' • 'quite good finish, very black with two applications; performed well in rain, shower, and swimming pool' • 'went on really well, loved the flexible brush; lovely natural effect, lashes looking longer, thicker and a little glossier; definitely showerproof and quite easy to remove: I am impressed and will buy again'.

Guerlain Le 2 de Guerlain Waterproof Mascara

7.4/10 Inspired by Creative Director Olivier Echaudemaison's use of two brushes for applying mascara, Guerlain's dual-ended winning entry offers a dinky short brush for accessing corner lashes and (at the opposite end of the wand) a medium-length brush to sweep the polymer-rich formula top and bottom. (Also in non-waterproof, see We Love….)

Comments: 'I've tested a lot of mascaras in the past 18 months and this is the only expensive one I would buy; survived onion-chopping sessions and lashes look defined, longer and thicker without being overdone' • 'eyes looked finished and "refined"' • 'gave very natural look for waterproof mascara' • 'loved the design; the little wand is fantastic' • 'unsure I'd use both wands but now I like them – but too long to fit in my make-up bag!'.

L'Oréal Telescopic Waterproof Mascara

7.12/10 With a huge range to choose from it's easy to get bamboozled by the mascaras in L'Oréal's range alone (let alone the other brands out there) – but our panellists singled this out for its endurance powers. Again, it has a flexible elastomer 'multi-comb' wand, for enhanced curling and 'stretching' of lashes.

Comments: 'No clumping; good lash lengthening and thickening, loved the results! Didn't budge in shower; only problem was having to rub lashes to get it off; great for special occasions' • 'excellent wand; I have insignificant lashes and this gave the length I like without too much bulk' • 'doesn't clump, so easy to get in close and for lower lashes' • 'removed easily with Clinique's Take the Day Off Makeup Remover for Lids Lashes & Lips'.

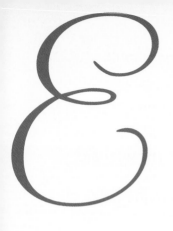

Lash-boosting treatments: *our award winners*

This is an entire new treatment category. Just a couple of years ago, there were one or two contenders – and now there's a couple of dozen lash-boosting options out there. Do they work? Our diligent Beauty Bible testers put them through their paces over a period of months, observing ongoing benefits as well as instant effects. We were cynical before we saw the results – but these award winners, which work in different ways, are a bit of an eye-opener. (Scores for the other lash-boosting products were much less impressive)

AT A GLANCE

Elizabeth Arden Lash Optimizer – Primer with Conditioners

RevitaLash Eyelash Conditioner

REVIEWS

Elizabeth Arden Lash Optimizer – Primer with Conditioners

You know about make-up primers. Well, this is a lash-primer (white in colour) to enhance the effect of your mascara so lashes look thicker and longer. Yes, yet another step in your beauty routine – but this is designed to make your mascara stay put and at the same time make lashes softer, healthier-looking and more supple, with less breakage. Our testers awarded it a pretty impressive score; here are their comments.

Comments: 'Really liked this product, easy to use, didn't flake/crumble/smudge/clump, and made my lashes look longer' • 'mascara-style wand made it easy to coat the conditioner on your eyelashes' • 'lashes considerably longer and seemed to improve staying power of my mascara; as I used this for longer, I started to see more benefits with lashes softer and in better condition' • 'really good at lash-lengthening and lashes were also thicker, just had to make sure I covered all the white'.

RevitaLash Eyelash Conditioner

This product is different to the one above: not an instant fix but a product formulated to amplify lashes over time. There's a poignant story behind RevitaLash: it was developed by an American ophthalmologist, Dr Michael Brinkenhoff, for his wife Gayle – who'd lost most of her lashes through treatment for breast cancer; seeing the results, they agreed the product should be shared more widely. With an ultra-fine brush, you paint one stroke of RevitaLash along the lash-line before bedtime. It's pricey, although a tube is said to last three to five months – and a portion of the profits go to breast cancer research and education charities. Most testers scored this highly but one low mark brought the average down.

Comments: 'I was rather sceptical about this but lashes are so much more plentiful and now look completely false with mascara on! Forget about buying expensive mascaras: buy a cheap one and this product' • 'once lashes are at full impact, you don't need to use daily, just every second or third night'• 'I am in awe of this product – it really works. Love putting on my mascara now and even curl my lashes daily; I can feel my lashes fluttering on my specs, which I love!' • 'my short stubby sparse lashes are now about three times as long as before and they're also starting to curl instead of sticking straight out; also thicker' • 'after several weeks, my lashes are thicker and denser; my husband felt there was a change too'.

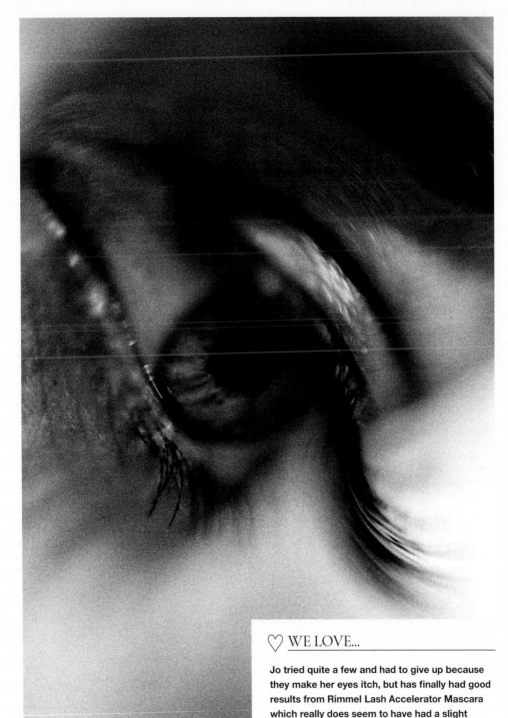

♡ WE LOVE...

Jo tried quite a few and had to give up because they make her eyes itch, but has finally had good results from Rimmel Lash Accelerator Mascara which really does seem to have had a slight lash-thickening effect. Sarah admits to being too lazy to remember to paint on the longer-term ones daily; of the quick fixes, she agrees with testers that the Elizabeth Arden Lash Optimizer is very effective. And don't forget that Joan Collins swears Vaseline is the best lash conditioner ever!

TIP

We have supersensitive eyes and have suffered dreadfully from some eye products. The big companies have to be incredibly careful with testing but may we suggest you observe the following advice:

● Make absolutely sure the conditioner is ophthalmologically-tested (it will say so on the packaging), and ideally is endorsed by eye-care professionals.

● Stop immediately if you do experience irritation. It's not normal for eyes to be irritated or for you to experience any form of blurred vision. If this does happen, we suggest you contact the manufacturer immediately, and press for a refund.

● Be careful! Most products are swept along the lash-line using a fine brush; take care not to get the product into the corner of your eyes, and don't apply if you're wearing contact lenses. If you're using lash conditioner in the morning, allow it to dry 100 per cent before applying anything else.

● Have patience. Most lash conditioners suggest nightly application for maximum results. Use as ritually as you would a cleanser, toner or moisturiser.

'Wrinkles don't
scare me;
they are a part
of LIFE and I
will and do
EMBRACE them.
But I look at
surgery and that
scares me'

Christy Turlington

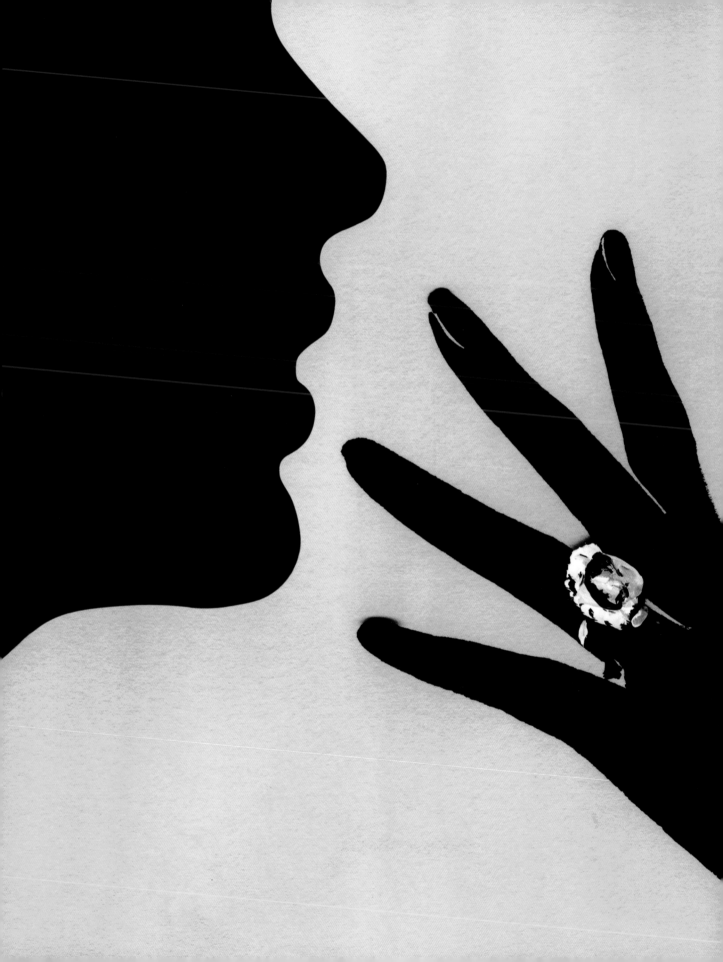

Get glowing – by recharging your skin

A visit to a facialist for a skin-reviving treatment is a rare indulgence for most of us – but in this book we show you the amazing masks, scrubs, creams, oils and transforming techniques that you can use at home to give your skin a real boost…plus insider tips from the experts

There are several ways to wake up your face fast. You can go the professional route: trek to a salon, have your face massaged (or needled as in acupuncture – see page 155), be slathered with creams (and lie there hoping you're not getting a parking ticket). Or you can go the D-I-Y route, which is infinitely cheaper and more accessible. Now, that's not to say we don't love a facial – see a list below for some of our favourite facialists. But realistically, who has the money or, just as importantly, the time to indulge more than once in a blue moon…?

Your daily regime is one thing. But it's easy to be lulled – out of sheer inertia and/or laziness – into doing the same routine for your skin, day in, night out. So we really, really can't encourage you too strongly to try some of the products and the face-transforming techniques in this book.

You can achieve a huge amount – near-miraculous, actually – with a simple, at-home, two-step blitz: a gentle-but-effective exfoliation, followed by a mask. On the next pages, you'll find our diligent testers' top facial scrubs and masks – the skincare wonders that, over the space of 18 months' research for this book, they identified as being the most effective on the market. And on page 212 you'll also find our rundown of the best 'instant face-revivers', packed with glow-getting ingredients that boost skin circulation, and are absolutely fantastic for emergencies (hangovers, jet-lag, or after a cold or flu, when skin can look positively grey). They're as close to eight hours' sleep-in-a-jar as you're going to get.

Throughout this mini-section of the book, we've also included some 'trade secrets': insider tips to try at home, from facialists who we rate and revere – and who, if we had a lunching-lady sort of life, we might see more often ourselves. But even though we're beauty editors, we can't justify that sort of indulgence as frequently as we might like.

But try the products, too, and prepare to be amazed.

5-MINUTE FIX FOR TIRED FACES!

Facialist Suzie Mitchell (who's local to Jo in Hastings) is something of a miracle-worker for tired faces. She has this tip for temporarily 'ironing' away lines from the face and boosting glow.

● Put a little facial oil in one palm and rub hands together, then smooth over face, neck and bosom.
● Rather than fingertips, use the big muscle in the cushion at the base of your thumb, always working upwards.
● Start by fanning out over and round your neck, then work round and up your jaw and cheekbones to the temples, then across and up your forehead to your hairline.
● Repeat, covering the whole face for five minutes. The oil will be absorbed, skin velvety, and your face look rosy and 'lifted'.

'You only perceive the *real beauty* in a person as they get OLDER'

Anouk Aimée

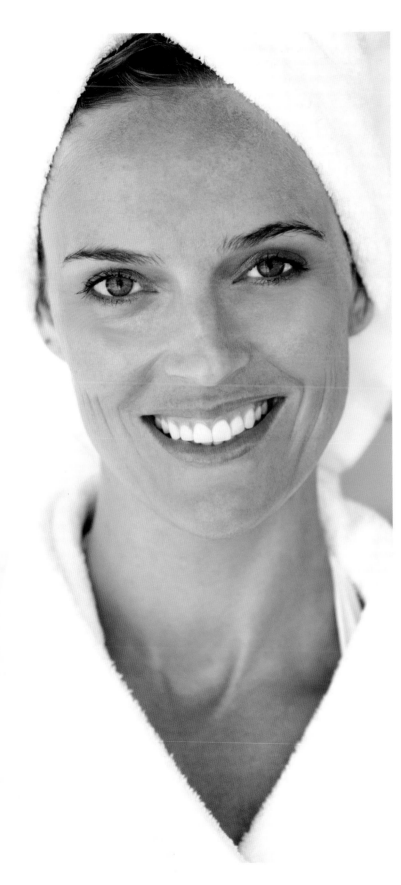

IF YOU HAVE 15 MINUTES OR MORE, TRY THIS!

We adore acupuncturist Annee de Mamiel's facial acupuncture treatment, which she combines with massage. If you can't get to see her (or anyone else), just try this…. Then look in the mirror and go, 'Wow!'.

● Smooth your favourite facial oil over your entire face and neck.
● Cup your hands over the nose and mouth, breathe in and out deeply.
● Tug your earlobes with thumb and index finger. Then with fingertips, use firm, circular movements to massage from behind ears to base of neck.
● From the point of your chin, work up and outwards along the jaw to your ear; then from the corners of your mouth over the cheeks to the ear; then from the base of the nose to the top of the ear. Repeat the whole sequence three times.
● Sweep your fingertips firmly over your eyebrows, then under, then gently pinch along them. Repeat twice.
● Pressing firmly with your middle fingers, circle the eyes beginning above the inner corners and working outwards. Repeat three times.
● From the centre of your forehead, just above the nose, zigzag middle fingers in small, firm motions out to the temples; repeat working up the forehead.
● With the side of your index finger (held vertically), smooth skin from centre of face outwards, beginning with your forehead, then sides of nose, middle of mouth and centre of chin.
● Finish by breathing deeply, hands cupped over your mouth and nose.

OUR FAVOURITE AGE-DEFYING FACIALISTS...

Amanda Lacey
Anastasia Achilleos
Annee de Mamiel (see her massage tips above)
Emma Hardie (not your typical facial – no products, but seriously 'lifting')
Ole Henriksen
Sarah Chapman
Vaishaly Patel
Plus: Bliss Triple Oxygen Facial

Facial scrubs: our award winners

Dry, dull surface skin cells are the key issue lying between many a woman's complexion and a youthful radiance. When cell turnover slows, the dead surface skin cells don't reflect the light in the same way as a twentysomething's naturally fresh, dewy skin – but the good news is that a gentle exfoliator can go a long, long way towards restoring a healthy glow

TIP

To avoid overdoing the use of a scrub on the face, use your ring fingers to massage in, using circular movements. The touch of this finger is naturally more delicate than with the index or second finger, all but eliminating the risk of over-zealous application.

G-E-N-T-L-E is our watchword, though – it's important to avoid anything that scratches or over-buffs the skin – so in our quest to discover the most effective facial scrubs, we dispatched several dozen to our panels of testers (ten for each product, as normal). They had truly glowing praise for some. PS Try using a facial scrub before applying a mask for maximum effectiveness.

REVIEWS

Darphin Age-Defying Dermabrasion

 Darphin (originally a French brand, now owned by Estée Lauder) promise this very high-scoring product is kind enough even for sensitive skins, with buffing particles of jojoba, silica, pearl and lava to refine skin texture, plus a corn-derived ingredient to target age spots. Gentian and bisabolol have been added for a soothing action, and Darphin say this can be used as often as every other day. (Though we advise: try it once a week first, and assess results. That may be enough to keep you radiant.) Luxuriously-textured and luxuriously-priced.
Comments: 'Love this, the rich, creamy, lush texture and my glowing, cleaner, brighter skin after; you can use it without water but if it dries out a little, just add a touch then you can really massage it in; a small amount goes a long way' • 'skin never felt taut or dry after' • 'very fine grains exfoliate skin gently, lovely fresh smell, skin looks polished and

fresh, clearer and brighter after; people say how good my skin looks' • 'super product that does brilliant job of exfoliating in the most gentle way – really lovely' • 'skin felt so soft and smooth and moisturised, it was wonderful, looks brighter'.

Dermalogica Daily Microfoliant

 As the name suggests, Dermalogica tell us this rice-based enzyme powder can be used every day – but please read the comments we make for Darphin about frequent use, above, before you do that. The powder formula – which shakes out of the container into the hand – activates when you mix it with water, releasing papain (a skin-brightening enzyme), salicylic acid and rice to smooth and boost cellular renewal. To add to its brightening power, bearberry, liquorice and grapefruit are incorporated, along with a skin-calming blend of green tea, ginkgo and oatmeal.
Comments: 'Not grainy at all, felt really soft and gentle, very easy to apply; skin looked really fresh and glowing, and felt unbelievably soft and smooth; people say I look very well; after a month skin looks glowing and refreshed' • 'can't believe people spend a fortune on expensive facial treatments when they could use this! I use it twice weekly, which is enough, but you could use it daily – a lovely comforting treatment without any harsh abrasiveness' • 'using this regularly has reduced my fine wrinkles and enlarged pores, made skin smoother and my skin feels so much nicer – a very

♡ WE LOVE...

Personally, thanks to diligent use of a muslin cloth at night-time, we go easy on facial scrubs – reserving them for an occasional blitz. For Jo, favourites include Liz Earle Naturally Active Gentle Face Exfoliator (yes, it truly IS gentle) and Origins Modern Friction (ditto), which has done well previously in our trials for *The Green Beauty Bible*. Sarah uses a flannel at night and in the morning to remove cleanser and virtually never exfoliates – though reading the reviews here, she's beetling off to the beauty cupboard!

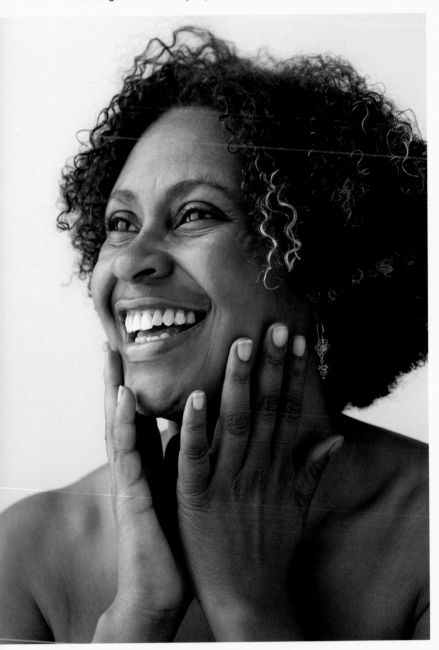

lovely product, and moisturiser goes on much better' • 'husband says my skin looks brighter and fresher, and he's been trying it too and is very impressed!' • 'after a month, skin looks a lot smoother, brighter and more toned'.

Clinique 7 Day Scrub Cream Rinse-Off Formula

8.57/10 A 'second generation' version of a product that's been a pillar of the Clinique range for years, with gentle exfoliating beads that enliven skin after just 30 seconds of massage. It can then be easily swooshed away with water but may also be tissued off, Clinique tell us.

Comments: 'Quite grainy, gritty texture but not unpleasant; very easy to apply and skin looks glowing and much healthier, much smoother and softer – very gentle on my skin' • 'top marks! Really nice creamy texture, feels like it is doing its job, doesn't dry skin at all, after a month skin looks really great, and there's been a noticeable reduction in spots' • 'my combination skin looks much better and the product lasts ages as you only need a 5p-sized amount' • 'looks rich and creamy – a bit like toothpaste!; pleasant herby smell, and skin looks fresh and smooth, with a lovely healthy glow after a month of use'.

Oskia Micro-Exfoliating Balm

8.5/10 The name of the niche Oskia brand comes from the Greek for 'delivering beauty'. Here, this balm-style exfoliator delivers beauty with a fusion of pure MSM and silica granules, redness-reducing zinc glycine complex and vitamin A, in a base of shea butter, sweet almond and sesame oils, together with omega-3 and -6 (from rosehip seed and kukui nut oils). It's the most natural of the award winners in this category.

Comments: 'Skin felt very clean and soft, perfectly moisturised, feels healthy' • 'brightened and improved tone, felt very smooth, softer and a little plumper; my friend says my skin looks brighter – though no mention of younger! I think there is a slight effect on facial lines' • 'so easy to use' • 'gorgeous creamy luxurious balm, skin felt pampered, soft and plump, skintone more even and pores smaller; no irritation! After a month my skin is definitely improved – a joy to use' • 'the claims that it refines, restores radiance and enhances softness are all true'.

Anti-ageing face masks: our award winners

We love, love, love face masks. The ritual of slapping on a mask once a week can be a rare moment of pampering in a hectic life. But more than this, we like the results that many masks swiftly deliver: brightening, smoothing, plumping and delivering a surge of dewy moisture to thirsty skins. Plus some now feature specific 'anti-ageing' ingredients, such as skin-brightening enzymes. Our diligent panellists lay back and relaxed while trialling an incredibly wide selection of masks – and their top choices, featured here, include two from Elemis. No mean achievement

AT A GLANCE

Guerlain Orchidée Impériale Exceptional Complete Care Mask

Elemis Fruit Active Rejuvenating Mask

Elemis Pro-Collagen Quartz Lift Mask

Clarins Super Restorative Replenishing Comfort Mask

REVIEWS

Guerlain Orchidée Impériale Exceptional Complete Care Mask

 9.11/10 A truly fantastic score for this mega-luxurious mask, in its blue glass and gold pot and with an utterly heavenly 'signature' Guerlain scent. The Imperial Orchid Molecular Complex features in many of Guerlain's deluxe options, with its firming extracts, microcirculation-boosting ingredients – and a natural sugar, ribose, to boost skin's oxygen levels. It comes with a special brush for perfect application, as well as instructions for a 'face-draining' massage – and is recommended for use twice-weekly.
Comments: 'I used this overnight and woke up looking ten years younger! Fine lines disappeared, face plumper, skin glowing and radiant' • 'immediately gave a real moisture boost, uplifted and plumped out my face, definitely softened and filled out some quite deep wrinkles on my forehead, albeit temporarily; gorgeous to use' • 'a luxury product for a real treat; very special – skin softer, more hydrated and a bit tighter though not taut' • 'skin took on a glow with that slight sheen of youth, seemed more resilient and firmer, even and smoother-looking; felt like applying satin! Can I give it 16/10?' • 'reduced look of pore size' • 'thank you for allowing me to feel this special, even opening the jar made me smile!'.

Elemis Fruit Active Rejuvenating Mask

 8.86/10 The first of two award winners from Elemis in this category, this mask contains strawberry and kiwi for radiance-boosting, macadamia nut oil, shea butter – and kaolin clay, which is deep-cleansing, helping to refine the skin and banish dullness. (Interestingly, they recommend it for smokers – which we don't recommend! – because of the circulation-boosting effect.) It's not tight, but it does 'set' more than the other winning masks.
Comments: 'Top score for a perfect mask! My skin looked fresher, less puffy, more "perky", dreamy texture, smells like a fruit smoothie, my face was rejuvenated – result!' • 'skin looked fresh and smooth, definitely brighter, which improved with regular use' • 'loved this creamy, light mask which felt a little tingly but not uncomfy, skintone improved, definitely healthier, and could actually see the difference' • 'skin softer to the touch and dewier-looking, gives a clearer-looking complexion than my usual nourishing mask' • 'make-up went on like a dream and stayed put so I felt far more confident after just one treatment'.

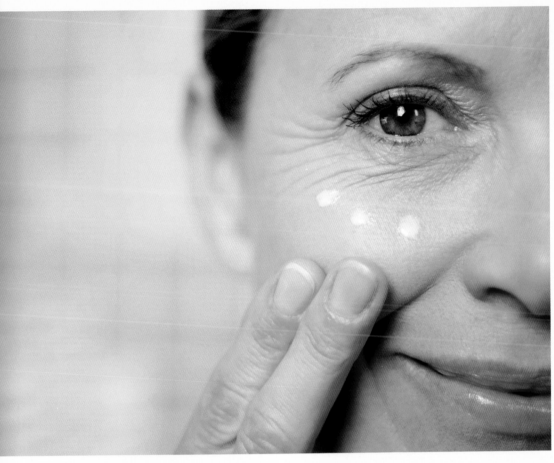

Elemis Pro-Collagen Quartz Lift Mask

 Much richer and creamier than the first Elemis entry above (and pricier, too), this is from the spa brand's state-of-the-art Quartz Lift collection. Quartz, they tell us, enhances cell communication, while argan offers a 'facelifting effect' – and two other botanicals (padina pavonica and noni) relax and smooth the skin. There's also an 'anti-pollution complex', and Elemis call this 'the take-home facial'. As for our testers…?

Comments: 'Top marks! Instantly lifted and toned my skin, revealing a more radiant complexion, felt glorious and beautiful smell; left with such a soft, glowing skin and fine lines smoothed out, really hydrated and plumped out skin' • 'usually have salon treatments but this could persuade me to do it at home; skin very much rejuvenated, glowing, smooth, soft and tight – seemed to contour it' • 'skin did feel as if I'd had a salon facial – glowing and not taut at all' • 'pleasingly moisturising, left skin very soft and more toned without feeling tight in

any way' • 'skin looked brighter and clearer, pores tighter'.

Clarins Super Restorative Replenishing Comfort Mask

Clarins have done consistently well throughout this book, with another winner here: a rich, cocooning pump-action mask which in ten minutes replenishes skin, restoring radiance and suppleness. 'Youth-giving' plant extracts include mango oil, shea butter, a collagen-activating ivy derivative and parsley, to brighten and even skintone.

Comments: 'I loved this! Top marks, it made me feel pampered; skin felt just gorgeous after, really smooth and soft, very dry areas looked great, slight tightening effect – which lasted about a few days, even more once I used it every week' • 'skin looked more hydrated, plumped up and glowing, brighter and less aged – benefits lasted a couple of days; the best I have used' • 'smelt expensive and indulgent' • 'skintone looked more even, effects lasted most of the week'.

♡ WE LOVE…

Jo's bathroom shelf is somewhat crowded with face masks: Neal's Yard Remedies White Tea Enriching Facial Mask (for general skin-brightening), their Nourishing Orange Flower Facial Mask (leave on overnight when skin's super-dry), Les Fleurs de Bach Anti-Stress Mask (instantly de-frazzling for the spirits, quenching for the skin) – but for the fastest pick-you-up of all, the two-minute miracle worker that is camphor-rich Liz Earle Brightening Treatment. Sarah's right there with Les Fleurs de Bach and Liz Earle's offerings but her big miracle-worker is Darphin's Youthful Radiance Camellia Mask, which plumps up skin and makes it more even-toned and, yes, radiant!

Facial oils: *our award winners*

The best facial oils sink softly into skin, plumping and nourishing without ever feeling tacky or greasy. Specific ingredients are often chosen for their age-defying properties, helping to brighten skin or lessen wrinkles. We asked our beauty sleuths to help narrow down the choices for you – and here are their top choices, all natural, from around 80 oils that were tested, including the highest-scoring product we've ever trialled for any of our books

We love oils, for mature skins. (And yes, they can even work to balance oilier complexions, with the right blend of essential oils.) They're also ideal for touchy skins, which may react to synthetic preservatives: oils are naturally self-preserving, so don't need anything extra to extend their life. As Geraldine Howard, of Aromatherapy Associates, observes: 'Think of facial oils as "food" for the skin, and moisturisers as the water. Skin needs both to keep it soft and supple.'

A few drops is all it takes. While they're sometimes expensive (because of the cost of the concentrated botanicals in the blends), a bottle of facial oil typically lasts for much longer than a jar of cream. Only use as much as your skin needs: usually three or four small drops is enough. It should sink in quickly, so if skin looks greasy ten minutes later, you've used too much.

Try layering, under face cream. We like to apply facial oil under night cream, for a double-whammy of effectiveness. Great for skins prone to dryness at any time – or in winter, when central heating wicks the moisture out of skin. Alternatively, put a little cream into your hands and blend it with facial oil using your fingers, before applying. We're great believers in 'customising' our treatments to deliver what our skin needs at any point in time, and this is a great way to make a not-quite-moisturising-enough night cream a bit richer.

You can make your own blends. (Shameless plug: in Jo's book *The Ultimate Natural Beauty Book* there are many recipes.) Or you can opt for one of the pre-blended oils which are increasingly widely available, many of which we trialled for this book. Once the exclusive preserve of Frenchwomen, who learned early on how powerfully skin-caring facial oils can be, there are now dozens and dozens of options on the market – which is why we've put them through their paces.

REVIEWS

Nude Replenishing Night Oil ✿ ✿

 Wow. We have waited fourteen years for a product to notch up a mark this staggeringly high – averaged across ten testers (mostly they gave it a ten). So yes, Nude Replenishing Night Oil – from the range developed in tandem with Ali Hewson (aka 'Mrs Bono') – has just ever-so-slightly nudged ahead of our previous long-standing highest scorer, Liz Earle Cleanse & Polish, and we have no reason to believe Nude Replenishing Night Oil won't also go on to become one of the great beauty classics. With its blend of active oils (including macadamia, raspberry and cranberry seeds, apricot kernel and kukui), this is super-rich in omegas 3, 6, 7 and 9. The pump-action bottle is sculpted from eco-plastic, and it is 100 per cent natural.

Comments: 'Absolutely enhanced radiance, I felt and looked ten years younger – smoother, less

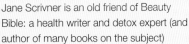

lined, brighter, this is serious skincare' • 'makes my dry crêpey skin and flaky patches softer and more dewy, and didn't aggravate at all, which is a miracle in itself' • 'my combination skin was definitely plumper, smoother, more moisturised and younger-looking, within 24 hours of first using' • 'my dry sensitive skin was much smoother, I would absolutely buy' • 'a real anti-age product, a must-have for mature skin'.

Liz Earle Superskin Concentrate ❀ ❀

 9.15/10 This previously came top of the facial oils category in *The Green Beauty Bible*, but when we sent it out to our mature testers again for this book, they awarded it a micro-mark higher than its previous score (which was 9.1/10, in that case). Which, to us, just goes to confirm what we know: that our trials are incredibly consistent! This is Jo's favourite (see We Love…).

Comments: 'Skin was immediately much smoother and after four weeks the difference was quite dramatic, my skin was more toned and firm' • 'my combination/dry skin looks youthful and I think the aromatherapy oils help me unwind and sleep better' • 'I'm 45 with slight wrinkles, dry skin, tightness, sun damage – and this product makes me look younger! Definitely plumped my skin, made jaw line more toned and helped my lines on my forehead' • 'my sensitive skin is smooth and soft; particularly liked the instruction to inhale the fragrance, which seemed to calm my mind before bed'.

Vaishaly Night Nourisher (Dry/Sensitive) ❀ ❀

 8.78/10 The Normal/Combination version of this also appeared in *The Green Beauty Bible*, but with our anti-ageing testing panel it was Vaishaly's blend for drier skins which wowed. The skin-cocooning oils include jojoba and macadamia nut, plus Arctic raspberry seed extract and grapeseed.

Comments: 'This is luxurious to use and makes me feel pampered: I followed the massage technique from the leaflet and my skin feels plump and hydrated, soothed and comfy; make-up stays put the next day too' • 'people say my skin is glowing, it feels intensively moisturised and really smooth, also fewer hormonal breakouts' • 'feels wonderful to massage your face with this, even nicer if you can get someone to do it for you!' • 'my dry/normal skin loved this – looked amazing! So soft and plump' • 'I didn't have that sinking feeling when I looked in the mirror in the morning!'.

Jane Scrivner Balance Skin Elixir ❀ ❀

8.6/10 Jane Scrivner is an old friend of Beauty Bible: a health writer and detox expert (and author of many books on the subject) who's finally brought out her own range. And testers loved Jane's golden jojoba oil, with its heavenly blend of essential oils: sweet orange, lavender, sandalwood, ylang-ylang, myrrh, frankincense and elemi. As Jane points out, it actually balances skin, so oily-skinned women shouldn't be afraid to use this blend.

Comments: 'My combination skin was brighter and looking better within 24 hours; absolutely divine smell; in the morning after using at night skin looks radiant and "alert" – wide awake!' • 'as a beauty elixir/pick-me-up, it's heaven; I use it all the time now and have noticed a definite improvement in skintone' • 'generous size lasts up to six months, has improved my combination skin by balancing and normalising it' • 'after a few days, skin felt softer and well-moisturised, with a healthy-looking bloom' • 'definite thumbs-up for brighter, plumper skin, which feels smooth and less dry, but didn't love the smell'.

Ila Beyond Organic Face Oil for Glowing Radiance ❀ ❀

 8.55/10 Luxe spa brand Ila harnesses the power of delectably-scented rosa damascena flower oil for this dropper-bottled facial oil, which also features argan oil, rosehip seed oil, sandalwood and vitamin E oil. More than 92.5 per cent of the blend is organically-certified, but the final product doesn't carry a certifier's symbol – so only two daisies in our 'daisy rating', not three. As so often with rose products we trial, testers were enraptured by the fragrance. Some testers, while liking the product, didn't quite feel it lived up to its name – though others absolutely did…

Comments: 'My skin seemed to radiate after using this: so bright and fresh – not sure it gets rid of lines, but a glowing look knocks years off – a real tonic in a bottle' • 'my skin laps the oil up and I can see/feel that it's plumper, smoother and brighter'• 'thought my face would look greasy but it sinks in very quickly' • 'my mature, dry skin is rehydrated and plumper; I also feel I get a better night's sleep, which is anti-ageing!' • 'plumpness is the first thing I noticed – which gave a better look to the more wrinkled parts of my sad old face!; smooth, soft skin from first application; glorious smell!'.

Learn the new foundation rules

As your face changes, so should your approach to creating a flawless canvas…

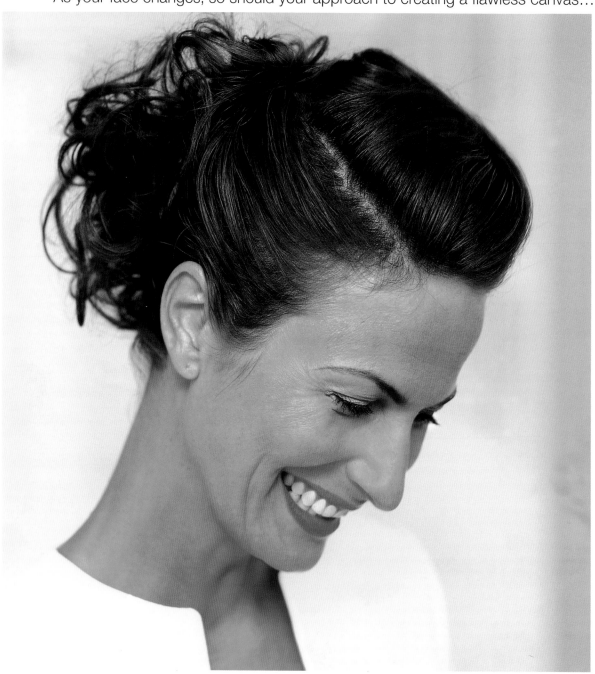

*T*hroughout this book, we're very prescriptive about what works and what doesn't – because we know what really works, and we're giving you the inside info. (That's what we're about.)

However, there are two areas of make-up – foundation (aka base) and eyeshadow – where we can't be totally prescriptive, and where you'll need to experiment to see which of our various proposed options work for you. Some will, some won't.

We suggest setting aside a little playtime to experiment with the different techniques (and maybe even products), to see which give you the best results. We don't have a webcam on your computer so we can't look and tell you which works, which looks best – but if you use two mirrors (one hand mirror, to get a side view), you should be able to judge for yourself. If you're not certain, ask a friend who you trust.

What we know for certain, though, is that the products you've been using through your twenties and thirties are pretty unlikely to make you look fabulous once you hit forty – let alone beyond…

As Trish McEvoy says: 'As we get older, we lose evenness (principally due to cumulative sun damage), clarity, colour and definition. That's the difference between a young face and an older one. Your aim should be to recreate these as naturally as possible.'

HOW TO APPLY YOUR BASE

The better your skin, the lighter the foundation.
That's the rule – according to Mary Greenwell and other make-up pros we respect. But she adds: 'Every woman over forty has to wear foundation. Ironically, up until that point it can sometimes be ageing.'

Echoes Terry de Gunzburg: 'I could get away without foundation until my forties, but no longer. Skin doesn't look neat – or even clean, in some cases – because the skintone is no longer uniform (which also makes you look tired). Your complexion may be a bit red, or look a little shadowy and grey or sallow. But this doesn't mean just applying more of the foundation you've always worn (if you have). Layers of heavy foundation make all lines look worse. If you have always worn quite a lot of base, you probably need to use less and with a lighter touch. You want uniformity – but you don't want a mask-like effect.' Never use your base as an all-over corrector/concealer. If you have flaws, use a corrector/concealer sparingly, just where it's needed. For the best effect, you need to learn to 'layer' products (as we explain here).

● **So: start your 'layers' with a primer.** (See page 89 for more information, and which ones our testers liked best.) Applied after your moisturiser (and don't forget to let this sink in for at least five minutes) and/or serum, a primer adds softness and luminosity, can go some way towards evening skintone, and helps turbo-charge the staying power of your make-up.

● **Rethink your foundation.** 'Nothing too matt, nothing too heavy,' is Mary's wisdom (she likes cream bases best). Our recommendations for Anti-Ageing Foundations, see page 90, are another good place to start. The 'finish' should not be too matt; a little dewiness or 'light' is flattering, but not so much that you look shiny. If you have oily skin, go for oil-free; dry skin, choose one labelled 'moisturising'. The big new option is mineral powder foundations, which many experts including Trish McEvoy and Jane Iredale (the pioneer of mineral make-up) recommend, particularly for conditions such as acne and rosacea. See page 92 for more.

● **Test the foundation shade on your neck.** 'Just below the jaw is the right place,' says Mary Greenwell. 'Your base should match your neck, not your face or even the jawline itself, and should "disappear" to avoid that tell-tale join line.' Be brave, and check it out in bright daylight, adds Barbara Daly.

● **Try a foundation brush.** We're big fans of these, and so is Terry de Gunzburg. 'I don't like sponges but I do like brushes,' she says. 'You can control the quantity that you apply and you can "layer" the foundation on a little at a time, using the brush to make tiny feathery strokes that tap it into the skin and pores. Apply a little foundation to the back of your (clean) hand, and pick the foundation up from there with the brush, a little at a time. You can always add, but it's harder to take away. Then use the warmth of your fingers to "press" the foundation into the skin, which makes it look natural.' (NB: we're big fans of all the products in Terry's By Terry make-up range: after all, she is the woman who created the legendary Touche Eclat/Radiant Touch for YSL, and there is probably nobody who understands light-reflecting particles and how to introduce radiance into make-up products better than her. She's very funny about her line, insisting: 'I created it for women who want to look as good as their daughters. Or their husband's mistress.' A very French approach…!)

Alternatively, use your fingers to smooth in your foundation, from the word 'go'. Fingers are Mary Greenwell's preferred 'tools', also Barbara Daly's. 'They

Can you fix an open pore? We know these bug you from the number of emails to www.beautybible.com, over the years. Pores tend to 'stretch' as we age, especially for those who've had oily skin in the past. Conversely, they can be very obvious on dry skin. The old advice was to avoid moisturising the affected area – but first, that's not practical and also we'd rather you protected your face with an SPF. And actually we suggest reading the comments made about award winners in our Miracle Treatments, Serums and Night Creams section as many testers observed improvements in tightness of pores as a result of using certain products featured there; ditto, the clay-based mask in our Face Masks section. But do avoid toners which can over-stimulate sebaceous glands. For a quick fix, try patting on a primer or line-filler – they can make pores vanish in a flash (albeit temporarily) and are your fast track to pore perfection.

are warm, and so help "meld" foundation into skin,' Mary says. (We say: try a brush, try your fingers, and see which gives you the best effect. Sarah favours fingers most mornings – with brushwork for dress-up days – but Jo finds fingers take off as much as she's putting on so uses a brush. So the mantra is 'experiment'!) Don't feel you have to apply it all over your face, says Barbara Daly. 'Start from the centre and blend out, so by the time you get to the fine hairs at the side (don't worry – everyone has them), there's nothing there.'

Remember, your base is not a corrector or concealer. So, once you've applied your foundation, stand back and take a look. If you still have flaws you want to hide, such as brown spots, red cheeks, scars or dark circles under your eyes, read on.

COVERING REDNESS, AGE SPOTS AND OTHER FLAWS

While Trish McEvoy believes every woman of a certain age should own a corrector, concealer (see below for the difference) and luminiser, they are certainly essential for camouflaging hyperpigmentation (brown spots), redness and other blemishes. Her advice: 'After you've primed skin, take your corrector (always matt, yellow- or peach-based, with deeper peach for women of colour), and dot it on with a little brush, then press it in. Very important to dot and press, do not sweep it on. If it needs more blending use a little make-up sponge.' You can then apply cream/liquid foundation, or brush on mineral powder base if you need it. Setting with translucent powder over liquid foundation is optional. 'Technology has advanced so tremendously that many formulas today are long wear and don't need powder,' says Trish.

'My grandmothers lived long into old age and they were always BEAUTIFUL to me. They *loved life* and it showed in their faces'

Penélope Cruz

And what's the difference between a corrector and concealer? Sometimes very little: though generally correctors are lighter and aim to correct colour and tone on very red cheeks or rosacea – rather than a concealer which sits on a blemish such as under-eye dark circles or a scar to conceal it. For more pronounced flaws, you might want to use a corrector followed by a concealer. (For more camouflage advice on covering rosacea and acne scarring, see page 168.)

For frown lines, try patting on a silicone-based filler, which will soften the edges (more on page 94).

Brighten up with a luminiser. Aka a light-reflecting pen (see page 56). These magic wands add luminosity to your high planes: cheekbones, upper brow, forehead – and you can dab a tad on your bosom and shoulders. As well as accentuating the positive, they draw attention away from the negative areas.

Set your make-up with face powder. This will definitely make it stay in place longer. (Disappearing make-up is a perennial problem for thirsty skins, and also anyone who's experiencing hot flushes.) But it has to be the right powder – feather-light and barely-there – and it must be used judiciously on the areas that need it rather than all over the face. A finely-milled, translucent loose powder will reduce pore appearance too, says Barbara Daly.

Apply face powder with a fat eyeshadow brush. (Yes, really.) Mary Greenwell advises using an eyeshadow brush (albeit the largest of these you can find) to target powder on the areas of the face that tend to shine: nose, chin, centre of forehead. Also try putting it on very lightly over your eyelids before you apply make-up. Leave the rest of your face naked of powder: you want to see the radiance, and powder may dull that.

One exception to the rule: By Terry Voile Poudre Eclat. This whisper-light, transparent face powder has the subtlest light-reflecting pigments which correct and even out skintone, mattifying while still leaving skin luminous. It also seems to add a veil of 'softness' to the skin. (Like all of the By Terry products it is far from cheap but a pot will last you just about for ever.) Rose Lumière is a colour that works on all skintones except black and Asian. To set your make-up for a long evening out, an all-over dusting of Terry's powder is the key. But this time, use a large round-headed brush, please.

Make-up primers: *our award winners*

We challenge you to discover the difference that a cosmetic primer can make to how well your make-up lasts and how much smoother your complexion appears

REVIEWS

Guerlain Météorites Perles Light Diffusing Perfecting Primer

 Delicate petal pink pearls are suspended in this gel primer, and diffuse when massaged into the skin to give a radiant glow without – miraculously – adding shininess. (In fact, there are absorbing powders to neutralise sebum.) It has the usual signature Guerlain violet-y fragrance (which we love, love, LOVE…though some testers didn't.) **Comments:** 'Really loved this product, easy to use, fantastic packaging, sank in quickly and made my skin feel like silk; enhanced radiance and an excellent base for make-up, which lasted longer – my skin glowed through the day' • 'gives a gentle, pretty glow which lasts all day' • 'make-up looks satin-smooth on top of this smooth, light serum, which left a sheen on my skin, and my friend said how good it looked; I like the ingenious pearls' • 'gave a much more smooth and professional look, fabulous fragrance, foundation glided on'.

Clarins Instant Smooth Perfecting Touch

 Clarins do tell us that this little pot of silky-smooth skin perfector CAN be used all over the skin – over day cream and under foundation/powder – but the dinky size of the jar means you might get through it quite quickly, even though you need very little. (It can also be used on specifically lined areas, as an instant smoother.) Has a 'Line Minimiser Pigment' for soft-focus effect, plus 'Acacia Micro-Pearls' which plump up to fill lines. **Comments:** 'Rich, silky texture is very easy to apply and sank in immediately; definitely enhanced radiance and is an excellent base of foundation – the glow lasted throughout the day; this little pot can work wonders' • 'you need to apply just a little then let it sit for a few minutes before applying

AT A GLANCE

Guerlain Météorites Perles Light Diffusing Perfecting Primer

Clarins Instant Smooth Perfecting Touch

Elizabeth Arden Good Morning Skin Serum

Cosmetics à la Carte Rose Dew

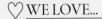

♡ WE LOVE…

Somewhat to her shame, Jo often does her make-up on the train, first using a sponge to smooth in Cosmetics à la Carte Skin Veil to turbo-charge the staying power of her make-up. For home use, she likes the Sue Devitt Microquatic Blue Anti-Aging SPF30 Protection Primer: it helps neutralise redness and creates a good base for make-up. Sarah is devoted to Trish McEvoy Even Skin Face Primer, which does indeed even out skintone and helps foundation create a (more or less) flawless finish.

foundation or else it gets mixed in; made skin look brighter and smoother and has encouraged me to use a primer more regularly'.

Elizabeth Arden Good Morning Skin Serum

 A slim glass bottle of serum featuring 'energising' botanicals and vitamin A, in what feels like a silicone-rich base. (Silicones do have a fabulously skin-smoothing effect and are widely used in primers.) **Comments:** 'Easy to apply, blended smoothly and made skin really velvety; evened skintone and gave complexion a fresh look; make-up did go on more smoothly and evenly' • 'left skin feeling silky and looking quite flawless, am convinced pores looked smoother after applying it; my husband said I looked lovely!' • 'skin was much more radiant; seemed to smooth red and dry patches and give a more even skintone, great base for make-up; I almost lost the "frazzled teacher" look!' • 'had a brilliant effect on my skin, lessened the redness of acne scars and my mum said I looked like I'd had a good night's sleep'.

Cosmetics à la Carte Rose Dew

 From a much-loved Knightsbridge make-up school and beauty emporium, this non-greasy primer features aloe and witch hazel for a skin-firming effect. The heavenly rose scent of this makes morning application a total pleasure. They recommend applying after moisturiser, 15 minutes before foundation. **Comments:** 'Brilliant base for make-up – mineral foundation and blusher – skin did not shine so I looked better!' • 'wonderful fragrance, worth buying it for that alone' • 'quite runny but rich too, and wonderful; a dream to apply, gives skin a glow; let it dry, apply make-up – and it makes skin look and feel fabulous' • 'enhanced radiance and made make-up last longer; the rose smell is adorable'.

Anti-ageing foundations: *four award winners*

Now there are foundations designed specifically for older skin that give good coverage to hide imperfections and create a more radiant, even tone

AT A GLANCE

Diorskin Nude Natural Glow Hydrating Makeup

Estée Lauder Re-Nutriv Ultimate Radiance Makeup SPF15

Clarins Super Restorative Foundation SPF15

Lancôme Teint Rénergie Lift R.A.R.E. SPF20

TIP

The most important thing with foundation is still the right colour: but don't try it on the back of your hand – the skintone is invariably dramatically different. Use a Q-tip to try it just below your jawline. If it disappears, it's the right shade.

In the past few years, a whole new category of foundations has emerged to cater to the wannabe-fabulous-at-forty-plus market. Anti-ageing foundations mostly do double-duty: instantly evening out skintone (one of the most instantly de-ageing tricks) plus moisturising, and some contain ingredients to help perfect skin over the longer term (firming/plumping/damage-limiting, etc.) The snag is that foundation should only be applied where you need it – definitely not as an all-over 'mask' – so there's a limit to what can be achieved in terms of serious ongoing improvements. Nevertheless, we felt this growing category of foundations targeted at older skins was important enough to research with the help of our testers – and here are the high-scoring bases which seriously impressed them.

REVIEWS

Diorskin Nude Natural Glow Hydrating Makeup

9/10 This is some score, when you consider that it's an average of ten women's opinions. In their own research, Dior observed that when using Diorskin Nude for a month, 70 per cent of women felt their skin 'became more beautiful over time, even without make-up'. Read on for our testers' views of this glamorously-packaged, lightweight liquid base, which is enriched with minerals, vitamins C and E, a silk derivative – and 'micro-droplets of water', creating a 'moisturising and energising cocktail for the skin'. There's a moderate SPF10.

Comments: 'I really, really love this foundation! Like a second skin on your face, really easy to apply and blend smoothly, sheer but covers small veins, large open pores, blemishes – and evens out skin – don't need concealer or powder, plus it lasts' • 'felt light and not greasy in any way, blended well, very good coverage, prevented shine, perfect for evenings' • 'even covered my red cheeks after being out in sun' • 'I found a foundation brush gave perfect coverage,

brown spots disappeared; worth taking the little extra time to apply and I received a couple of compliments about my complexion'.

Estée Lauder Re-Nutriv Ultimate Radiance Makeup SPF15

8.85/10 Lauder, of course, are known for their anti-ageing technology, and the Re-Nutriv range is their most serious (and luxurious) treatment range. Alongside hyaluronic acid, vitamin E and broad-spectrum UV protection, this contains a 'micro-fine crystal mesh of precious gemstones and crystals' for radiance (and an SPF15). It's fragrance-free.

Comments: '10/10! Gave just the right coverage, not heavy or thick, looked very natural, made skin younger-looking and brighter instantly and improved over time, with fine lines diminishing; made my skin feel lovely and light' • 'sheer coverage but you can build it up; looked glowing and smoothed my complexion, all tiredness disappeared instantly, worth every penny!' • 'could go through all day and into evening without reapplying' • 'balanced skintone very well, made it look more radiant due to light-reflecting particles, definitely evened my skintone, smoothed lines and reduced the look of imperfections'.

Clarins Super Restorative Foundation SPF15

8.56/10 Clarins offer a couple of anti-ageing foundations, of which our testers preferred this velvety, fluid cream, with a 100 per cent mineral SPF (so no chemical sunscreens), and firming pine extract. Created to brighten and 'lift' skin, there are 'Soft Focus Pigments' to blur lines. It's for all skin types (and especially from age 50+) seeking medium-to-full coverage, with an SPF15. A more mixed bag of marks, but a good average.

Comments: 'Very pleased with the finish; my sister told me my skin looked clear and smooth – very good product which I would buy' • 'gave lovely dewy finish, very natural sheer coverage, which suited my fair complexion perfectly' • 'lovely thin silky texture, excellent coverage for redness and spots, evened my skintone well – didn't need concealer, more dewy than powdery' • 'this genuinely makes me feel a lot more confident as it improves the look of my skin so much, is really quick to apply and I love the SPF'.

Lancôme Teint Rénergie Lift R.A.R.E. SPF 20

7.81/10 This uses the same R.A.R.E. ('Retightening and Repositioning Effect'!) oligopeptide technology as Lancôme's similarly-named creams, for a firming, radiance-enhancing effect. Used over time, they promise an actual firming action, but in the short-term what you get is good, natural-looking coverage – and SPF20 protection, on the areas of face it's blended into. Testers were more divided on the longer-term benefits though.
Comments: 'Natural finish and dewy radiant look; two female colleagues asked if I'd done a week's detox!' • 'skin looked immediately rejuvenated, and it fulfilled its claims to smooth wrinkles and lift skin in a month!' • 'finish looked natural and enhanced complexion rather than disguising it, balanced skintone but didn't cover all imperfections' • 'added luminosity, not certain if it lifted and firmed, but I do like it' • 'with daily use wrinkles appear reduced and skin feels firmer but still needed concealer and powder'.

♡ WE LOVE...

Jo is a huge convert to By Terry Teint Lumière Veloutée, an ultra-moisturising formulation which offers good coverage – just what she needs for an English rose skin somewhat plagued by red veins. Another extravagant but velvety-finished favourite is La Prairie Skin Caviar Concealer Foundation SPF15, which cleverly comes with a matching cream concealer tucked inside the silvery lid, and a fabulous tiny synthetic brush that's brilliant for spot-targeted foundation, so you can use the barest minimum required. Sarah favours the finish and coverage of Clinique Even Better Makeup SPF15, which promises to help combat hyperpigmentation and give brighter skin and even skintone, and, for really dry days, the light super-dewy finish of new Lancôme Teint Miracle.

Concealers: *our award winners*

Many cream concealers (usually a little thicker than cream foundation) we've tried are not suitable for under-eyes, as they can look cake-y – but the top scoring products here do claim to work well for dark circles. So, depending on your needs, you may only have to invest in one double-duty concealer for your make-up bag.

Benefit Erase Paste

8.62/10 A seriously spectacular score for a product from a pretty light-hearted brand – which actually does serious products. This concentrated creamy formula principally targets discolourations and flaws but can also be used on dark circles, as the three shades are specifically 'brightening'.
Comments: '10/10 for thread veins, small blemishes and pigmentation, also made wrinkles look less obvious – but not enough for scars; blends in very well and looked natural' • 'I used it on moles, blemishes, scars, wrinkles, pigmentation and it covered them. I also used it on my daughter who has acne – it was incredible to see the difference'.

Estée Lauder Double Wear Stay-in-Place Concealer SPF10

7.45/10 A 15-hour 'life' is an extravagant promise for any concealer, but this comes from the Stay-in-Place collection – Lauder's Duracell-bunny-of-a-range. This lightweight formulation is easy to blend and again may be used under the eyes.
Comments: 'Very easy to apply and blend in; good coverage' • 'not cake-y or drying and looked so natural it was unnoticeable' • 'excellent for redness and thread veins around nostrils, good on my dark circles'.

Susan Posnick ColorCorrect

7.1/10 Something different: this is a creamy, double-ended stubby pencil with subtly different textures of product at either end. One end works to neutralise discolouration – redness, sun spots, etc – while the other features brightening pigments, to soften lines or fill in the under-eye area.
Comments: '10/10! Blended brilliantly and liked having the two colours' excellent staying power, didn't need constant retouching on red spots' • 'surprisingly easy to apply and blended very well; great for thread veins, red bits round my nose and small scars, but felt uneasy using it under my eyes'.

♡ WE LOVE...

To erase redness, Jo dips her finger in the product that collects around the neck of her foundation bottle (By Terry Teint Lumière Veloutée) – which makes for a perfectly matched shade, in a slightly thicker and more covering format (because some of the water's evaporated from the formula). Sarah doesn't use much concealer but for the odd blemish, pigmented spot/ patch and redness is delighted by By Terry VIP Touch-Expert Advanced, which does the trick beautifully.

Try a mineral foundation

Mineral make-up has been a huge beauty buzz over the past few years, and many women around our age are converts. But it does require a new set of make-up skills, so if you're going to try a mineral foundation, we want to ensure you optimise your chances of great results

Two things we'd say: the first is that provided you use a good product and follow this advice, you will get great coverage – one friend used Susan Posnick's ColorFlo to camouflage the flaming redness after she had her face lasered (and went out dancing, she was so confident). Second, mineral make-up need not look dry or caked if you start here…

Moisturise your face first. The mineral powder will adhere to the natural oils of your skin, but as there's no natural moisture in a mineral foundation you need to add some extra. If skin's too dry, the powder will end up looking just like that – powder. (As usual, wait ten minutes for moisturiser to sink in before applying make-up.)

Use a specific mineral foundation brush. Some of these are 'kabuki-style': stubby and short-handled. Because they're almost circular, they work for the 'swirl and buff' movement that's best for applying this type of make-up (see below for details). Some brands – such as Susan Posnick – have the powder in the handle of the brush, so of course you use that.

Tip a little of the powder into the lid of the jar. If the powder is loose (rather than contained in the brush handle), never, never dip your brush directly into the mineral make-up – you'll pick up way too much. A little is all you need. If you require more, gently tip a tad more into the lid, and swirl your brush in that. But all you'll need is a pinch or so.

Then tap the brush. This dusts off any excess powder.

Swirl and buff. You apply mineral foundation by holding the brush at right angles to your skin, not at a sloping angle. Then rub the brush on to your skin using circular movements, particularly focusing on areas you want to conceal. You can gradually build coverage this way, until it's the level you want. This isn't like normal face powder where you want to skim it over the surface: you're really aiming to buff and push the powder into the skin. As with all foundation techniques, it takes a little practice, but is worth persevering.

Spot-target any veins, etc, with a fingertip dipped in

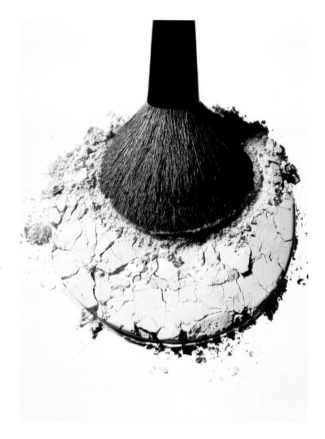

powder. This is a great tip we picked up: rather than continuing to layer on mineral powder, you can put a dab on the end of your finger and press it on to something you want to conceal (a broken vein, an age spot). The heat of your finger helps the powder to meld into skin.

Try a setting powder if you find your mineral make-up disappears. In general, women report to us that mineral make-up lasts for longer than regular foundation. But if that's not the case with you, try a specific mineral setting powder (such as Bare Minerals Mineral Veil). Do not, however, try setting mineral make-up with your regular face powder: the textures don't work well together.

Mineral make-up: *our award winners*

Mineral make-up appeals to women for two reasons: in powder form, it's easy to swirl on to the face (though you may need a bit of practise, see our how-to, left), and many users like the fact it's 'natural'. All mineral foundations aren't created equal, though. If you are looking for a truly 100 per cent natural product, check out the daisy rating of the award winners listed here (for more about this see page 7): two daisies are the sign that the product is all-mineral, with no synthetic or chemical 'fillers'. One daisy? Mostly mined mineral pigments. It's your call. NB: we list other excellent mineral make-up products in our book *The Green Beauty Bible*, but not all those were tested on mature skins – unlike these winners…

Youngblood Mineral Cosmetics Natural Mineral Foundation

8/10 From California, an attractively-packaged mineral range (they aren't all!), which is 100 per cent pure mineral powder and no 'fillers'. Comes in a wide screw-top plastic jar, which is helpful when it comes to swirling your brush in the lid, and there's a clever dispenser which releases just the right amount of powder at the tap of a finger. In 16 shades – from pale to Mahogany (great for black skins); our testers received Neutral, one of the light-to-mid tones. Testers were a bit mixed in their reactions – mainly novices, because they needed time to practise.

Comments: 'Once I got the hang of using this, it wasn't messy, and lasts well: after years of using liquid base, I'll always use mineral powder now for great natural coverage' • 'once blended it looks good, and I felt like I was wearing no make-up – but it did take me a quite lot of work' • 'looked sheer but covered well, especially open pores and small blemishes; I would buy' • 'concealed my open pores and gave a dewy glow' • 'very impressed, but I had to learn how to apply'.

MAC Mineralize Skinfinish Natural

7.95/10 This does well for sheer ease – it's a pressed powder compact (eliminating any risk of spillage, which can be a factor with some mineral powders) – but it's not 100 per cent natural if that's a concern for you. (No mirror in the compact, or sponge, which lost it marks.) The powder delivers a matt radiance, and would also be good for 'setting' a liquid foundation. Eight shades (we had pure golden beige Light/Medium) – and be sure to go for the Skinfinish Natural option, as the original Skinfinish is seriously frosted.

AT A GLANCE

Youngblood Mineral Cosmetics Natural Mineral Foundation

MAC Mineralize Skinfinish Natural

Cosmetics à la Carte Cover Tint

Origins Multi-Grain Makeup SPF14

♡ WE LOVE…

For sheer ease, Jo chooses Susan Posnick Colorflo – less messy than most, because the powder's contained in a see-thru tube with a built-in brush, which makes for easy swirling while gradually building coverage. And she's very impressed with the way this can easily cover her red veins.

Comments: 'My first experience but it was easy to apply with my own sponge; gave sheer coverage which you could build up without looking overdone; concealed open pores and small blemishes but needed concealer on thread veins; brilliant product' • 'lovely sheer natural finish which covered well without looking cake-y' • 'used my own brush which gave a sheer natural finish, minimised the open pores on my cheeks' • 'loved this fine texture, fantastic at evening out my skintone and didn't sit in fine lines'.

Cosmetics à la Carte Cover Tint

7.71/10 For easy application, the mineral powder in this 100 per cent natural powder features a built-in sponge; you swipe it over the surface of your skin for the lightest coverage, and 'press' it into your complexion where more help's required. Again, spill-proof – and we like the built-in mirror on the lid. Nine shades and we trialled Vanilla.

Comments: 'Ten out of ten! Fantastic to use, blended really well and no mess; natural even finish that balanced all redness – a powder that felt like a cream foundation' • 'felt like silk and covered all flaws without concealer' • 'gave a warm glow, even coverage, balanced skintone, covered small flaws'.

Origins Multi-Grain Makeup SPF14

7.55/10 Despite being a lightweight powder, Origins' option features a touch of shea butter for a skin-melting texture, with organic oats, tapioca, soy, rice flour and barley micro-grains plus silica to absorb oil, and antioxidant from goji berry and pomegranate. Of course it's also based on titanium dioxide – the principal mineral in this category of make-up, which offers some measure of an SPF (but only where you apply it…). We tested Light/Medium of the five shades. NB: this product divided testers into Love and Dislike. Here are the ones who loved it.

Comments: 'Unbeatable for daytime; had several comments saying how well I look, despite moving house, and it's great not to have loads of heavy make-up to remove; it improved my skin too, with fewer spots' • 'my first experience of mineral make-up and I am very impressed; I expected it to be very powdery but skin looks glowing and even without looking as if I am wearing anything'.

*F*Wave a magic wand over your lines

Fact: most of us are cowards when it comes to physical invasion of our one and only face with a syringe. (And we say: that's no bad thing.) But as an alternative to Botox and line-filling injections, there is a new generation of cosmetic wonder products which make lines vanish in a flash

You may have decided, like us, that doctor-administered fillers aren't for you. But after a certain stage can there be a woman among us who hasn't glanced in the mirror and wondered what we'd look like if a magic wand was waved over this furrow, or that laugh line, or the annoying little groove – or 'marionette' line – that's just started to run from mouth to chin? Yes, we've all been there…

Which is why we are very, very, VERY excited about the latest trend to hit the beauty scene. Call them 'faux fillers', if you like – but what they really amount to is Polyfilla for faces: products that you apply to your lines and hey, presto! They're gone. Of course, it's all an illusion. But who really cares? Because isn't that what make-up is actually all about? (And personally we love them!)

Bear in mind, of course, that topical fillers will never be as effective as those applied with a syringe by a cosmetic doctor. True volume can only be created when the 'volumiser' is applied deep in the skin's fat layer, and that's not going to happen when you merely pat something on. (If you really want to go down that route, see page 46 to arm yourself with all the right questions to ask before anyone comes waving a syringe in your direction...)

Choose your product. There are two categories of these products (known to insiders as 'optics'). The first is purely cosmetic: the Polyfilla-types – called 'line-smoothers' or 'line-fillers', which have a temporary effect only. As well as delivering those blink-of-an-eye results, the second category of these line-diffusing fillers also offers anti-ageing benefits, which claim to work with regular continuous use to fight those pesky grooves.

Essentially, how do they work? According to Steven Hasher, Vice-President of Research and Development for GoodSkin Labs (an exciting and somewhat hush-hush new division of Estée Lauder Worldwide), 'Imagine a cloaking device – similar to the technology used to make planes invisible to radar.' He goes on to explain in more detail that by taking different sizes of spherical particles – including nylon, talc and silicones – and matching them to the skin's own 'refractive index' (that's the way light naturally bounces off the skin), you can hide and veil the wrinkles… We would add that although this type of line-concealer has anti-ageing benefits, we'd say you also need a 'miracle' cream, or

an eye treatment product – rather than relying on a faux filler alone to treat lines and wrinkles.

Remember: practice makes perfect. Unlike a face cream, there's a little bit of extra work involved in applying these fillers – and just maybe, a bit of experimentation, while you establish which technique works best for you. (Persevere. It's worth it.) Here's our advice:

● Most of these products have tiny nozzles or pen-style applicators which dispense just a little product – and with those, we've found that squeezing the product along the length of the line, then patting it in lightly with the ring finger, delivers the best turn-back-the-clock results.
● Try this over make-up, but also underneath: some fillers won't shift if you apply foundation over the top, although we recommend leaving the 'filler' for a minute or two before applying base. There's really no way round it: you need to experiment.
● Carry the product round in your kit for on-the-go touch-ups since our experience is that none of them – yet – endure from breakfast to dinner without a little repair work.

So which to choose – 'Polyfilla' (for instant results only), or with the addition of precision-targeted anti-ageing ingredients…? We can't make up your mind for you. So we suggest you read our testers' comments on both types of line-filler, opposite.

Line-fillers: *our award winners*

AT A GLANCE

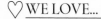

Cosmetics à la Carte Skin Veil

TRI-AKTILINE Instant Deep Wrinkle Filler

Monu Line Smoothing Skin Perfector

♡ WE LOVE...

Jo is hugely impressed by two line-smoothers. First, TRI-AKTILINE Instant Deep Wrinkle Filler (which our testers also rated highly): the tiny nozzle makes it easy to target specific deeper lines and wrinkles, Jo finds. (When she demo-ed this to a group of friends, they were so impressed everyone went out and bought it next day.) Second, L'Oréal Paris Studio Secrets Smoothing Resurfacing Primer, with an almost jelly-like texture that blurs lines astonishingly well, when patted over make-up – almost as if a gauze was drawn across them. Sarah has also been a long-time fan of the TRI-AKTILINE filler, and has now added Bremenn Instant Forehead Smoother to her must-haves – cos it just does what it says on the pot!

For anyone troubled by lines, wrinkles and grooves, these are utter magic. We've even managed to dissuade women from opting into Botox treatments by demo-ing the instantly line-blurring power of some of these 'line-fillers', which work by depositing optical pigments, silicones and synthetic ingredients like nylon into lines to minimise (and in some cases, even eliminate) their appearance. As a bonus, some of these also contain anti-ageing ingredients which target the lines themselves, over time. There are now dozens of options within this category, of which our testers rated these highest. (Most others, they observed, performed far less well, with plenty languishing in the line-filling doldrums…)

Cosmetics à la Carte Skin Veil

 A product that Jo, too, rates highly: a sleek silver mirrored compact, this is super-easy to use: it features a velvety sponge which you can swipe over lines and wrinkles, under or over make-up (most testers preferred the latter). The optical pigments also work to minimise the appearance of open pores (great around the nose), and it can also be used all over the face as an under make-up primer. Skin Veil comes in three shades: Original (untinted for any skintone, which our lot received); Vanilla (for paler complexions) or Honey (for medium-to-dark skintones) – although none deliver actual coverage. Very easy to use.

Comments: 'The texture is like a creamy/satiny foundation which goes on invisibly and gives a fabulously smooth, luminous quality, with the illusion of flawlessness; I am totally addicted!' • 'I applied with fingers, and my foundation went on easily over it; all seemed to blend together to cover and plump' • 'fine lines seemed to disappear, worked best under mineral powder foundation, made my skin look air-brushed! Loved it as a primer' • 'this really gave a very natural look that lasted all day'.

TRI-AKTILINE Instant Deep Wrinkle Filler

 Point the teeny nozzle at your lines, and squeeze – then pat the squiggle of line-diffusing cream into furrows and wrinkles, and watch them d-i-s-a-p-p-e-a-r… Over time TRI-AKTILINE is also said to offer skincare benefits, helping to boost collagen production – but this score is mostly for the instant results it delivers, with a plumping action from avocado oil, shea butter and hyaluronic acid, as well as ultra-light spherical optical diffusers. Jo uses it over make-up; they say it can also be used beneath.

Comments: 'I was surprised at how effective this was, I noticed an immediate improvement in the appearance of fine lines and wrinkles, particularly on my forehead, which has increased in the six weeks I've been using it' • 'my husband asked me what I was using and if he could use it!' • 'would definitely buy again, worked quickly and effortlessly, fine lines and wrinkles definitely less pronounced and plumped, appeared to blend seamlessly into my skin' • 'fine lines seemed to be filled and disappear' • 'definitely blurred wrinkles, and I needed less make-up, in fact if I applied too much there was a "cake-y" effect; I was really sceptical about this but I did notice a difference and my mood improved immensely!'.

Monu Line Smoothing Skin Perfector

 A generous tube of silkiness, this silicone-rich weightless formula can be used all over the face as a make-up primer – or on specific areas where you're troubled by lines. (For more on primers, see page 89.) The polysaccharides form an instant 'veil', and there's nourishment from omega-6 essential fatty acids. With a very pretty, slightly tropical fragrance, it's paraben-free – but we have to point out that there are plenty of synthetics in the Monu range, which doesn't quite live up to its 'pure and natural' label.

Comments: 'Simple to apply this gel-like cream with fingers; really seemed to blur out fine lines and smooth skin, then applied make-up over the top for a very natural, even, radiant finish! Worked really well and easily' • 'very impressed, lifted the area, looked completely natural, made me feel younger and more confident; would definitely buy' • 'needed very little, and fine lines were plumped, skin more lifted and looked more radiant, lasted all day – people have been commenting on how well I look; will certainly buy more'.

Score boxes: 7.87/10, 7.83/10, 7.05/10

Be very, very nice to your feet

…every single day. We put more stress on our feet than any other part of the body. And, as leading podiatrist Margaret Dabbs says, 'Foot pain shows on your face.' (Like any pain actually)

Feet are the foundations of the body: when they go wrong, it impacts on our whole being. Plus we want our tootsies in the best possible shape, not just to look good but to take us walking, which is nature's greatest medicine – good for our heart and lungs, and for improving bone density (of our lower half), doesn't strain the joints – and gets us from A to B absolutely free. Walking can also work as a weight-loss technique, if you put in the miles regularly and vigorously.

All of which means that after about 35, we need to think of our feet in terms of much more than ways to show off fabulous shoes and glam nail polishes. Foot problems before that aren't unknown, of course – though they're usually shoe-related (corns and bunions, in particular). But as we age, feet become more problematic. And our experience is that whenever we stop walking regularly – because of illness, injury or simply painful feet (Jo was once almost crippled by an allergic reaction to MSG, Sarah by an ingrowing toenail) – then it's not long before everything feels like it's falling apart.

Remember: foot 'wellbeing' is vital. Overleaf, you'll find answers from one of the most respected 'foot pros' that we know, to help you tackle specific foot problems. Because unless feet are happy, the rest of you is going to be miserable – and that's going to add ten years to how you look. Give them some daily 'foot love' and you'll float along, looking like a spring chick!

Treat yourself to some sexy, comfy shoes. Once upon a time, comfy shoes equalled 'old lady' shoes. Well, baby, look at the comfortable shoe selection NOW! The reason's simple: as the population ages, we're just not giving up on fabulous shoes. We're both absolutely fetishistic about shoe/foot comfort because we walk wherever we can, and we now have a wider-than-ever choice of shoes which look great – but, very importantly, cushion our feet. (This is crucial because the collagen in the sole of the foot dwindles, along with the collagen in our faces.)

Look for these brands we love: Taryn Rose, Clarks (don't write them off because they've been seriously jazzed up), Ecco (ditto), Terra Plana, ShoeTherapy pumps (with posture-correcting soles), Aerosoles, FitFlops and Chie Mihara, a fantastically funky but wearable Spanish brand Jo recently discovered, which is increasingly widely available. And Sarah adores her Ugg boots! All these have extra 'padding' beneath the ball of the foot. (NB: we find those 'party feet' gel insoles squish your toes, putting pressure on the top, so aren't ideal for everyday wear – although fine for the occasional cocktail *soirée*.)

Buff, buff, buff. One of the basic but avoidable ways feet become painful is through the build-up of hard skin – on the balls of the feet, the big toes, and/or heels. A minute of daily exfoliation is literally all it takes to prevent this. (See below for our thoughts on medi-pedis, to get you started.) Lightly whisk a foot file (see page 101 for recommendations) across areas of hard skin. Do not use pressure because this 'compacts' the layers of skin, making the problem worse, according to medi-pedi guru Bastien Gonzalez. NB: we like to buff dry or slightly damp feet, rather than wet ones – on a towel to avoid unalluring 'foot dandruff'.

Massage, massage, massage. Bastien's other critical piece of advice is to use a moisturiser every single night to keep feet soft and comfy. And really, really work that balm or butter into hard skin areas with your fingers like a deep-tissue massage so it breaks down any 'compacted' skin.

Treat yourself to a medi-pedi. This isn't about polish and paint (though you can sometimes tag those on to the end): it's about ultra-efficient removal of hard skin, correct trimming of toenails (to avoid ingrown nails), nail-buffing, cuticle TLC and diagnosis of any problems, which can then be professionally addressed. Once you've had a medi-pedi (we have them every couple of months), it is much, much easier to do the maintenance at home. In fact, given the choice between having our face and our feet attended to, we'd choose feet every time.

Go mad with a nail polish. This is one area where you don't have to worry at all about being 'age-appropriate'. So go a little wild: crazy metallic jade; pillar-box red; Chanel's classic vampy burgundy/black Rouge Noir. It'll make people smile. Especially you. (And that takes ten years off.)

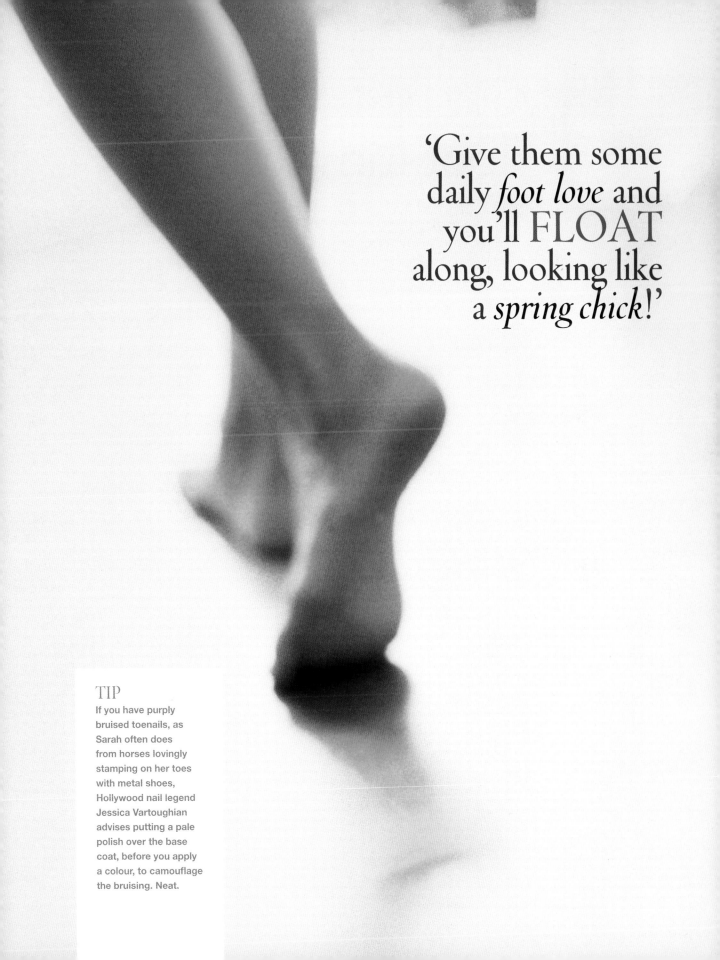

'Give them some daily *foot love* and you'll FLOAT along, looking like a *spring chick*!'

TIP
If you have purply bruised toenails, as Sarah often does from horses lovingly stamping on her toes with metal shoes, Hollywood nail legend Jessica Vartoughian advises putting a pale polish over the base coat, before you apply a colour, to camouflage the bruising. Neat.

Put your best foot forward

... and treat any foot woes. Podiatrist Margaret Dabbs's London clinic is where beauty editors (and many other foot-aware folk) head, when feet need not just a treat but actual treatment. So we turned to Margaret for some sole-searching advice on how to stop common foot problems in their tracks

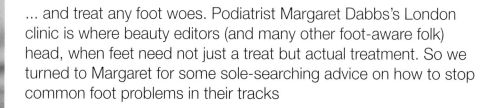

Actually, the biggest problem that Margaret sees in older feet, she says, is dehydration. As we age, the skin thins, we lose subcutaneous (just-under-the-surface) fat, and our tootsies become as dry as the desert. Fascinatingly, that's partly a side effect of the circulatory system preferentially looking after the female organs, and directing blood there. 'Your feet are the end of the road,' explains Margaret. The rest, though, is down to us not looking after them – so, if we may repeat earlier advice, it's vital to moisturise every night.

What's more, it's important not to wear closed-in shoes without socks or tights: 'The moisture from your feet drains into the shoes, drying out the skin – and your feet and shoes are liable to get a tad whiffy, too,' says Margaret. (Open sandals with bare feet are fine because they let your feet breathe.) Now deal with…

Calluses and corns. A callus is a thickening of the surface layer of the skin – hard skin, in other words – which usually forms in response to pressure, often on the ball of the foot, the heel and/or the underside of the big toe. Well-fitting shoes, plenty of moisturising and regular buffing should keep calluses in check, while seeing a podiatrist for regular treatments is also a boon. For corns, professional attention is vital – ideally, as soon as you get one.

A corn is a tiny, cone-shaped mass of

hard skin with a visible centre; it can be excruciatingly painful. The key is to consult a podiatrist who's experienced in biomechanics (the action of how you walk) to find the cause – which could be tight shoes, toe deformities, sticking-out bony bits or an unbalanced gait. As well as treating the corn, you should get advice in order to prevent a reccurrence; they may suggest supportive inserts called orthotics, which can be individually made (expensive) or, increasingly, off-the-shelf (much cheaper).

Warts. These small, rough lumps on the skin, caused by a virus, occur mostly on feet (where they're called verrucas) and hands. Most clear up spontaneously in time (could be a long process though). But since they're contagious and unsightly, treatment is worth exploring. Margaret Dabbs uses a 'holistic' combination of cryosurgery (freezing) and acupuncture: 'It's really successful over about three sessions,' she reports. Pharmacist Shabir Daya, who specialises in natural remedies, recommends this regime: twice daily, apply Manuka Paint, which contains a powerful antifungal and antiviral herb called horopito plus antibacterial manuka (tea tree). Cover with a plaster. Also take L-Lysine 1000 mg, one tablet twice daily on an empty stomach, to help prevent the virus multiplying, plus the herb astragalus (an effective immune enhancer).

Thick toenails. This is a perennial problem for Sarah, again due to horses stamping affectionately on her toes! Medically called 'onychogryphosis', it's also known as Ram's Horn Nail. It's safe to file thick toenails down with a sturdy emery board or foot file, advises Margaret, adding that podiatrists can reduce them speedily with a diamond file. But the damage to the nail bed is likely to be long-term, so don't expect nails to grow back quite normally.

Morton's neuroma. Women over forty sometimes get a shooting pain in one foot

when they get up in the morning. This may be down to a condition called Morton's neuroma, where a nerve is compressed, usually in the space between the third and fourth toes. Acupuncture can help, but in some cases surgery may be necessary.

Plantar fasciitis (PF). Inflammation of the plantar fascia, a band of tissue that stretches from your heel to your middle foot bones, causing intense pain. One thing we know: FitFlop sandals help this foot condition (and many others). Among fans is Olympic long-jumper Jade Johnson who had PF; she was given foot exercises to do in sand by her physiotherapist but found she got 'the same effect from wearing FitFlops for 20 minutes daily. They were really helpful in getting my feet working and pain-free quickly.'

Bunions. These inflamed and painful bumps on the side of your big toe joint afflict about one woman in three in the West. The moment you notice a problem, consult a qualified podiatrist specialising in biomechanics and human movement. The underlying cause is usually the foot shape you inherit, but looking after your feet – and in particular wearing roomy, softer, foot-shaped shoes (eg, trainers) – may help. Wearing toe separators round the house may also be helpful (check out Beech Sandals, which are a specific type of footwear that separates the toes). Avoid high heels and pointed toes except briefly

for glam occasions, and don't wear flip-flops continuously. If you need surgery, make sure the surgeon is really experienced: we've heard horror stories of general orthopaedic surgeons (who do just a few bunions a year at most) taking out too much bone. Sometimes, says Margaret, the problem is actually arthritis on the joint: this can be cleaned out via keyhole surgery, but may need repeating.

THE BEST EXCUSE WE KNOW TO BUY NEW SHOES

It's not just the pointy-toed and heeled Jimmy Choos that may be putting pressure on your feet. (Actually, we're rather keen on wearing flimsy, pretty shoes because it means you have to keep your feet looking good.) Supportive footwear – from Birkenstocks to trainers, via FitFlops and MBTs – may all cause problems if you don't replace them annually. 'They definitely benefit your feet, building to an optimum in about six weeks,' says Margaret Dabbs. 'Then you need to wear them to maintain the improvements. But be aware that the footwear itself will wear down over time – so you'll begin to notice hard skin building up. The bottom line is: don't over-wear supportive footwear – and buy a fresh pair regularly.' Experts also recommend not wearing the same shoes two days running – both for your feet's sake and because leather needs a rest.

TIP

'Always cut toenails straight across: don't curve and dig down into the outer corners,' advises Margaret. A poor pedicure resulted in a sore toe for Sarah when the therapist dug down one side of the nail, causing a small but very painful build-up of hard skin. It was only diagnosed when she had a pedicure at the fantastic Beverly Hills salon of the 'Hollywood queen of nails', Jessica Vartoughian. We think it pays to invest in your feet: good shoes, good pedicurists and podiatrists, top-notch salons.

Foot treats: our award winners

First you buff (see opposite for foot files), then you slather. That's our mantra for soft, supportive, supple feet. After a certain age, feet cry out for richer emollients to deal with cracked heels and hard skin, which can ultimately have a wider impact on health, affecting how we walk. At the same time, we want products to put the spring back into our step – that's where reviving botanicals (think camphor, rosemary, mint) can work mini-miracles. So, good news: the foot treats listed here had our valiant testers skipping with delight

AT A GLANCE

Aveda Foot Relief

Botanicals Natural Foot Scrub

Barefoot Botanicals Refreshing Foot Balm

Eucerin Dry Skin Intensive Foot Cream

REVIEWS

Aveda Foot Relief

8.72/10 Already a seriously high-scorer in our books, we dispatched this to a fresh panel of ten mature, foot-weary testers who awarded it similarly stellar marks. The lavender and rosemary oils deliver instant welcome refreshment, there's a moisture surge from castor and jojoba oils, and all the while, salicylic acid (from willow bark) and lactic acid help gently soften calluses and rough patches. We're elevating this to the Beauty Bible Hall of Fame.

Comments: '10/10! I've used this product on my very dry feet twice daily; it's creamy and I love the fragrance; worked exceptionally well, feet feel refreshed, cool and silky soft; the most amazing cream I have ever used' • 'I get a lot of hard skin on my feet, leaves them soft and smooth, as well as cooling and refreshing; it's expensive but you only need a little dab: I'm a reflexologist so I know about feet!' • 'a really refreshing effect – lovely cooling sensation that lasted a long time – and liked the faint menthol fragrance; left skin soft and moisturised' • 'really loved this rich cream which left my feet and legs comfy all day; will certainly buy'.

Botanicals Natural Foot Scrub

7.95/10 The 'sister' product to Jo's fave foot balm (see We Love...), from a small British apothecary brand: Dead Sea salts and Himalayan mineral crystals are blended into a solid base of organic shea butter, sunflower and castor oil, with a lively lemongrass and mandarin scent, plus a drop of antiseptic tea tree oil. When sluiced away, it leaves skin softly moisturised – so no need for additional foot cream.

Comments: 'Loved this product and the lemongrass smell and smooth scrub texture, refreshed wonderfully and reduced soreness; a week in and feet were noticeably smoother' • 'feet felt wonderfully revived after a long day walking and standing; longer term it helps my hard(ish) skin' • 'smelt like Lemsip, worked well and skin feels revived and soft' • 'easy to apply, if a little messy, you can feel the cleansing salt crystals; very refreshing, reduced swelling and tenderness, left feet soft, clean and incredibly pampered – a real treat for the feet: love it!'.

Barefoot Botanicals Refreshing Foot Balm

7.86/10 One of the downsides of older feet can be dry, cracking heels – which this sense-waking foot balm sets out to soothe with generous amounts of shea butter and jojoba. It's also infused with reviving grapefruit, lime, Himalayan cedarwood and peppermint essential oils to truly put the spring back in your step.

Comments: 'A real pamper treat: perfect for anyone who stands all day, legs felt less tired and tender, refreshed and revitalised – the smell reminded my kids of Polos!' • 'feet felt really soft and pampered; it also helped my

ANTI-AGEING AWARD WINNERS BEAUTY BIBLE

very dry hands' • 'I use it every evening after bathing on the very dry cracked skin on feet, especially heels, and it does a really good job, feet feel wonderful, refreshed, soft and no redness; especially good for cracked skin – also helped my mother's psoriasis on her feet immediately and she didn't need to use her prescription cream'.

Eucerin Dry Skin Intensive Foot Cream

 7.74/10 Intensively moisturising ingredients – including glycerine and skin-compatible lipids – have been specially combined with 10 per cent urea (legendary for its moisturisation power) and gentle skin-softening lactic acid to combat rough, scaly skin and calluses. It's fragrance-free, so doesn't have the aromatic 'zing' of the other award-winning foot treats showcased here, but is definitely worth seeking out by anyone with dry, hard skin on feet and heels.

Comments: 'Really liked this, does exactly what it says it will, instructions are clear and concise, brilliant value; extremely effective moisturiser with instant effect, easier to rub in and better absorbed than my usual high-street brand' • 'excellent on dry skin: quite rich but not too greasy, very pleasant to use; extremely good at moisturising hard skin – heels felt almost soft for once!' • 'calming and soothing, left feet soft and cared for' • 'over time made a vast improvement to the rough, dry skin on my feet, much smoother and small cracks on the soles have disappeared; I would buy again'.

♡ WE LOVE...

For Jo, it's a new-ish discovery made while we were judging the UK Soil Association's Health & Beauty Awards in 2010: Botanicals Natural Foot Balm, lush with shea butter and with foot-reawakening (and antibacterial) oils of peppermint, spearmint and tea tree. She is also a convert to just about all of the many, many products in a targeted range called All About Feet from a (slightly-strangely-named) company called Upper Canada Soap. The whole ritual takes some time, but is very foot-perkifying. Sarah revives her feet with a scrub such as Yes to Carrots Feel the C Pampering Hand & Nail Spa, then massages in (really important to do this thoroughly) a butter or balm; currently its Neal's Yard Remedies Rose Body Cream – which leaves them baby-soft and delightful.

Foot files: *our award winners*

Hard skin is Public Enemy Number One when it comes to happy feet. Rather than an occasional blitz, we prescribe a nightly buffing session when that day's skin build-up can be lightly scuffed away. (For serious hard-skin removal after a long period of neglect, there's nothing to beat a professional pedicure, or a visit to the chiropodist – or a medi-pedicurist, those brilliant hybrids of the two which are popping up here and there.) The key with a foot file is to find one that is hand-friendly, so it's comfortable to hold and allows for the perfect 'angle' when you access your soles and heels. These high-scoring award winners were several steps ahead of the competition. NB: if you have diabetes it's always best to consult your health professional before using anything like this.

Tweezerman Pedro Callus Stone

 8.87/10 Tweezerman recommend using this wet for best results; first the rough side (for removing calluses), then the fine side (for smoothing).

Comments: '10/10 for this double-sided rough pad, which whisked away rough skin so it was soft and smooth with no irritating bits left!' • 'resounding yes to this: the smoother side was also excellent for rough elbows'.

Marks & Spencer Miracle Foot File

 8.87/10 This tied for first place with Tweezerman's. It also has two sides: the top for hard skin zones, the underneath for general sloughing.

Comments: 'Exceptionally well designed, left skin lovely and smooth' • 'easy and comfy to use and removes all dead dry skin quickly'.

Space NK Foot File

 8.5/10 The contender from renowned beautique Space NK is very lightweight – but ready for heavy-duty action. It's fashioned from stainless steel with a white plastic and an abrasive metal 'paddle' at one end. Compared to the other two featured here it's quite dinky – which we find makes it nicely manoeuvrable, for accessing the whole foot.

Comments: 'This is FANTASTIC!!!! I suffer hard, dry skin and this worked so effectively. I now have great feet and the most wonderful heels!' • 'handle and head perfect size and shape; one of the easiest files I've ever used'.

♡ WE LOVE...

In our opinion, Alida's Foot File can't be beaten, for three reasons. First, because it was designed for elderly and disabled people, it's incredibly ergonomic – so fits in the hand beautifully making it easy-peasy to access the soles. The two sides – coarse and fine – really do subtly shave away even the toughest hard skin. And last, the holes make for easy cleaning (we think that's rather important for anything to do with feet…). It is, in fact, almost identical to the Marks & Spencer Miracle Foot File, but we prefer the feel of Alida's own handle: a soft, cushiony rubber.

Maybe, just maybe, switch your fragrance

Most of us by now have acquired a 'perfume wardrobe' (as a couple of scent-o-philes, ours are more walk-in closets, actually). Or maybe you're one of those women who've worn a 'signature scent' all these years. Well: don't be surprised if gradually your favourite fragrance smells different on your skin. Or, which is also very common, fades faster...

You are not hallucinating. There's a reason. As Roja Dove (the oft-quoted *professeur de parfums*, who is an old and valued friend of ours) points out, 'Skin tends to become drier from perimenopause onwards and that affects fragrance – because it interacts with the oils in your skin. Less oil means there's nothing for the fragrance to "grip" on to.'

As a result, evaporation is speeded up, which also fast-forwards the process of the fragrance's development. So the base notes swoop in much sooner, and you'll get a more fleeting encounter with the top and heart notes.

But you should also be aware that there's another reason why fragrance may not smell on you as it once did: the formulation may have changed. New laws and guidelines governing fragrance ingredients have led to many ingredients being withdrawn – either for reasons of potential irritancy or for environmental conservation reasons – which has forced fragrance brands to tweak some legendary confections.

We do suggest trying Roja's tips, right. Then you may well find that your favourite fragrances smell 'right' on you again. Or if not, then he's come up with a shortlist of scents (which we echo) to explore now you are *d'un certain âge*. (You can feel a little bit smug that on younger women, most of them smell way too grown-up and elegant – a bit like a little girl trying on mummy's shoes.)

ROJA DOVE'S TIPS FOR HELPING FRAGRANCE

Use a pH-neutral body wash. This won't strip away your skin's natural oils, which are already in shorter supply than they were. (Many body washes trumpet their pH-neutrality on the label, but as a short cut, you'll find them in ranges including Dr Hauschka and Garnier.)

Apply moisturiser before you apply your scent. This gives the scent something to 'cling' to. On your body, use either a totally unscented lotion (or oil), or the 'matching' body lotion to your usual fragrance. (Most neck creams aren't so scented that they'll interfere with your fragrance choice, but they will help by counterbalancing dryness.) 'Layering' the body lotion or oil that matches your scent, in our experience, actually 'time-releases' the scent during the day as you warm up (which you may well do quite a lot!) and cool down.

Try something new. If the advice above doesn't help with your current scent, look for something different – it could be a wonderful discovery! Don't rely on scent-strips in stores (except for eliminating things you really aren't ever going to like); it's crucial to know how something's going to smell on your skin. Apply to your well-moisturised pulse-points, allow a few hours to develop – and don't be rushed. Which means that duty free is not the place to find your new 'signature scent'; go to a department store, an independent perfumery or a specialist fragrance store – there are more and more of these, showcasing fabulous 'niche' brands in which there are some truly sublime creations.

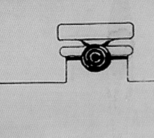

N°5

CHANEL

PARIS

10 *FABULOUS* FRAGRANCES FOR *FABULOUS* OLDER WOMEN

This list – compiled by Roja Dove – features some of the most divine fragrances, which, if you don't already know them, are worthy of at least a brief encounter, but we suspect might have you falling in love…

GUERLAIN *Shalimar*

GUERLAIN *Mitsouko*

JEAN-CHARLES BROSSEAU *Ombre Rose*

LANVIN *Arpège*

CHANEL *No. 5*

HOUBIGANT *Quelques Fleurs*

YSL *Rive Gauche*

ESTÉE LAUDER *Private Collection*

CHRISTIAN DIOR *Diorella*

NINA RICCI *L'Air du Temps*

SEM

'ATTITUDE
is *everything*'

Diane Von Furstenberg

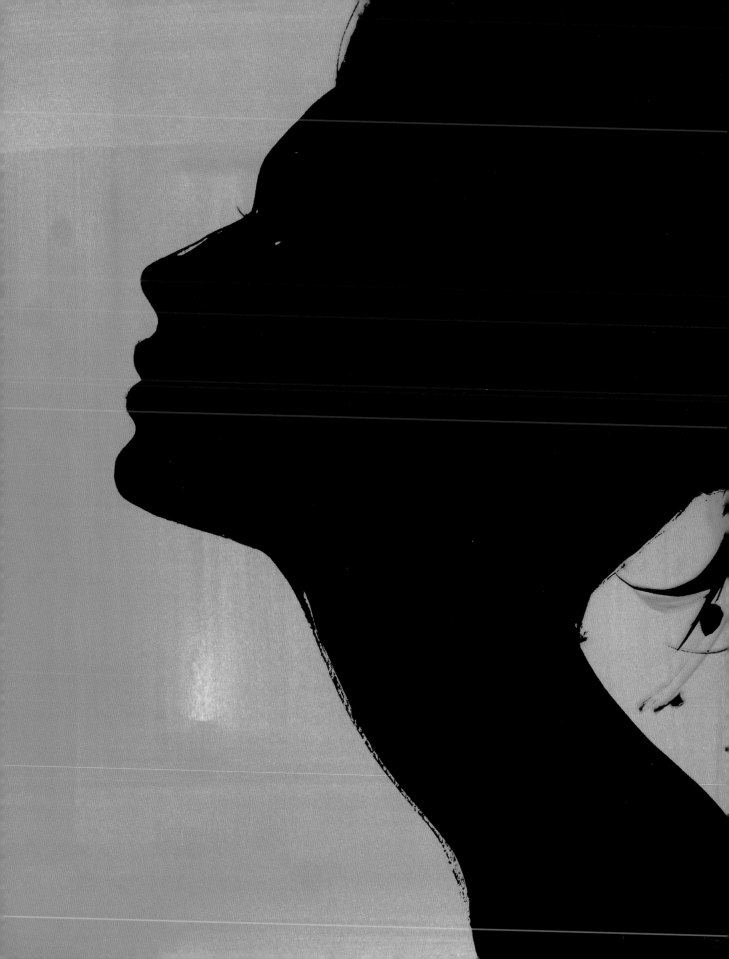

Get a great hairstyle

(And if you like, tear up the rule book into a million pieces)

We may be bossy about how to clean your face or apply foundation so that it takes years off you, but we don't feel that anyone should be prescriptive about what hairstyle suits who at what age. That's because – as legendary Manhattan stylist John Barrett says – today, almost anything goes for older women. Pixie short-cuts. A bob. A funky-chunky textured cut. Long hair. Think: is Julianne Moore cutting her hair short and getting a perm? Is Daryl Hannah or Joanna Lumley? No way. And nor do you have to. But there is *one* absolute rule: you've got to keep it in fantastic nick.

What we've done is to create a montage of some fabulous-looking hairstyles. Use it as your inspiration if you don't feel your current style is working for you and you need ideas. You might also want to keep your own cuttings folder of women whose hair you think looks fabulous. Tearsheets aren't just for teens: they're a great communication tool at any age. Don't be shy to take this into your present stylist – or to a new one: please don't be afraid to divorce your current hair beau if they can't give you a good hair year – and workshop the ideas with them. (Actually, at this age, you really don't need to be shy about anything, any more…)

Personally, we recommend opting for the very best cut you can afford (also colour, see overleaf). We prioritise hair over clothes, because unlike even the most favourite jacket or pair of shoes, your hair is something you wear every single day of your life. Going around with good hair makes you feel amazing, whatever else is iffy. And it can make such an impression on other people.

If you've had the same hairstyle for years, think about this: is this your 'signature' style? In which case that's absolutely fine. We know plenty of women who've had the same style for-flipping-ever, and we can't imagine them any other way – think Goldie Hawn, for instance. With those visual markers in place, your actual age can be almost unnoticed. What may need to change, however, is your colour.

If you spot someone with a great haircut, ask them who looks after their hair. We do it. Our friend Lulu does it. Honestly, that person will just be flattered.

Don't decide on a new cut while you're wearing a salon robe. The style should suit the type of clothes you wear, and your stylist should

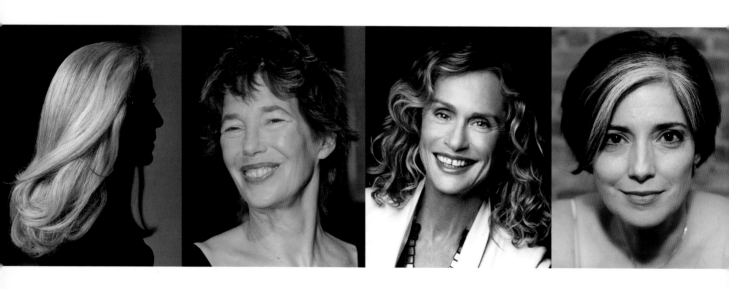

always, always see you in your 'everyday' clothes before cutting your hair for the first time. They should also take into account the texture of your hair, which is the ultimate deciding factor for any style. Never trust a stylist who decides on how to cut your hair having only ever seen you after a shampoo; Jo once walked out of a New York salon – with dripping hair – when this happened to her.

Which means: ideally, schedule a consultation before you get your hair cut. Use this face-to-face (which you should never be charged for) to give your stylist a potted history of styles you've loved – and hated – so they can get an idea of your favourite looks. Let them run their fingers through your hair, and feel its weight and texture.

Be truthful with your hairdresser about the amount of time you have for upkeep. Can you wash and blow-dry it every day? If you opt for a short, precise cut, have you got time and funds to have it trimmed every three to four weeks? If you want to dedicate your life to your hair, that's your call, but if you want low-maintenance hair so that you can get on with everything else you want/have to do, you're going to need a style that can be tousled dry with some styling product, or tied back, or pinned up simply. Honesty pays. What do we do? Jo takes her shortish layered style to the hairdresser once a week, and has a blow-dry, then goes again a week later. Sarah mostly does her own (she does live in the wilds) with an occasional 'treat' when she's going out. She actually finds long hair's easier (except for the time

it takes to condition and dry) because she can tie it back for riding, etc – and it only needs trimming every six weeks.

Avoid razor cuts like the plague. Sarah spent months in recovery after an attack! Always, always talk through with your hairdresser how they're going to 'texturise' the ends, if that's part of the look you're going for, or thin out very thick hair. Razors can roughen the cuticle and the tips; the hair appears more dull because you've disturbed the reflective surface, and it can go as flat as a crêpe Suzette. That's our experience (and that of others) – and if anyone comes within 20 paces brandishing a razor in the direction of our hair, we're outta there.

If you have very curly hair, go very short – or go very long. Anything in-between is unbelievably high-maintenance and can have a massive 'broom' effect. (Or you could consider a Brazilian keratin hair-straightening treatment, though be aware that in tandem with banishing the frizz, it can flatten your previously fulsome hair. The results can be temporary – but one friend nearly had a nervous breakdown; nothing gave her back the volume she'd taken for granted, not rollers, not thickening lotion, not backcombing – nuffin!)

And for more on which cut suits which face shape... Visit www.beautybible.com/faceshapes. We have archived on our website some drawings from our previous book, *Feel Fab Forever*, which offer guidance about cuts and styles that suit particular face shapes. You might find it useful.

TIPS

'Use a little light-textured hand cream to add a non-greasy texture to short hair. It works brilliantly.' – Trevor Sorbie

'Use a shower cap as a portable hood dryer for quick styling. Put Velcro rollers in, put the shower cap on, and tuck the nozzle of the dryer in the corner of the cap. This creates an even heat over the hair for much faster setting.' – Charles Worthington

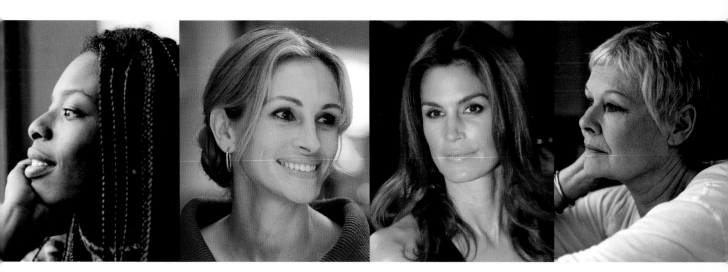

Learn to speak the language of hair colour

If it sometimes seems as if your colourist is speaking another language – well, he (or she) is. So here are all the key terms translated into real-life words – which should help you achieve the look you want, whether you're having your hair coloured in a salon or doing it yourself

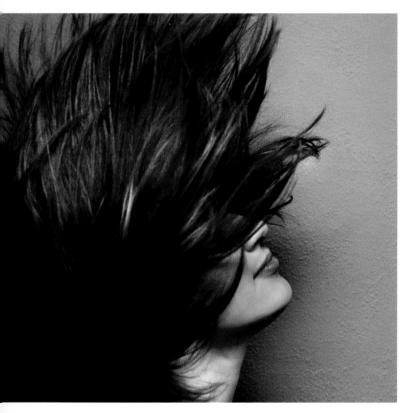

TIP

After colouring, never shampoo before 24 hours. This will help the colour to 'set', so it takes perfectly.

We truly, truly recommend, though – if at all possible – that as you start to develop grey, you have your hair coloured professionally at least once, and then at least occasionally. We know that hair colouring can be pricey and can carve huge chunks out of your diary to maintain. A sympathetic colourist, however, will be able to advise you on the best shade for your skintone. If they're really generous-spirited, they may be able to point you in the direction of a particular shade in a drugstore/chemist brand that might work for you, or at least tell you where on the Hair Colour Level Charts you are (see right), and what level of shade would work best with your (undyed) colour.

HAIR COLOUR GLOSSARY

Baliage (aka balayage) The technique of painting highlights directly on to the hair without using foils (see Highlights, right); this can enable a colourist to get closer to the parting/ roots with the bleach. Can give a 'beachy' look and lessens the occurrence of unwanted regrowth lines sometimes associated with foil highlights or those pulled through a cap – but best left to true hair colour artists.

Demi-permanent colour Lasts up to 28 shampoos. Contains lower levels of peroxide (which means it's less harsh and drying) than permanent colour. It's great for creating natural-looking tone changes (such as taking brown hair to a rich auburn shade) and will cover grey. Gradually fades back to the underlying shade.

Double process A technical term for having single process colour (all-over colouring of the hair, see single process, below), at the same hair colouring session as having your highlights done.

Glaze (aka Gloss) A pigment-laden or clear liquid used to enhance a hair colour temporarily.

Highlights Streaks or chunks of lighter colour (created through the use of ammonia/hydrogen peroxide), applied through the hair – usually using foils or pulled through a cap.

Permanent colour This doesn't wash out, and requires the roots touching up every four to six weeks. It contains both ammonia and peroxide, so it can lighten, darken and/or completely change your hair colour; it can also cover grey.

Peroxide Otherwise known as hydrogen peroxide, extensively used in hair colouring as a 'developer' or 'activator'. Its role is to open up the cuticle and allow bleach or colour into the cortex of the hair.

Rinse See temporary colour, below.

Semi-permanent colour Washes out after six to 12 shampoos. This enhances natural hair colour but won't lighten it and won't cover grey, although it can soften its appearance. (NB: the reason hair colouring companies cite the number of washes rather than a time-frame is that some of us wash our hair every day, others as occasionally as once a week.)

Semi-temporary Not to be confused with semi-permanent: this colour lasts from four to six washes, contains no ammonia and isn't mixed with a 'developer' such as hydrogen peroxide.

Single process All-over colouring of the hair, from the roots at the scalp right through to the ends, in one step.

Temporary colour Simply coats the hair shaft and rinses out after one shampoo. These cannot lighten hair, but only temporarily brighten or darken.

Tint May sound subtle, but this is an alternative phrase used by hairdressers to describe permanent colour.

Tone-on-tone colour Another phrase for demi-permanent, see left.

HAIR COLOUR LEVEL CHARTS

Now you've mastered this, get your head around Hair colour Level Charts. This is why so many women head for the salon to have colour done (and that includes us). There is an absolutely fiendish system for numbering hair colour: there are 12 levels, with one representing black and

Home hair colouring can be incredibly messy. We are very, very impressed by some new innovations – including Precision Foam Colour from the John Frieda brand – which are 'mousse-like' once they have been mixed, rather than liquid. This means they are drip-free, don't wreck all your towels and there is no need to cover every surface in the bathroom before applying – because unlike most, they don't splatter all over the place. A truly welcome haircare revolution.

12 representing ultra-light blonde. As a general rule, the first number on the label of a box of hair colour will tell you the colour level of that product. However, your own base colour – and where it falls in that spectrum from one to 12 – will affect the final shade on you personally. This is why colourists advise that you don't stray more than one or two shades lighter or darker than your current natural hair colour, for optimum results.

But remember: no matter what the language of hair colour, one picture speaks a thousand words. It's all very well being able to speaka da lingo when it comes to knowing your semi-permanents from your demi-permanents – but in our experience, the biggest challenge can be successfully communicating actual shades and colours to a salon colourist. So: you say 'brown'. Your colourist could be thinking: anything from milk chocolate to dark chocolate. At the same time, what's 'red' to you might be pillarbox to a colouring professional. (Yikes.) This, we think, is where photographs truly come into their own: brandishing a cutting torn from a glossy of the colour that you are hoping for, in front of your hairdresser, can save an awful lot of confusion. (And, potentially, tears.) We recommend keeping tearsheets of anyone whose hair colour you'd love to emulate. You can then talk through what's actually achievable and – crucially – what the upkeep would be.

HAIR COLOUR LORE

The golden rule of hair colour is this: don't stray more than one or two shades from your natural colour. It won't suit your skintone, and will be a nightmare of upkeep. Now read on! When it comes to covering a whole head of grey, don't go darker. Not only does it showcase greys and regrowth, but it can look opaque, like you painted your head with shoe polish. Generally, you should request a single process (see our GLOSSARY) and highlights that bring your natural hair colour one shade lighter, because it will add dimension and disguise the greys, and flatter your complexion. If you're thinking of going blonder, a shade or two lighter can be very flattering – especially because skin gets sallower with age, and a few fine streaks can wake it up. But going too light can be just as ageing as going too dark. Here's a quick way to tell, from Manhattan colour maestro Louis Licari: 'If you have to put on more make-up to make your new colour work, you've picked the wrong shade. The one colour you should absolutely avoid when you're over 40 is raven black. It will sap life and colour from your face.'

Coloured haircare: our award winners

Statistically, most women colour their hair from mid-life onwards (and many of us, of course, start much earlier). But we know that many of you don't take advantage of the growing number of products specifically created to put back some of the shine and life that colouring can take out, as well as preventing colour fade

It's a fast-growing section of the haircare market, and our testers trialled shampoos and conditioners for all shades of coloured hair – and also for blonde, brunette and auburn-tinted mops. (While blondes can enjoy the top-scoring product, the brunettes only liked a conditioner, and redheads nothing – so do consider the general coloured hair options.)

SHAMPOO REVIEWS

Aveda Camomile Shampoo

8.78/10 Aveda's high-scoring colour care products feature deeply conditioning babassu oil, which not only leaves hair silky but helps to revive colour. The formulas are infused with plant-derived ingredients to refresh colour naturally – in this instance, chamomile and calendula, enriched with beta-carotene to enhance golden tones. It was trialled by blonde testers, who loved both this and the 'matching' conditioner (opposite).
Comments: 'Great product, left hair feeling light and clean, helped brighten and freshen up my blonde highlights' • 'good gloss on my ashy-blonde hair, and made it more manageable and a bit more golden' • 'made my dry blonde hair blonder, softer and more shiny: I would buy' • 'fantastic results: I give it ten!' • 'great shine – best for golden blondes rather than grey blonde'.

Green People Intensive Repair Shampoo (Coloured/Treated Hair)

8.36/10 Based on organic aloe vera, jojoba oil and pineapple extract (to ease scalp irritation), this organically-certified shampoo for all coloured hair also features panthenol and beer yeast, known for their strengthening action, along with horsetail and green tea. Rose geranium, orange, lavender and sandalwood essential oils not only boost shine, but (we think) smell divine.
Comments: 'Gave a natural, healthy gloss and bounce, hair hangs better and seems to be more moisturised; usually slightly parched and frizzy but this has persuaded me to buy a natural shampoo for the first time' • 'very easy to work through hair, lathered well, easy to rinse and didn't sting eyes; hair looked glossy, colour brightened definitely, also much softer and easier to style: looked younger!'.

Pureology Hydrate Shampoo

8.19/10 Pureology – a new-ish botanically-rich vegan colour-care range under the L'Oréal umbrella – has done well in our anti-ageing hair categories, here with a highly concentrated shampoo (each bottle is said to last 80 washes), which is zero-sulfate and delivers their 'anti-fade' complex, to optimise colour protection for any shade of coloured hair.
Comments: 'Prolongs the brightness of my colour, delivered a beautiful gloss and shine, improved manageability and the overall look of hair, so yes, it's anti-ageing!' • 'no problems with scalp irritation which is important because I occasionally get psoriasis on my scalp; helped to keep colour "truer" for longer and hair is in much better condition' • 'very impressed, this nourished my hair so colour became brighter and lasted longer'.

Jo Hansford Colour Care Everyday Shampoo

7.88/10 Another suitable-for-all-shades option from a colourist who's a London legend, with an A-list (and royal) clientele. Sunflower

extract, keratin amino acids, vitamins A and E and UV filters (to protect against environmental damage) feature in a formula gentle enough to use every day.
Comments: 'Gave hair a nice healthy sheen and it's much easier to style, feels light, soft and clean; made hair very shiny, silky and easy to manage: hairdresser said it wasn't as dry as on my last visit' • 'lovely simple packaging, nice citrus fragrance, lathered really well and didn't irritate' • 'gave a nice shiny result to my coloured, dryish hair' • 'made my coarse coloured hair very smooth and soft'.

CONDITIONER REVIEWS

Aveda Camomile Conditioner

8.78/10
The 'matching' conditioner to the winning shampoo (for blondes and lighter shades of hair). By popular demand, Aveda's colour-care range also comes in one litre bottles.
Comments: 'Works best if used as instructed! Leaving in for five minutes or longer gave great shine to my grey-blonde hair' • 'excellent for brightening and freshening blonde highlights/colour but probably not rich enough for people with very dry ends' • 'gave good gloss and manageability to my ashy-blonde hair' • 'easier to get a brush through, and made my dry hair softer, more shiny, easier to straighten' • 'pleased that my hair colour was more even and the grey-blonde is brighter'.

Jo Hansford Colour Care Everyday Conditioner

8.37/10
This is the conditioner to complement the Jo Hansford shampoo, and the pair was trialled by our testers in tandem. Two testers gave it 10/10.
Comments: 'Loved using this conditioner, divine smell, hair is very shiny, with highlights standing out more, and healthy-looking, and behaves better than usual, excellent results: definite 10/10' • 'left hair soft and well-conditioned, easy to style, no frizzy flyaways or weighty build-up after washing daily' • 'I've ordered more supplies of this and the matching shampoo, and masque for fine hair – I love it! My hair has been a nightmare for so long it's worth being in your trial just to discover this'.

Green People Intensive Repair Conditioner (Coloured/Treated Hair)

8.33/10
The 'complementary' conditioner for Green People's winning shampoo, which notched up an almost identical mark from our team.

Comments: 'Gave high-gloss shine and bounce; revived colour so hair didn't look dull, seemed to hang better and didn't seem so "parched", made a real difference to the moisturisation' • 'like the fact that it's an all-natural product' • 'very nice fresh, green smell, easy to work through hair, which was much softer, smoother and glossier, shine made colour look brighter, style was easier to manage' • 'makes colour look more vibrant' • 'brightens up hair and prolongs the colour; I have already bought more shampoo and conditioner'.

Pureology Pure Hydrate Conditioner

8.19/10
For more about the range, see the shampoo write-up; meanwhile, here's the feedback from testers.
Comments: 'Hair looked really shiny and healthy after first use, definitely brightened hair, easy to comb through and didn't dry frizzy before blow-drying; hair felt great, not heavy, and in far better condition despite using straighteners, etc' • 'I used these products just after having my hair coloured and I do think they have improved the colour for longer, very impressed by gloss, shine, manageability – and hair seemed to stay cleaner for longer too' • 'seriously noticeable defrizz effect, I have dreadfully frizzy hair and while using this I could omit my usual leave-in conditioner – which is a real result! Plus it's over three months since I had my highlights done and they should look like they're screaming for help but the colour still looks good!'.

Lee Stafford Blinding Brunette Conditioner

7.62/10
We separately trialled the companion shampoo which, on its own, didn't impress testers greatly. However, it seems that combining the two could be a great marriage! So, if your tresses are brown, this duo – which feature a 'Pro-Brunette System Pigment' (oh, how we love beautyspeak) – might be your best bet to add warmth and depth to colour. (Some testers liked the effect, others felt it was OTT.)
Comments: 'Not really glossy but did seem to enhance and deepen the colour' • 'friend said my thick, extremely coarse hair looked shinier than usual and was much softer, which my husband agreed with; think it did slow down the fading process a bit' • 'high gloss and much more manageable, but slightly weighed down my fine, flat hair' • 'delivered a super gloss and shine, hair felt softer and was easier to style, brought out highlights and I would definitely buy it'.

Moisturising haircare: our award winners

We get so many emails from readers concerned about dull, dry hair. The dryness can be linked with hair colouring, or simply be a manifestation of the fact that as we get older, everything seems to desiccate a bit. A mini-revolution in the haircare market has seen a raft of haircare products calling themselves 'moisturising' – so we wanted to know: how hair-quenching are they, really…?

Here's the low-down, on both shampoos and conditioners. (NB: normally we're cynical about the need to use 'matching' products, but it does seem to have paid dividends for our testers, as with coloured haircare.)

SHAMPOO REVIEWS

Sebastian Professional Strengthening and Repair Shampoo

 8.39/10 Sexy, sleek packaging – but that's not what swayed our testers, who highly rated this shampoo, designed to repair, strengthen and protect hair. It's also 'colour safe', Sebastian tells us, so could have been trialled in that category – but was primarily judged by our ten-strong panel for its moisturising qualities.

Comments: 'Hair looks better than it has in years; I thought I would always have greasy hair and scalp but not any more' • 'very easy to apply, delicate fragrance and user-friendly packaging, lathered well, and got hair clean with one shampoo; left hair really shiny and manageable, tangle-free and easier to style; I could leave it for a day or two longer than usual' • 'left hair clean but not stripped of natural oils' • 'fab rich product which made hair a bit shinier, lighter and softer than usual'.

Matrix Biolage Réjuvathérapie Age Rejuvenating Shampoo

 8.22/10 Promising 'optimal suppleness, resilience and renewed radiance, all without weighing hair down', key ingredients in this specifically anti-ageing range (also recommended for long hair) include antioxidant lycopene, elasticity-boosting rice protein and 'weightless' omega-3 fatty acids from camelina flower seed.

Comments: 'Rich product that gave glossy, easy-to-manage, healthy-looking hair' • 'I would seriously recommend this product; it kept my coloured hair from going too dry and didn't leave any residue; could leave it for two days instead of washing daily' • 'made hair look glossy and hydrated without being heavy, so I guess this counts as anti-ageing' • 'made my slightly coarse hair feel very sleek and soft and easier to style'.

Alterna Caviar Anti-Aging Seasilk Moisture Shampoo

 8.16/10 Caviar by name and somewhat caviar-ish by price, a specific range created to counteract the ageing, damaging effects of blow-drying, heat-styling and environmental stress. It's rich in marine botanicals, omega-3 fatty acids, proteins, vitamins and minerals and a 'Color Hold' technology, designed to soothe the scalp. Fine-haired testers didn't feel it gave much body.

Comments: 'Great! Worked perfectly, gave a lovely shiny gloss, long hair was so soft after, very easy to comb through, felt wonderful: definitely felt and looked younger' • 'made hair look very healthy and nourished, gave shine, body and bounce, might not always need a conditioner with it, and didn't need any extra styling products' • 'pricey but the benefits to my increasingly dry, brittle, lacklustre hair (previously my crowning glory) make it worth the investment; even my hairdresser has complimented me on its condition, with softness, bounce, vibrant colour – and top marks for gloss'.

Head & Shoulders Hydrating Smooth & Silky Shampoo

 7.8/10 Well, knock us down with a blow-dryer. We never expected a dandruff shampoo to do so well in an anti-ageing category, but this option from the legendary dry-scalp-treatment range proved a moisturising pick-me-up for hair, with its specifically replenishing, softening twist on the globally best-selling formulation.

Comments: 'Great lather, very little needed, rinsed out easily and didn't sting; gave a good glossy finish on my silver hair, as good as my expensive shampoo and I will buy' • 'I enjoyed using this and will buy again' • 'left scalp feeling comfortable and clean – this is completely different from the old Head & Shoulders of my youth!' • 'I have a big problem with sensitive scalp and this was great, as was the conditioner; great value'.

CONDITIONER REVIEWS

Matrix Biolage Réjuvathérapie Age Rejuvenating Conditioner

 8.72/10 In the conditioning category, the Matrix entry nudged slightly ahead of Sebastian. The key ingredients in the Réjuvathérapie shampoo and conditioner – used as a duo – are the same. Really high scores and delighted reviews.

Comments: 'Amazing to see such a visible difference in my coarse hair; it shines, is definitely smoother and keeps its shape well; a noticeable improvement in condition – a real stand-out product' • 'gave my hair a good shine, and it's healthy and moisturised-looking, improved my colour too' • 'really impressed with this conditioner which works well with the matching shampoo'.

Sebastian Professional Strengthening and Repair Conditioner

 8.14/10 The conditioner which 'matches' the top-scoring shampoo in this moisturising category (see that review for more info). Again this attracted several top marks and made for very happy, glossy testers.

Comments: 'Getting a glossy result outside the hairdressers is a challenge on my thick, coarse, coloured hair but this worked! Impressive manageability, this performed really well in all ways;

nice surprise!' • 'creamy and easy to apply, fresh fruit fragrance, this transformed my hair: my daughter couldn't stop touching it and saying how shiny it looks; also bouncy, full and manageable' • 'I needed a minimal amount to get my very fine hair glossy, shiny, frizz-free and manageable'.

Alterna Caviar Moisture Conditioner

 8.05/10 For more about the Caviar Moisture range, see our shampoo review – while for testers' comments on the conditioner, just read on. Lots more happy testers!

Comments: 'There is always one miracle product in the Beauty Bible testing packs and this was it! Quite expensive but I will definitely buy it as it transformed my hair. Amazing! Gave lovely shine, so soft it was a miracle' • 'gave me soft, shiny locks that smell divine; seems to protect from colour fade as well' • 'worth investing in as the ensuing boost to self-esteem is priceless!'.

Head & Shoulders Hydrating Smooth & Silky Conditioner

 7.8/10 As with the shampoo, this super-affordable conditioner wowed our testers.

Comments: 'I suffer from bad itching, and my very thick silver hair is big and frizzy after washing but not with this: it was rich and lovely to work through hair, felt more expensive – gave a nice glossy sheen. I shall continue to use this' • 'very easy to use, not too thick or runny; gave nice gloss for my very long, frizzy hair, even my mother-in-law commented on it' • 'I really liked this product and the matching shampoo and have bought more'.

Bumble and Bumble Mending Conditioner

 7.78/10 We've added one last conditioner to the list of award winners on the strength of its performance. For 'hair that's truly damaged', it targets weakened hair with a blend of cuticle-smoothing ingredients 'like Polyfilla on a damaged wall', as they put it. Panthenol-derived ingredients also help with the mending action, with silicones to smooth fly-aways.

Comments: 'Dream to apply, to say I love it is an understatement: it ticks every box for my "candyfloss" hair, easy to use, mild fresh scent and fantastic long-lasting results: I am a total convert' • 'glides on to hair, smoothed the knots as it went, hair looked very shiny and felt supersoft but with a bit of body, also calmed the frizzy ends' • 'I enjoyed using this, could I have a big bottle please?'.

Give yourself more hair

– by pumping up the volume. Hair 'oomph' is a real issue. In general, it becomes a little thinner as we age – and with less of it, volume's even more important if you don't want your locks to look skimpy…

Thinning hair is a very common beauty woe shared by women from forty-something-plus. We're not necessarily talking full-blown, hormone-related/stress-related hair loss: simply the fact that over time, there seems to be less to play with – and most of us could do with a little extra oomph in the hair department.

So we asked stylist Andreas Wild (from the John Frieda salon in Mayfair, London) – who looks after both our mops quite wonderfully! – for his advice on dealing with fine and/or thinning hair.

Have your blood checked to see if you're missing any nutrients. If thinning is associated with the menopause, it could be that you're missing some nutrients – in particular, iron. Women often lose hair around the hairline in pregnancy but it grows back – whereas menopause-related hair loss seldom does.

Work with what you've got. Talk to your stylist about the best cut for your face and shape – and the amount of hair you have. Take pictures with you of styles you like (as with any haircut, frankly), but in particular talk to your stylist about how practical that style might be for you, with your individual volume of hair (or lack of…).

● Shorter hair is almost always easier to manage – and looks younger and fresher; in addition, length weighs the hair down, so shorter may equal bouncier. Shorter-than-chin-length bobs or more gamine cuts may suit heart-shaped faces with a 'right-angled' jaw-line (think Judi Dench), but won't suit anyone with a longer face.

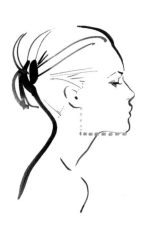

● Actually, there is a simple equation to see if short hair will work for you (see illustration, left). If the measurement from your ear lobe straight down to the level of your chin is more than 5.5cm/2in, you probably won't suit shorter hair. Truly!

● A chin-length bob often works well for women with finer hair (but do remember hair will 'lift' when it's dry, so it should be a good centimetre below your chin when wet).

● If you are tall, broad-shouldered and anything less than slender, bear in mind that you need enough hair on your head to balance your body shape.
(PS Look on our website – www.beautybible.com/hairstyles – to find drawings of which styles work best for which face shapes.)

Camouflage any hair loss at the hairline. The hairline is the first thing people notice about you, so if your hairline is receding, try a soft, graduated fringe – side-swept if you like. Damp hair down in the morning and pop a couple of big rollers in it to keep the oomph up (or use heated rollers).

Don't try to put too much volume in. On some heads, all that extra va-va-voom will just go flat after a couple of hours; better to choose a sleeker, lower-maintenance style requiring less wrist action.

Prep hair for styling with a volumising shampoo and conditioner. We trialled some of these (see overleaf), to help you identify those which work best. Then use a specific thickening lotion or volumising mousse.

Apply a regular strengthening treatment. Kérastase has a dedicated 'Extreme Strengthening' range which many stylists (including Andreas) recommend.

Never overuse heated hair appliances. Dryers, straighteners, curling tongs, etc will damage and weaken hair. When drying, towel hair to damp then lift the roots with a smallish brush or your fingers. Put medium-sized Velcro rollers on and around the top, let hair dry while you do your make-up. Remove rollers and finger-comb or brush smooth.

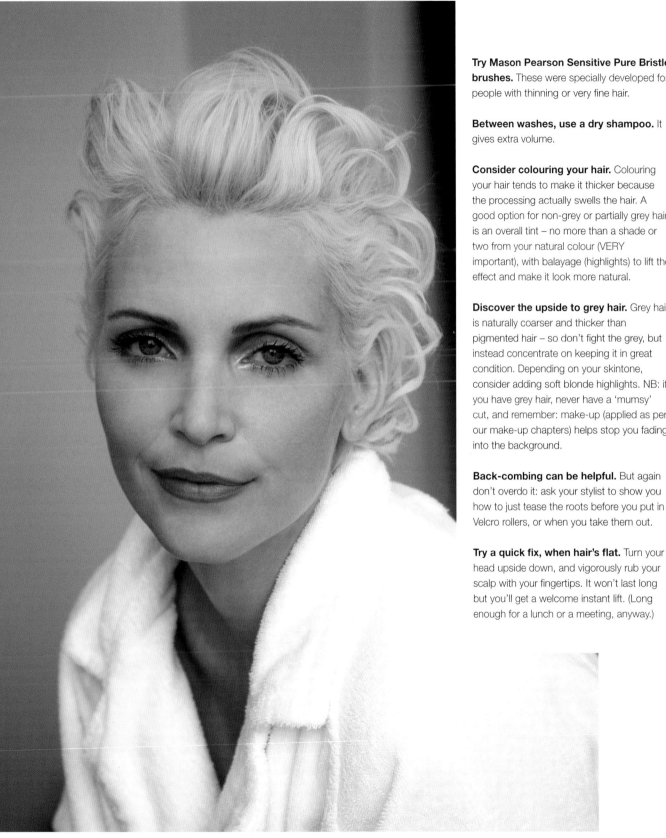

Try Mason Pearson Sensitive Pure Bristle brushes. These were specially developed for people with thinning or very fine hair.

Between washes, use a dry shampoo. It gives extra volume.

Consider colouring your hair. Colouring your hair tends to make it thicker because the processing actually swells the hair. A good option for non-grey or partially grey hair is an overall tint – no more than a shade or two from your natural colour (VERY important), with balayage (highlights) to lift the effect and make it look more natural.

Discover the upside to grey hair. Grey hair is naturally coarser and thicker than pigmented hair – so don't fight the grey, but instead concentrate on keeping it in great condition. Depending on your skintone, consider adding soft blonde highlights. NB: if you have grey hair, never have a 'mumsy' cut, and remember: make-up (applied as per our make-up chapters) helps stop you fading into the background.

Back-combing can be helpful. But again don't overdo it: ask your stylist to show you how to just tease the roots before you put in Velcro rollers, or when you take them out.

Try a quick fix, when hair's flat. Turn your head upside down, and vigorously rub your scalp with your fingertips. It won't last long but you'll get a welcome instant lift. (Long enough for a lunch or a meeting, anyway.)

Volumising haircare: our award winners

For hair that's starting to look thin, there are formulas to help create greater fullness...

Happily, the haircare industry recognises this and is lavishing hundreds of millions of research dollars (and euros) into creating products which give hair extra body, bounce and root-lift. Our more flat-haired testers trialled a couple of dozen shampoos and conditioners in this category, and got pretty pumped up about the following. The shampoos tended to score higher than the conditioners – which may reflect that conditioner can sometimes weigh hair down a tad...

SHAMPOO REVIEWS

Yes to Tomatoes Tempting Tomato Daily Volumizing Shampoo ❀❀

9.12/10 YTC (as we call them) have done very well in previous books (and our iPhone App!) – and here earned an incredibly impressive score for this whacking great bottle of daily shampoo, with 26 Dead Sea minerals to boost volume and combat wear and tear, plus antioxidant ginkgo and lycopene (from organic tomatoes).
Comments: 'This worked brilliantly and over the years I've tried just about everything on the market; very practical and easy to use; left hair shinier than it's ever been with significant increase in volume after a few uses, which lasts until next wash; very easy to style and manage – the best shampoo I have ever used' • 'does exactly what it says it will do' • 'liked the light fragrance, and made hair and scalp very squeaky-clean; hair is thicker and fuller, soft and healthy; I had to use the conditioner too for detangling and am very impressed with the range: would highly recommend' • 'added volume to my fine hair and curls were more defined – would definitely buy'.

Phil Smith Be Gorgeous Big It Up Shampoo

8.19/10 A supermarket range, at supermarket prices (from an award-winning UK hairdresser): the thickening ingredient in this fruitily-scented shampoo is derived from wheat proteins.
Comments: 'Not so much a bouffant effect more a subtle change in hair texture and workability so that it lays more uniformly and therefore looks smoother and thicker' • 'no wispy separate flyaway straggles where my side parting used to lay, hair feels entirely more manageable and I haven't had to use a dozen styling products to get it to look good' • 'can't believe such a cheap shampoo works so well – no miracle cures for thin hair, just a hardworking shampoo that does your hair good' • 'light bounced off it giving a lovely sheen, hair felt fuller and smoother'.

Pureology Pure Volume Shampoo

7.4/10 The Pureology range is actually a colour-care range (it did well in our specific trials for that category, too) – but they offer a volumising option, with a protein complex from soy, oat and wheat, all fragranced very sophisticatedly with amber, mandarin and ylang-ylang. It's sulphate-free, with an 'anti-fade complex'. Your best choice if you have coloured hair that needs oomph.
Comments: 'I love this product, good smell and made my hair feel clean and soft, I use it every wash and my hair is noticeably better and fuller' • 'like this product very much, made hair soft and full, without being flyaway; it's very concentrated and lasts for ages' • 'hair was bouncy and I was very pleased with this, lovely lather, hair felt clean

and looked shiny after use; also I usually get slight itching and/or dandruff after having my colour done, this was the first time for ages that I didn't'.

Aveda Pure Abundance Volumizing Shampoo

7.3/10 Aveda – who have so many different haircare options available – have done well across our hair trials (and we did test LOTS of other brands!). Key ingredients here are acacia gum, babassu, calendula, honey and marshmallow, with a signature Aveda-esque aroma from organic peppermint, ylang-ylang, palmarosa and jasmine.

Comments: 'Gloss was very high and people commented; worked the product into root and scalp and it really plumped up my hair quite significantly, which lasted approximately three days after washing; hair felt in better condition – fab product' • 'gave some extra volume, both with the first wash and over time; did a good job of getting my hair clean though not much lather; no irritation at all and hair felt good' • 'worked well without the conditioner; more gloss and volumising – really beneficial and pleasant to use' • 'my hair was immediately abundant – I couldn't stop admiring it; very manageable and easier to style: I used both shampoo and conditioner and have never been more surprised! The shampoo really is the 'amber nectar' of the hair world'.

CONDITIONER REVIEWS

Yes to Tomatoes Tempting Tomato Daily Volumizing Conditioner

8.94/10 This was trialled by the same group as the YTC shampoo, notching up almost as high a score. The key high-performance ingredients in the conditioner are the same – and the bottle's equally generous.

Comments: 'Hair was very glossy, shiny and felt thicker, but my thin fine hair wasn't too slippy, I could style it easily and it seemed slightly bulked out' • 'felt really luxurious to use, coated every shaft of hair and rinsed out easily, could comb through hair easily and was a joy to use' • 'gave extra volume, fair gloss, was less knotty and easier to brush, liked the fruity fragrance' • 'left my hair a better texture' • 'my hair is shinier than it has been in years and gave lots of added volume – looked fuller; much easier to manage and style'.

Phil Smith Be Gorgeous Big It Up Conditioner

7.87/10 One panel trialled the Big It Up duo, and this winning conditioner has similar ingredients/fragrance to the shampoo; we needn't add much, except that they didn't rate the conditioner quite as highly (although it still did much better than most volumising conditioners we trialled).

Comments: 'Good volumising results, after only one use my hair felt fuller; a big bonus for me; I did need to use more product than with other conditioners, even though I was careful to apply it only on the ends' • 'hair in worse condition than usual but this smoothed through very well and gave slight sheen (almost unfair to test shine with state of hair), used with shampoo and gave definite lift; would buy' • 'I'd stopped using conditioners as they just made my hair lank and greasy but I am astounded by this smooth, light cream, which left hair smooth, light, glossy, manageable and bouncy: no startling big hair but an overall effect of smoother volumised hair which kept its style'.

Lulu Operation Glam Larger-Than-Life Conditioner

7/10 We're not really surprised this conditioner earned a place in this book: the Operation Glam range (from singer Lulu's signature line) was developed by the chemist genius who used to work for John Frieda and brought you products such as Sheer Blonde and Funky Chunky (a late-lamented product for flat-haired women). This ultra-light conditioner contains a panthenol blend that thickens without weighing hair down. However, testers were divided about its effects: some thought it was fab, others weren't impressed.

Comments: 'The large tube is very practical in the shower, and it was easy to work the product through hair; gave a very healthy gloss with added volume which lasted a day or two; it was easier to style and definitely helped with the frizz factor. Improved the condition of my hair and made it shinier' • 'lots of added volume, very impressed! Hair was shiny and light after, maybe because it provides colour care: my hair is highlighted so to have two effects in one is definitely a bonus!' • 'twice as good as my normal conditioner' • 'the pink packaging with zebra stripes is really fun and I liked the tongue-in-cheek copy'.

Hair masks: our award winners

File this under 'essential weekly maintenance', whatever your age. Packed with replenishing oils, nourishing botanicals – and sometimes shine-boosting silicones – we've long believed that hair masks are a must for every woman. More and more women agree with us, and in response the hair industry now offers multiple mask choices. Our testers used these once a week over a period of time, giving us feedback on instant and longer-term benefits, and awarding some pretty stellar scores

AT A GLANCE

Kérastase Masquintense

Louise Galvin Sacred Locks Treatment Masque for Fine Hair

Kiehl's Olive Fruit Oil Nourishing Conditioner

Kevin Murphy Born Again Masque

TIP

Any hair mask will work better if you apply some heat. Wrapping hair in a hot towel is one way. The only problem is that the heat doesn't last long – so instead, our friend Philip B applies conditioner to hair and then blasts it with a hairdryer for 15 minutes, 'twisting' the hair. This is particularly good with oil treatments, though these are best applied before shampooing.

REVIEWS

Kérastase Masquintense

 9.37/10 Kérastase are renowned for their salon treatments, which are now more widely available (via websites) for the at-home user. This is something of a beauty classic, and scored incredibly well: the key re-glossing, strengthening ingredient is their 'GlucoActive Complexe', with lipids and proteins to overcome dryness. It comes in a version for fine or thick hair (our testers had the latter). If you have time though, we can't recommend too highly an occasional Kérastase treatment in a salon, where the stylist will prescribe the exact mask in the range for you. Hair bliss.

Comments: 'Simple to use and delivered a healthy gloss; hair looked full-bodied and shiny, became more silky and easier to shape and style, I would buy' • 'massaged two hazelnut-size blobs through my hair, and it did give a shine and gloss to my blonde hair – which is very hard to do; hair so silky it was much easier to blow-dry, and gave a super-smooth result' • 'definite de-frizz factor with this wonderful conditioner; didn't weigh hair down, it was lighter, softer and more swingy!' • 'one of the most effective hair conditioners I have ever used'.

Louise Galvin Sacred Locks Treatment Masque for Fine Hair ❀

 8.75/10 This luxurious winning mask targets fine hair, which can so often be weighed down by conditioning treatments. Louise's products have done very well in our previous books, including *The Green Beauty Bible*, as they use naturally-derived ingredients in place of synthetics/polymers/petrochemicals/silicones, etc. The treatment masque deploys a form of honey combined with wheat proteins, with twice-weekly treatments recommended.

Comments: 'Very easy to work through wet hair; on first use, hair was glistening!' • 'helped keep my colour bright, hair stayed conditioned rather than becoming dry and brittle, definitely helped with smoothing and making it manageable' • 'loved this product, so easy to apply and divine smell; left hair squeaky clean, easy to manage and thicker – the first product I've found that really works well on a consistent basis' • 'hair much more manageable, smoother and nice shine'.

Kiehl's Olive Fruit Oil Nourishing Conditioner

 8.75/10 There's an even richer Hair Pak in this range (see Jo's We Love…), but our testers actually trialled this lavish conditioner as a hair mask, since it's designed for dehydrated, damaged hair. Replenishing ingredients include avocado oil, olive fruit oil and lemon extract, which gives an uplifting zestiness.

Comments: 'My coloured, rather dry hair was shinier and manageable – usually a wet bird's-nest after washing, really tangled and difficult, but this was one of the best conditioners I've used, it was easier to comb out, and left hair light and smooth' • 'delivered an incredible shine; the first time I used it hair was noticeably greasy but definitely a case of less is more for good results; tangle and static-free hair, light and shiny' • 'simple to use, sensible plastic tube, lovely product and very economical; my once-dry hair was softer and more shiny, easy to comb through and to style, which left me more in control'.

Kevin Murphy Born Again Masque

Aussie hairdresser Kevin Murphy's products score well in the style stakes, but also here for performance: a creamy mask blending babassu oil with mango and shea butters, vitamins, soy and wheat amino acids, to add strength and shine, plus – the Australian touch – kakadu plum and wattleseed extracts from their rainforest, which are packed with antioxidants.

Comments: 'Worked through hair easily, gave high gloss without greasiness, hair much easier to style, de-frizzed; product did a great job but please could they redo the packaging so it's easier to open?' • 'delicious sharp natural fragrance, gave high gloss, hair like satin and easier to style, less dry and flyaway; plus hair will now go a day longer without washing; didn't weigh it down at all' • 'fantastic product; has improved the condition of my hair tremendously; glossy and pliable with no static or frizz factor – hurray!'.

♡ WE LOVE...

How much space have we got...? Coloured hair is thirsty hair. So we follow our own slavish advice to use a hair mask once a week, and in Jo's case, that could be the super-effective Kiehl's Olive Fruit Oil Deeply Repairative Hair Pak (lovely lemony smell), generous lashings of the Liz Earle Botanical Shine Conditioner for Dry/Damaged Hair, or Christophe Robin Masque au Germe de Blé (that's wheatgerm), which she lugs back from Paris, created by one of that city's leading colourists. And a truly extraordinary deep treatment she uses once a month is Philip B Katira Hair Masque, based on an ingredient well-known to Persian women, which seems to 'fill in' the cuticle to reflect shine back. Sarah has two favourites: Ojon Restorative Hair Treatment, which is a solid oil that needs warming – a bit messy and takes time but gives great shine – but for speed and fantastic results, she loves Jason Intense Moisture Treatment Mint & Rose which really, really works on her superdry hair.

Hair shine sprays: *award winners*

We don't necessarily advise using these all the time, but for an instant boost when hair looks less-than-glossy, they're a boon. Long term, however, hair masks, moisturising haircare – plus hair-nourishing foods and supplements (oily fish and omega-3 supplements) – are more effective for improving the shine factor. The challenge is that some of these sprays make hair appear greasy rather than shiny. (Start off by using a little, applied to the ends of your hair from the back, so if it's too heavy for your hair, you'll get through the day without it all going lank.) Although there aren't a gazillion options out there, some did go down reasonably (if not spectacularly) well.

A word of warning: do use these sprays before getting dressed in anything you care about – one tester found three spots of shine spray on her T-shirt, and as she says: 'If it had been a new expensive outfit I would have been heart-broken.'

Aveda Brilliant Spray-On Shine ❀

Aveda have done exceptionally well in the haircare department in our book, here with a shine-boosting finishing mist which also tackles flyaways. For all hair types, there's vitamin E as well as Pro-vitamin B5 (to 'temporarily mend split ends').

Comments: 'Made my long hair – thin but lots of it – look good, nice and shiny with no flyaways; no greasiness and no residue at the end of the day' • 'shine lasted a long time; I would definitely buy. Brilliant' • 'amazing shine on my thick coarse grey/white hair which lasted all day'.

Paul Mitchell Soft Style The Shine Spray-On Polish

As well as instantly delivering gloss, this is recommended for use before straightening irons, with a protective shield offered by jojoba, aloe, henna and rosemary, plus silicones. (You can also apply it to bare skin for 'a touch of glamour', Paul Mitchell tell us.)

Comments: 'Gave my fine, wispy baby-like – awful! – hair a natural sheen/gloss that I liked and lasted through the day; no downsides and I love the packaging!' • 'surprised how light this spray is, hair wasn't damp/limp after use, and did stay in place longer' • 'good for my thick coarse coloured hair, which is dry and not responsive to my usual shampoo/conditioner'.

Label.m Shine Spray

Again, this can play a heat-protective as well as an instant shine role, with Label.m's 'Enviroshield Complex' helping to ward off UV damage. Label.m is brought to you by the team behind Toni & Guy, and this sexily-packaged bottle delivers a mist infused with extracts of bamboo, fig, echinacea and ginger.

Comments: 'My fine, salon-coloured hair – lots of it – was nicely shiny and "settled", it removed any fluffing miraculously, and it didn't weigh my hair down at all' • 'really worked so well that my naturally curly, very thick hair became instantly shiny and looked sensational' • 'left a pleasant sheen on my slightly frizzy hair and overall condition looked better'.

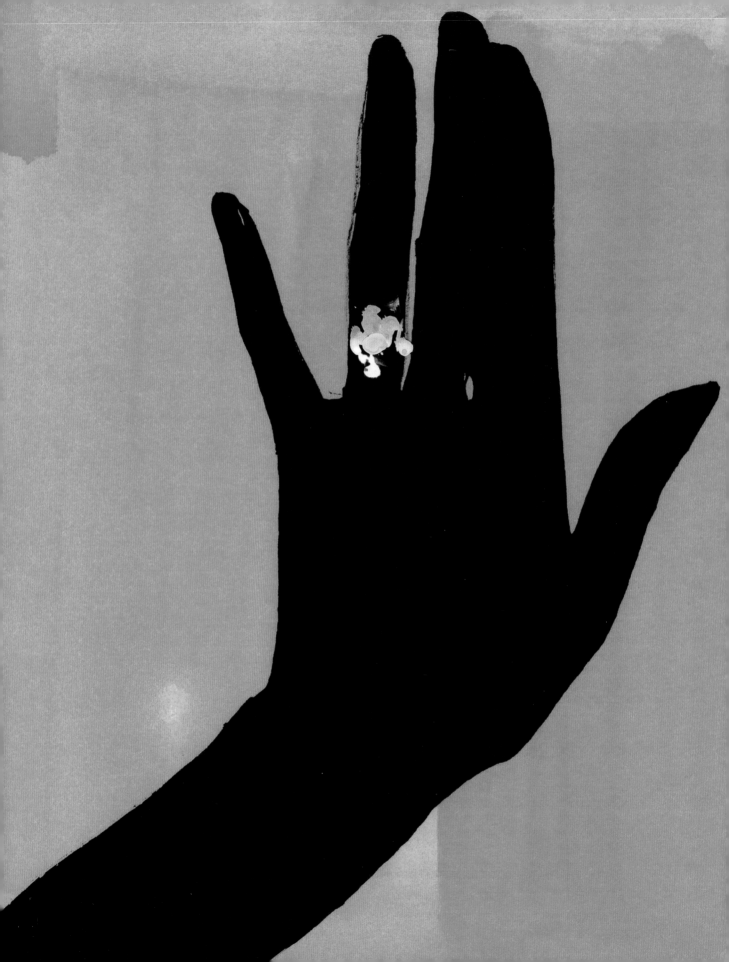

'I've been living
in this EXCELLENT
body for over 60 years.
I *LOVE IT* so much.
As long as it doesn't
get too fat, or too thin,
doesn't break –
I just think,
"*Thank goodness!*"'

Joanna Lumley

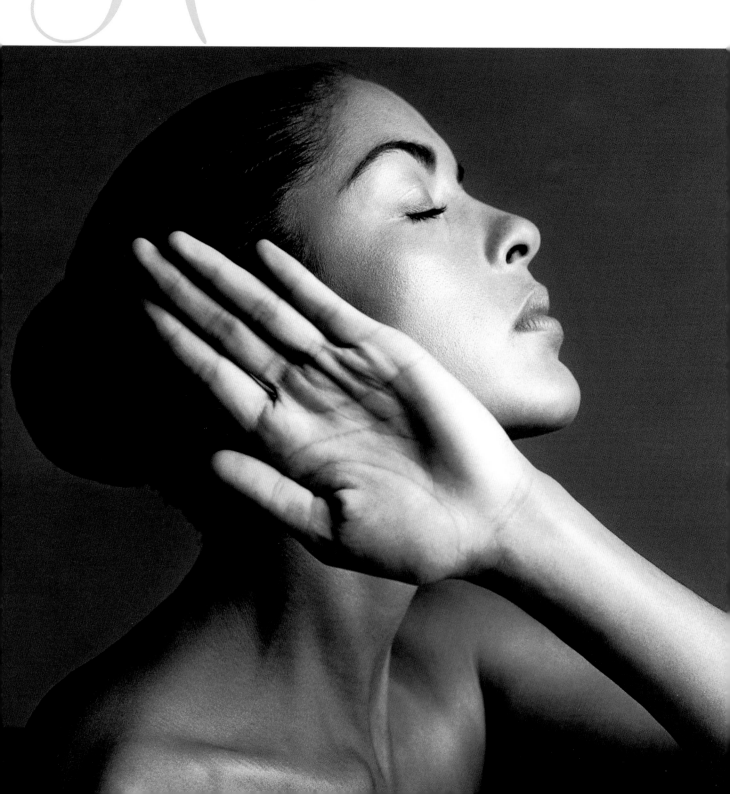

$\mathcal{H}$reat your hands with

the same care as your face

Every time Madonna's photographed with her hands on view, bitchy tabloids rush to point out that they haven't aged as well as her face. (Good tip: she often covers them up in gloves, long and lacy for evening, soft leather for day.) We don't go in for bitchiness, but if Madonna's hands are a better clue to her real age – fiftysomething-ish – than her very famous *visage*, she's not the first woman that's true for. There's a very, very simple rule to ensure ageing isn't fast-forwarded when it comes to hands. It is this: lavish them with the same attention as your face. (They are equally visible, after all, though that's so easily forgotten.) Which means…

Shield them from sun damage. Either use a body sunscreen on the backs of your hands and forearms, or a hand cream formulated with a built-in SPF. (There are still too few of these on the market for our liking. Ole Henriksen Hands Forward SPF15 is one of our top choices.) Remember to reapply after washing – so the tube needs to be neat enough to carry in your handbag. Basically, get in the habit of putting an SPF on your hands as part of your morning beauty ritual – post-sleep cleansing, moisturising, SPF-ing, etc. (Apparently it takes 16 to 21 times of performing a task to make it a habit. That's less than a month, for something which is truly going to keep the years at bay.)

Scrub, every week. Just as a once-a-week exfoliation does wonders for facial dinginess, so the same is true for hands. When you're exfoliating your face (and your body), scrub the backs of your hands. It helps treatment products penetrate quicker, while also instantly brightening by buffing away the surface cells. We'd also like to tell you about a product which is frankly a bit of a party trick of ours: Yes to Carrots Feel the C Pampering Hand & Nail Spa. We were turned on to this because it did incredibly well with testers in our book *Beauty Bible Beauty Steals* – and quite rightly so. It's a tub of Dead Sea salts blended into a skin-nurturing oil mixture, which you use as if washing your hands. We have yet to try this on anyone who isn't blown away by how bright, moisturised and incredibly soft hands are, in about 15 seconds flat. (One friend said she couldn't stop her beau holding her hand.)

TIP

Please don't forget the obvious: wear gloves whenever you're washing up, gardening, and maybe even handling paper – it makes nails as dry as the Sahara. If you can't bear to wear gloves while you work with papers (we can't), make sure you slosh on really oily hand and cuticle cream before and after. And don't use your nails as staple removers, to tighten Phillips screws, or dig out stones from horses' hooves…they were not designed for those purposes.

Slap on a mask. When you put a mask on your face, put it on the backs of your hands. Couldn't be simpler. (If you're in the bath, that means keeping them above the water-line. Er, obviously…)

Slather on a rich hand cream overnight. Last thing at night before switching off the light, uber-moisturise your hands with lashings of hand cream. For a shortlist of those which our testers found had anti-ageing powers, turn to page 126. Conventional beauty wisdom says that it helps to apply cotton gloves over the top, but we're not convinced: the cotton 'wicks' the cream off the hands, and they feel frankly odd to us. (Not to mention being total passion-killers.) In the same way that night creams and facial oils applied at night harness the body's skin-repairing mechanism, this is true with hand creams. Where the cotton gloves can be useful is if you're slathering on a cream while, say, watching a movie on telly; stops your greasy paws from getting all over everything.

Hand and nail problems – and the fixes...

Dry and ragged cuticles. This is just another manifestation of (not to put too fine a point on it) the gradual dessiccation of the body. A cuticle oil massaged into nails overnight will go a long way towards fixing this problem, while boosting blood flow to help encourage nail growth (yet another thing that slows with age). For specific recommendations of cuticle treatments, see page 128.

Flaking/splitting nails. The oil treatment mentioned above will help prevent flaking – not immediately, but over time. Submerging hands in water isn't helpful – but it's what rubber gloves were invented for (if you really can't bear the feel of them, try surgeons' latex gloves – provided you're not sensitive to latex – which feel like there's nothing there). Avoid acetone-based nail polishes – the only exception to this rule being the slightly-unlikely-at-this-stage-in-life event that you have fallen for a glitter nail polish: a quick blitz with an acetone-based polish remover is preferable to endless, endless rubbing and soaking with a regular polish remover to get the glitter off. And NEVER, EVER buff if your nails are weak. Oh goodness no, no, NO! – and don't let perfectionist manicurists do it either: shriek, jump out of your chair, run, whatever it takes to stop them, or your nails will suffer for months.

Nails that snap. Over-dry, brittle nails will simply break. Again, oil treatments help. Our testers review nail strengtheners on page 128, but the chemical types should be used for short bursts (not more than a month) – otherwise nails become over-strong, and prone to snapping rather than bending flexibly when challenged.

Ridges. Very, very common, these. Length-ways ridges can respond to very, very gentle buffing; your nails need to be naked for this (although again, as above, you can oil them first). Buff lengthways, but never to the point where you create 'heat'. (And note our caution about buffing above...). The quick-fix is a ridge-filling base coat; we recommend the excellent Diorlisse Pastel Ridge Filler, which comes in two pretty tones – one pinky and one apricot – that can be worn instead of polish (although you'll need a top coat); another good option is Essie Ridge Filling Base Coat. Occasionally, a ridge becomes a split, for which the best solution is a 'patch' applied at a nail salon, while it grows out, or a false acrylic nail. Yet again, you need to boost nail health while it's growing out with stimulating oil massage of the nail bed.

For all these, try nutritional supplements. Sarah is a bit of an oracle on weak nails – her weak spot – and sadly notorious with the manicurists at John Frieda, who are practically as relieved as she is when they grow at all. (Think horses, gardening – and, simply, fragile nails...) The thing that really, really works for her is Sun Chlorella (tiny pillules of food state green stuff, see page 176). Pharmacist Shabir Daya also recommends taking a magnesium

TIP

Taupes, oranges and frosted nail polishes can be desperately unflattering to older hands. (No matter how hard Chanel try to persuade us that they are this season's must-haves, and no matter how long the subsequent waiting-lists...) Ironically, mature women often choose taupes because they think this will distract from hands they feel self-conscious about, but instead pale pinks, soft crimson – and even deep berry/wine varnish, which has become a modern classic – will bring nails (and hands) back to life.

supplement at night (as important as calcium for bones, nails and teeth, plus it keeps you calm!) and, if budget permits, silica (aka horsetail), also an important compound for nails.

And eat good food. Try to consume oily fish (salmon, mackerel, sardines, tuna, etc) two to three times weekly for the omega-3 essential fatty acids, which help nails, skin and hair (not to mention brain and pretty well everything else...). If you don't like fish, try a supplement with fish oils, or plant oils if you're veggie. Also make sure you get enough protein for the iron content – iron deficiency is a common cause of flaking nails as well as thinning hair (Sarah finds a steak a week works a treat; veggies should consume lots of wholegrain cereals and flours, leafy green vegetables, blackstrap molasses, pulses such as lentils and kidney beans, dried apricots and figs). And everyone needs lots of multicoloured veg for the vitamin C which is vital for iron to be absorbed.

Camouflage sun spots on the back of hands. Try self-tanner on hands and forearms as this reduces the 'contrast' and thus the visibility of sun spots. Medical peels and lasers are a pricier – and potentially riskier – way to deal with sun spots: we suggest reading the advice on page 186 before you go there.

Veins. Ah, the Madonna problem. Many of us develop large, bulging veins on the backs of the hands, partly to do with the skin relaxing and thinning with age (as well as the gradual loss of fat), so they become more visible. It is, technically, possible to have the veins on the backs of the hands 'stripped out'. The surgery is akin to the way varicose veins are treated, but in general only one hand is operated on at a time as hands can be painful and swollen for the first few weeks after surgery and tender for some time after that. (For more advice which covers all forms of cosmetic surgery, see page 46.) Personally, we'd counsel an attempt at Zen-like acceptance of veins. Gratitude for the miraculous tasks our hands perform on a daily basis – from typing to texting, writing to playing the piano – helps, we find.

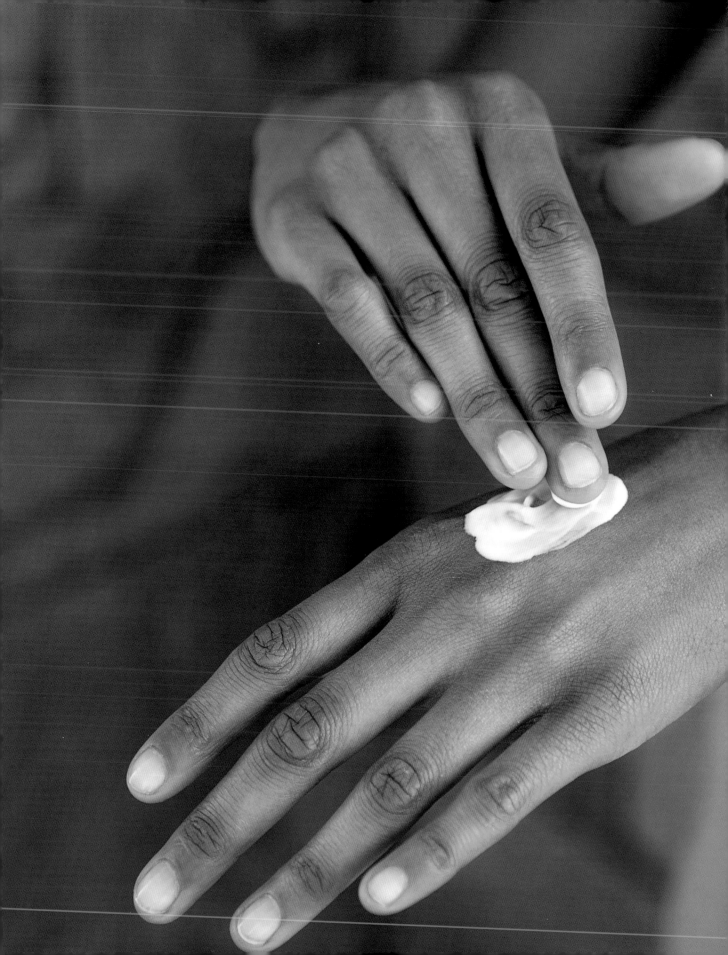

Anti-ageing hand creams: *our award winners*

Because hands give your age away faster than a glimpse in your passport. Because hand-creaming is one of our favourite (and most frequent) beauty activities. Because there is now a raft of creams which promise that as well as soften and moisturise, they help eliminate signs of ageing, by harnessing many of the same ingredients as facial care. For all those reasons, we assessed dozens of hand creams for specifically age-defying actions, rather than just something to leave hands smooth and velvety. Were our testers wowed…? You bet. And to our delight, the highest-scoring ones are all natural!

AT A GLANCE

Balance Me Super Moisturising Hand Cream

Jurlique Purely Age-Defying Hand Treatment

Trilogy Rose Hand Cream

Liz Earle Hand Repair

Weleda Pomegranate Regenerating Hand Cream

Barefoot Botanicals Rosa Fina Anti-Ageing Hand and Nail Cream

REVIEWS

Balance Me Super Moisturising Hand Cream ❀ ❀ ❀

 Shea butter, beeswax and sweet almond oil give Balance Me's organically-certified hand cream its mega-moisturising power, in a rich blend that also features healing benzoin and yarrow, patchouli for 'weathered skin' and kukui nut oil for suppleness. As we've come to expect from this niche aromatherapeutic brand, this also smells wonderful.

Comments: 'Fantastic: my hands felt and looked years younger, and my nails became less brittle; perfect creamy texture' • 'very quickly absorbed but hands felt hydrated for a long time; after overnight application they looked amazing, extremely smooth and silky' • 'loved the smell and other people did too; hands looked younger every day I used this' • 'my wrinkly hands look noticeably smoother and it worked wonders on my cuticles' • 'hands more supple and less crêpey, very soothing after weeding or cutting conifers!'.

Jurlique Purely Age-Defying Hand Treatment ❀ ❀

 Beauty Bible testers have previously awarded Jurlique hand creams very high marks, and this specifically anti-ageing addition to the range continues the winning streak. The non-greasy cream harnesses the anti-ageing power of botanicals such as liquorice (to combat redness and fade discolourations), turmeric extract, softening marshmallow and sunflower oil – and many ingredients are biodynamic, produced and harvested in rhythm with nature. It's lightly rose-scented, and we know from countless previous comments that many of you are enraptured by rose fragrances.

Comments: 'Thick, rich cream which is very easy to smooth in and not too sticky; after a month small age spots have almost gone, my nails are growing very quickly and hands are silky smooth until their first dunking in water' • 'fabulous results: hands instantly went several shades lighter and look five years younger, overnight it leaves them softer and brighter' • 'best as an overnight treatment as it can leave a slight residue – a good rescue cream for dry hands' • 'wonderful, far better than anything I've used before – love this'.

Trilogy Rose Hand Cream ✿ ✿

Another rose-scented award winner: New Zealand brand Trilogy call this a '60-second formula' – it works its rich, moisturising magic super-fast, and doesn't leave skin enduringly greasy. Key botanicals include rosehip and evening primrose oils, shea butter, calendula, horsetail (which is packed with nail-friendly silica) and anti-inflammatory marshmallow gel.

Comments: 'Brilliant! Am so impressed with this – quickly absorbed, immediate hydration, hands look smoother, more moisturised, more even-toned with regular use; very good results from overnight treatment – hands look younger' • 'love the very calming smell, fab overnight treatment' • 'hands felt very soft and looked very fresh, moisturised and soothed my hands after gardening'.

Liz Earle Hand Repair ✿ ✿

A personal favourite of ours which has performed well in previous trials. This time testers for *The Anti-Ageing Beauty Bible* put this through its paces specifically to assess its age-defying benefits – and Hand Repair rose to that challenge, too, with its instantly smoothing, botanically-powered formula. (Echinacea, hops, beta-carotene, vitamin E – and an essential-oil blend of bergamot, chamomile, neroli and lavender – all feature generously.) This comes in lots of different sizes and formats – pump-action, flip-top, etc – and we like the travel size for on-the-go hand pampering. You might also like to know that anecdotally, many users report it's great for eczema.

Comments: 'Wonderful stuff: absorbs easily and quickly yet still moisturises brilliantly; hands look much better, nails are much stronger too, yummy herbal scent' • 'made my hands supersoft and could notice a difference' • 'I work as a science technician and my hands are usually pretty wrecked but this moisturises them really effectively' • 'confession: I use this already, the smell is divine and it absorbs quicker than any other hand cream so you can carry on straight

away, without worrying about greasy handprints – a lovely product' • 'hands looked plumped up and less crêpey, with a nice sheen; also my nails got stronger'.

Weleda Pomegranate Regenerating Hand Cream ✿ ✿

Pomegranates star in Weleda's relatively new anti-ageing bodycare collection, including this 'intensive care' hand cream, which is based on the oil of that famously antioxidant fruit together with lashings of shea butter, avocado oil and olive oil. (Don't run away with the idea that it's greasy – although personally, we do like this best for pre-bedtime slathering.)

Comments: 'I have eczema and very dry skin and this is brilliant, the best hand cream I have ever used' • 'absorbed almost immediately and liked the slightly medicinal smell' • 'nice consistency and beautiful smell; any cream can have some positive effect used regularly – I looked forward to this one so half the battle is won!' • 'hands brighter and more hydrated, keeps hands soft and younger-looking, strong favourite now' • 'skin looks smoother and more supple'.

Barefoot Botanicals Rosa Fina Anti-Ageing Hand and Nail Cream ✿ ✿

Rosa mosqueta (rosehip seed oil) and tretinoin (a derivative of vitamin A) were chosen for their anti-ageing powers in this luscious cream, from a Brighton-based botanical brand founded by a respected homeopath. Cysteine (an amino acid) was added to strengthen nails, while mallow and macadamia nourish. And then there's the gorgeous rose (once again), frankincense and lavender scent... Testers generally felt it wasn't suitable for those with very, very dry hands.

Comments: 'Consistency just right, was absorbed immediately, no stickiness after; smell was adorable – I wanted to smooth it everywhere – and hands felt silky after, age spots lessened with regular use, dryness and nails improved gradually – an improvement on previous hand creams and the effects lasted' • 'seemed a bit runny at first but I was pleasantly surprised as it absorbed easily and quickly; hands felt soft and well-moisturised' • 'they use the words "satin gloves" on the label – spot on!'.

TIP

Right before bedtime, slather on a few drops of sesame oil, sunflower oil or sweet almond oil (or any body oil, come to that) and massage into skin. Layer your hand cream over the top and by morning, hands will be baby-soft and smooth.

Nail treatments: our award winners

There are different formulas for nail-boosting treatments. Oil treatments soften the cuticle area and help to nourish nails at the base, making for stronger and more flexible nails. Specifically nail-strengthening (chemically-based) products are painted on like nail varnish, and work to harden nails. (We don't counsel the use of those for more than a month as they can make nails brittle and likely to snap.) Some of these were trialled as cuticle treatments, some as nail strengtheners – and several rose to both challenges

AT A GLANCE

Nails Inc Vitamin E Oil Pen

Orly Cuticle Oil

Green Hands Organic Cuticle and Nail Oil

Essie Millionails Ultimate Nail Strengthener

Nails Inc A & E Treatment Base Coat

Qtica Solid Gold Cuticle Oil-Gel

REVIEWS

Nails Inc Vitamin E Oil Pen

 9.4/10 A sexy-looking beauty accessory, this: a shiny silver wand-style product with a brush at one end, which you 'prime' by twisting to deliver nourishing vitamin E. It was trialled as a cuticle treatment but used over time you should also observe strengthening benefits, with nails becoming strong but flexible. You'd do well to keep it in your handbag – to put bored moments to beautifying use…

Comments: 'Brilliant having the pen because I have no excuse now! Glides on with no mess, trialled it on my left hand, and the difference is clear: moisturises immediately so cuticles are less obvious instantly, and now soft enough to push down; nails look much stronger and healthier: thanks to this I have now started taking much better care of my hands' • 'nails and cuticles now look uber-glossy and in good health: would absolutely buy' • 'fantastic for strengthening my dry, brittle nails, cuticles softer and easier to push back, easy to do on the move – I am addicted!'.

Orly Cuticle Oil

8.12/10 This was tested as a cuticle treatment, not a specific nail strengthener – but again, if applied nightly, we believe it should be good for nail durability. There's a deliciously sweet, slightly citrus scent, thanks to orange blossom.

Comments: 'My dry, slightly brittle nails looked much healthier, did make a difference' • 'great product: very easy to apply, made my really dry, flaky nails and bad cuticles much stronger and healthier, and looked very hydrated' • 'I'm a nurse so wash my hands a lot, then put on lots of hand cream; this helped make my nails stronger so they don't break so much; you only need a drop per nail, so it lasts for ages' • very easy to apply' • 'my dry, scruffy cuticles are softer and in better condition, though nails no different' • 'love, love, love it! So easy to apply and splitting, breaking nails are soft and shiny, and raggedy cuticles look moisturised and very healthy'.

Green Hands Organic Cuticle and Nail Oil

8.06/10 This teensy bottle of Soil Association-certified blend of jojoba and apricot kernel oils (deliciously scented with frankincense and neroli) did well in *The Green Beauty Bible* – and really impressed a fresh set of testers when we sent it out for this new book. Actually, *two* sets of testers: one lot trialled it as a nail strengthener, with a separate group of ten putting it through its paces as a cuticle treatment. For double-duty, massage in and around nails before bedtime.

Comments: 'Nails were bad after false ones: this was a pleasure to use and smell, and I saw a great

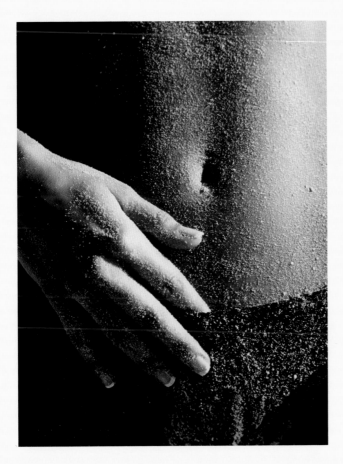

interested in my nails; I even liked the look with just this on' • 'very easy to apply, dries really quickly and I had to start using it on both hands instead of the trial one, as the nails on the first hand grew so much longer and it looked weird!' • 'a miracle for nails, only downside is when you remove it and the surface looks stripped'.

Nails Inc A & E Treatment Base Coat

7.57/10 A second winner from the successful British nail empire started by an ex-*Tatler* journalist, this nail strengthener is designed to be used either as a protective base coat under colour – or apply one coat of this to nails every day for a week, for treatment purposes. Remove after a week and continue the 'programme' for four weeks altogether.

Comments: 'Easy to apply and happily not nail-breaking to unpack! Fairly quick improvement in my snappy nails' • 'my slightly brittle nails were less prone to flaking and splitting' • 'very practical and straightforward to use, and I noticed a difference in strength within about ten days, and it lasted' • 'nails were 100 per cent stronger after two months' usage'.

Qtica Solid Gold Cuticle Oil-Gel

7.33/10 OK, so this is a cuticle oil. But our testers assessed its strengthening powers before awarding marks. The antibacterial, anti-fungal oil goes on like a gel, then becomes oily on skin – and confirms our belief that massaging oil into nails is best for boosting their strength.

Comments: 'My brittle, flaky nails were much more flexible and conditioned within one month; great for cuticles – I really like it and saw some improvement within days' • 'no cracks or splits for the month of testing, which is unusual; nails definitely softer and more supple, and love the way it oiled my cuticles; very easy to apply' • 'skin on my toenails has really improved; I put it on, then bedsocks (really glam!)'.

improvement in strengthening of nails in a month, plus softer cuticles' • 'nails more flexible and less prone to breaking; good for cuticles used once or twice daily: I liked this product and it does all I would expect' • 'really good at softening my very sore and dry cuticles, and my dry, weak nails became more flexible and smooth-looking within a month: really impressed with this oil'.

Essie Millionails Ultimate Nail Strengthener

7.83/10 This is part of a three-step nail-strengthening system – but used on its own put on a very good show. 'Positive results for weak, fragile nails are visible within days,' promise Essie. Ideally, paint on a fresh coat of this nail base – a bit like a nail lacquer – every other day, to benefit from the toughening effect of silk amino acids and iron.

Comments: 'My sad, neglected, flaky nails improved markedly, no breakages and the quality vastly better, but no discernible benefit to cuticles' • 'with this level of improvement, I became more

♡ WE LOVE...

Nail nourishment really works. Jo has an armoury of products that have defeated her previously flaky nails: divinely-scented Cowshed Apricot Nourishing Cuticle Oil and Body Shop Almond Nail & Cuticle Treatment (with its so-useful built-in hoof stick), as well as the Essie Cuticle Pen: this paints on cuticle-softening natural emollients through the brush tip, and features nail-boosting botanicals, too. Sarah relies on Seven Wonders Miracle Lotion, a hand and body product with sweet almond and olive oils which has transformed her dry, flaking nails – they take time to grow but look better instantly. And please don't forget to eat well – nails need lots of food as much as the rest of you.

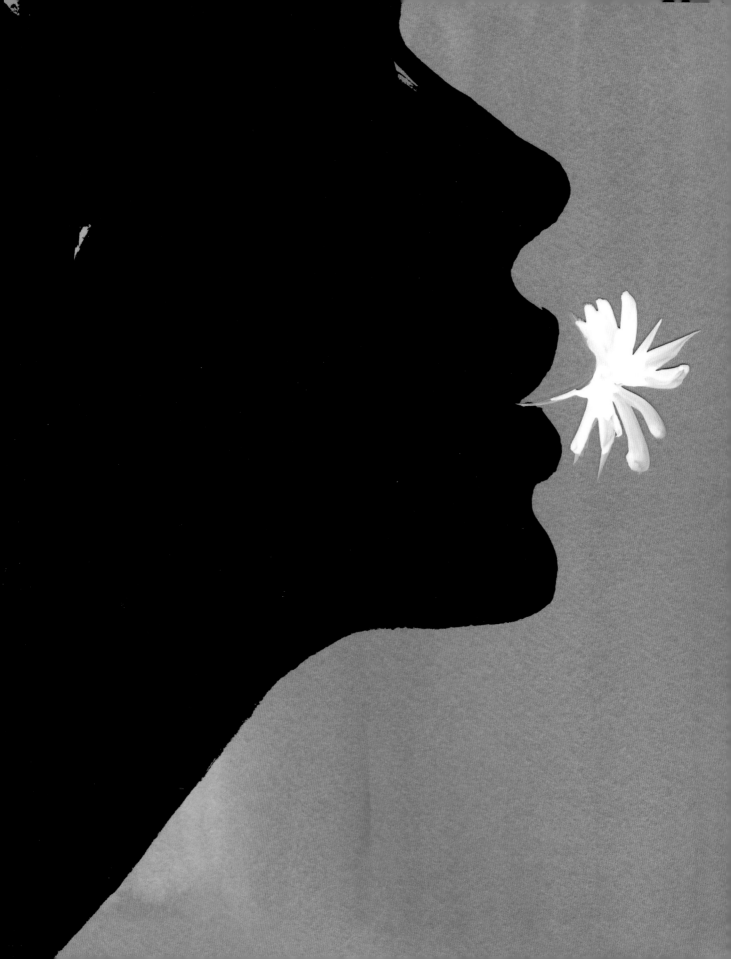

'Never stop
your *passion*.
Just keep going.
Be useful.
Stick up for what
you BELIEVE in.
Get *angry* about
what you
CARE about'

Jane Birkin

Learn a few lip tricks that put a smile on your face

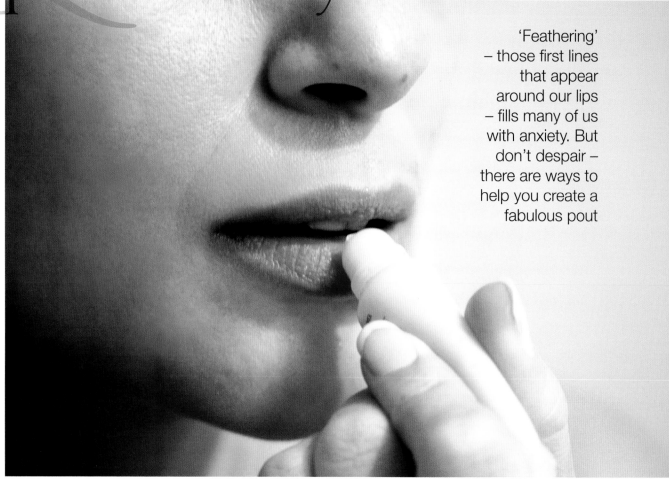

'Feathering' – those first lines that appear around our lips – fills many of us with anxiety. But don't despair – there are ways to help you create a fabulous pout

We speak, we laugh, we eat, we kiss! – so the lip zone gets a lot of action. No wonder, then, that fine lines and wrinkles – starting off with 'feathering' – develop around the lip contour not long after they show up in the eye zone, often causing women we know quite some distress (and beware, it happens earlier – much earlier – if you're a smoker. Skin really doesn't like the free radicals contained in smoke, or that puffing action). Over the next few pages you'll find your 'lip action plan': the treatments, the make-up, the tricks to make your pout fuller,

smoother, sexier – and, in turn, maybe just a little smilier. So your lips won't tell the world your real age…

Brush lips with a toothbrush to remove any flakiness. For perfect lip colour, you need a smooth base. To achieve this, we suggest regularly using an old, soft toothbrush – which you keep for this purpose – dabbed in balm: make gentle circular movements to buff away flakes and really push the balm into the lip skin, because it has no natural moisturisation of its own.

Give lips back their natural, rosy hue. Lips – like so much else – tend to fade as we age, and naturally rosy lips are rare. (Though if yours are really pale, do get your iron levels checked.) So we believe in giving them some help. 'As you get older, slightly brighter lips are important,' advises Trish McEvoy, 'but they shouldn't be opaque or matte. Outline the lips [see lip liner tips below], then fill in with sheer or semi-sheer lipstick.' Mid-rose toned lipsticks are, most make-up artists agree, the most flattering for women of forty-plus – think of the colour that lips naturally are, only a tiny, tiny bit stronger. If you choose a really sheer lipstick, you can go a bit darker – it'll just leave a slick of colour.

Use a nude lip pencil for a crisp, youthful outline. Choose a rose-y nude, not a brown-y nude, which should be as close to the natural colour of your lips as possible – and then, explains Terry de Gunzburg, 'You can draw your lipline at the outer edge of your lips and actually increase the apparent size of both the top and bottom lips.' (You have to make sure the line dovetails perfectly at the corners of your lips, though. Otherwise the ghastly spectre of Ronald McDonald swims into the imagination…) There should, of course, never be a gap between the pencil and your actual lip – but you can use the pencil to 'extend' the contour of the top and bottom lips.

Lip pencil will help prevent 'feathering'. The waxiness helps stop moisturising or lubricating ingredients in a lipstick formulation from travelling into tiny lines around the lip line (and we all have those too…).

Try lip pencil and gloss, or sheer/semi-sheer lippy. No matt lipstick ever. Outline lips, then fill in with pencil; top with gloss or balm (tinted if you like).

Feel free to use your daughter's lip gloss. (Or your goddaughter's.) When it comes to many make-up items, we're recommending that you 'shift' your buying habits towards make-up ranges which specifically target more mature skins. But lip gloss? You can get away with pretty much anything, so long as it's not over-shimmery, or too intense in colour. (Or too sticky if you have longer hair – that awful feeling of strands being glued to your lips.)

Having said that, try adding just a touch of

shimmer to the centre of your bottom lip. This really does help make lips look fuller. Apply the shimmer (or gloss) with your finger, and pat it in. (Terry de Gunzburg's By Terry Or de Rose balm is also perfect for this, as well as for an overnight lip treatment: it has tiny shimmering particles of real gold, which look super-flattering.)

Between 45 and 60, give up the statement red lipstick, says Mary Greenwell. Mary remembers the time when she was walking down Fifth Avenue in Manhattan and saw a pair of red lips on legs coming towards her. Then she realised it was a mirror, and that's the moment she gave up her red lipstick. For now. 'Somehow, on a woman at that stage in her life, a geranium or poppy or pillarbox red lipstick is all you see when you look at the face – and it doesn't look sexy. After sixty, you can take it up again – it becomes a glamorous "statement", a bit eccentric and rather divine.'

Also avoid shrieking orange or fuchsia, and very pale lipsticks, advises Barbara Daly, 'although pale gloss is fine'. But, says Barbara, 'bright, rich colour can look very chic at night'; she created silver-mopped fashion designer Betty Jackson's trademark soft, clear crimson especially for her. NB: the word is 'soft'…

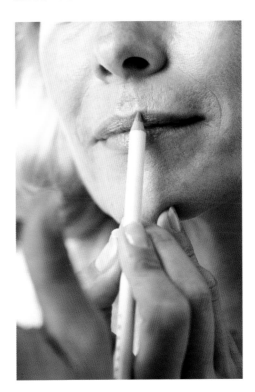

TIP

Remember that lips need sun protection just as much as the rest of your face. So either choose a lippy containing SPF15, or apply a separate product (balms with sun protection are great, and widely available) before your lipstick. NB: if you suffer from cold sores, an SPF lip product may help prevent them.

L Lip gloss: our award winners

Ah, lip gloss. Gorgeous, glamorous, makes-you-feel-girly-at-any-age lip gloss. What's more, it's possible to use lip gloss not just for a slick of sexy shine, but to create the illusion of a fuller pout. At this stage in life you're almost certainly looking for something that stays put that bit longer than the rest. Look no further, say our panellists

AT A GLANCE

New CID Cosmetics i-gloss

Lancôme Juicy Tubes Ultra Shiny Hydrating Lip Gloss

Yes to Carrots C Me Shine Lip Gloss

Chanel Aqualumière Gloss High Shine Sheer Concentrate

TIP

Applying lip gloss generously all over is fine for 15-year-olds, but there's a more age-appropriate technique for this stage in life. Add a dab to the centre of the bottom lip, swipe it side to side with your finger, and don't rub lips together – smack them like you're saying, 'Ma! Ma!' If you need more, repeat the process. (See our tips for applying lip pencil, page 133, as this gives gloss a base to 'cling' to and prevents gloss and lipstick travelling.)

REVIEWS

New CID Cosmetics i-gloss

 8.9/10 An awfully clever gizmo, this: at the touch of a button it lights up so that you can apply in the dark using a mirrored panel on the side of the wand (very useful for taxis). The colour which our testers received was Moonstone, a sort of holographic, crystalline pink, which is very fetching when lightly applied over a lipstick – but a bit too 'disco' if applied generously on its own.

Comments: 'Would I buy this? Yes, yes, yes and YES! It's easy to apply, very glossy, not sticky, moisturising, colour is just right and I love the shimmery finish – my lips looked like Angelina Jolie's!' • 'blown away by this glam glossy girlie high-tech product, wonderfully moisturising yet sheer; I've bought it for five girlfriends and my husband is bemused at how much time we have jabbered on about it' • 'gorgeous, gorgeous, gorgeous! Loads of comments from girls asking what it was, and men saying how lovely my lips looked' • 'inbuilt light and mirror are one of the most ingenious fab inventions for lippy lovers!'.

Lancôme Juicy Tubes Ultra Shiny Hydrating Lip Gloss

 8.34/10 With their angled tip (for ease of application), Juicy Tubes have become a cult, with limited-edition shades and fragrances. Our testers had Melon 22, a classic sheer rose pink with a melon-y scent. Super-shiny – and often fruit-scented – Juicy Tubes are a love-'em-or-hate'em product; for our testers, it was a Juicy love-in… (Though some did find the stickiness a problem.)

Comments: 'Lovely sheer flattering colour, and it's

so moisturising – gave dry, flaky lips immediate relief, also helped plumpness a little' • 'I like how instantly glam it makes me look' • 'impressed by the suitably scrumptious range of shades' • 'lasts well for a lip gloss: I'm never without it'.

Yes to Carrots C Me Shine Lip Gloss

 8/10 From a crazily-named natural brand that's done incredibly well in our previous books, this is a balm-like, all-natural, 98 per cent organic, lightly-shimmering gloss which packs a seriously minty, cooling punch. The slightly peachy shade which we sent to our testers – Carrot Kiss – would suit most skintones.

Comments: 'Feels lovely, not sticky at all; moisturises lips beautifully and lasts ages; gives lips a lovely wet look – my thin lips appear fuller' • 'very shiny but not gloopy; subtle colour; makes lips so soft I sometimes use it instead of a balm' • 'worked well over a nude lip liner, lips looked full and glossy – got a few compliments!' • 'gave a cool, confident gloss – I liked the lip tingle from the mint'.

Chanel Aqualumière Gloss High Shine Sheer Concentrate

7.88/10 Sweeps shimmeringly on to lips with a super-slim brush. This scored well for comfort, non-stickiness – and the sheer wash of colour delivered by the softly gleaming pink (73 Bonbon) which we sent out.

Comments: 'Very glossy, made me feel like going on a night out! Extremely moisturising and the shimmery effect is extremely appealing, made me feel a million dollars' • 'made lips feel comfy, smooth and sexy, and look fuller' • 'this is FAB! Very pretty pale pink shot through with a little sparkle, so moisturising, feels wonderful, light, just gorgeous!'.

Lip pencils:
our award winners

A must for the more mature make-up kit. As we've said, lip liner defines the lips (which become more 'blurry' as lines arrive). It helps prevent 'bleeding' by creating a waxy barrier that stops lipstick travelling and gives any lip colour something to 'cling' to, helping it stay put. These were all sent to ten women and had them beaming

REVIEWS

MAC Lip Pencil

The shade Spice, which was sent to our testers, is an absolute legend in the make-up world, probably the best-known lip liner of all time, as used by supermodels, super-make-up-artists, you name it… A perfect brown-y/pink lip colour, with vitamin E to condition lips, it glides on smoothly and stays put, too.
Comments: 'Soft creamy pencil which lined and filled in lips very easily, I loved using it all over lips with lip gloss, lasts for ages and makes the gloss last twice as long as normal' • 'smooth and easy to apply, looked good, and made other lip products last longer so saving me money – always a bonus!' • 'delighted with this pencil and how natural it looked – I used to dread the dark line around lips but this was excellent as liner and base colour'.

Inika Mineral Lip Liner ❀ ❀

This is a clever design: there's a pencil sharpener in the lid, so you push the pencil in, turn the cap – and hey, presto! One sharpened pencil. It's the most natural option that our testers rated, with a blend of certified organic plant waxes and oils, from an Australian mineral-based make-up brand which is vegan-certified. It was dispatched in Sugar Plum, a pink-y nude.
Comments: 'Really good texture and I was very pleased with outline; impressed with it as a base for lipstick, lasted several hours although I sip water or coffee all the time' • 'loved the sharpener in the lid, wish I had eye pencils like that: a very good idea'.

Sisley Phyto-Lèvres Perfect

From the luxury end of the make-up spectrum comes Sisley's winner: a deep rose/nude pencil (Rose Thé) enriched with kokum butter, aloe vera and jojoba oil for softness and hydration, plus beeswax for a long-wear finish. There's a brush at one end for softening the line you've smoothly created.
Comments: 'Simply the best lip liner I've ever tried; slightly creamy and goes on smoothly and precisely for a realistic outline; I used it as a lip liner, base and lipstick; the lip brush applicator at the other end was an excellent tool for blending' • 'nice smooth-textured soft pencil that went on easily and didn't smudge, the outline was not too hard so you don't look like an old woman!' • 'looked good all over my lips; didn't dry out lips'.

Revlon Colorstay Lipliner

Beauty Steal

Revlon's Colorstay range is designed to be especially 'budge-proof' – which, with a lip pencil, is a terrific boon, as it really will lengthen the lifetime of any lipstick applied over the top. The SoftFlex technology, which achieves this, means that while this twist-up pencil should be durable it's not uncomfortably hard or drying (though some testers pointed out that it's best to apply it on top of balm, as we always suggest). It comes in ten 'full coverage' shades, also five sheer and one clear. Our testers trialled Nude.
Comments: 'Very easy to apply smoothly and precisely, didn't drag' • 'great base for lipstick and really helped my usual colour to last; even when that faded, the lip liner lasted and looked fine' • 'I had a long lunch and my lips still looked great at the end – in my book that's pretty good going' • 'a good beauty "steal"'.

AT A GLANCE

MAC Lip Pencil

Inika Mineral Lip Liner

Sisley Phyto-Lèvres Perfect

Revlon Colorstay Lipliner

♡ WE LOVE…

Jo has a wide selection (Chanel, MyFace, Benefit) and is fairly unfussy about the brand, so long as the shade is right – a truly nude tone, since she's almost as afraid of VLL (Visible Lip Line) as VPL (Visible Panty Line) from a too-dark liner. Sarah favours Putty Lipliner by Valerie Beverly Hills, a creamy long-wearing pencil in a perfect neutral, both as lip liner and over well-conditioned lips.

TIP

Do condition lips before applying lip liner: even the creamiest can be a bit drying on dry lips! Apply balm and leave to sink in for a few moments before putting on lip product. (Actually do keep lips conditioned anyway, lip liner or not; see page 137 for lip treatments.)

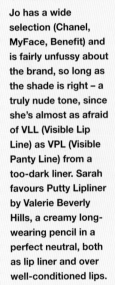

Lip-plumpers: our award winners

Nothing in a wand is going to give the plumping effect of something that comes in a cosmeto-dermatologist's syringe – but for millions of us who are happy to help nature along purely with cosmetics, a lip-plumper can be a useful addition to the beauty arsenal

AT A GLANCE

MAC Plushglass

Pixi Lip Booster

♡ WE LOVE...

The one that really works for Jo (so much that the tingle's almost painful!) is **Valerie Beverly Hills Bee Sting Lip Plump,** in a chic little silver mirrored compact. It's a cosmetic effect, rather than a long-term treatment – but definitely does make lips a touch more Bardot. Sarah almost never remembers to do it, but the Valerie lip-plumper certainly works – and it's fun!

True 'lip-plumpers' offer ingredients which actually increase the volume of the lips temporarily (such as capsicum, which works by bringing blood to the lips accounting for the tingle in the million or so nerve endings in the lips) – or for longer-term plumping contain ingredients to encourage the production of cushioning natural collagen in the lip area. Sad to report, this proved probably the most disappointing category in the book. Of more than 30 products we dispatched to our testers, just a couple proved worthy of inclusion – and reading testers' comments this was more to do with an instant optical illusion than any longer-term change. But do also see We Love…, left, and Lip Glosses on page 134: the message is that you can achieve a bee-stung look, albeit temporary (and rather a small bee…but better than a large trout we think).

REVIEWS

MAC Plushglass

 A sheer lip colour with a high-shine finish, MAC describe this as delivering 'a cool-warm vanilla buzz to the lips'. It features vitamin E and lip-conditioning ingredients, and is available in 13 shades (our testers received Ample Pink, a soft neutral). As we said above, although this was popular and gained a few high marks, the effect was transient. Testers differed widely on what they felt about the tingling!

Comments: 'Very effective for instant illusion of fullness – gave my lips a plump shimmery, sexy look – and stays on for ever. Loved it and will definitely buy' • 'instant tingle but not unpleasant, I re-applied every two hours and felt my lips were genuinely fuller and looked plumper within minutes of applying' • 'pale pink shade was very natural and youthful, subtle and beautiful; I re-applied every two hours' • 'the tingling made me think it was plumping out my lips and I think it did make them look a little fuller, but I wasn't keen on the "thick" feeling of the product' • 'created a genuinely puffy lips look but I found the "stinging" sensation uncomfortable' • 'pleasant sensation and I think the gloss made my lips look and feel slightly fuller and more youthful: a make-up bag staple'.

Pixi Lip Booster

 Pixi – a range started by a trio of Scandinavian sisters – is an old favourite of ours, and has done well here with a gloss designed to 'treat and restore lip vitality'. Over time, they claim this improves lip fullness by 40 per cent, decreases lines by 30 per cent and boosts lip moisture by 60 per cent. It's got a twist-up pen-style applicator with built-in brush to dispense the gloss; we dispatched in No 7 Daisy, a neutral.

Comments: 'A grown-up lip-plumper that is much better than other lip-plumping products I've tried; lips looked genuinely fuller within a few minutes; effect lasted about an hour' • 'modern exciting packaging, fruit fragrance, and lips did look plumper and smoother straight away – even if it's an optical illusion, it was very nice!' • 'a bit sticky but did work briefly and the brush was brilliant' • 'the bonus is that the gloss/colour made my teeth look white!'.

PS We would also point you in the direction of Rimmel Volume Booster Lip Plump Gloss, which did pretty well in our book *Beauty Bible Beauty Steals* (scoring 7.44/10). However, it wasn't re-submitted by Rimmel for this book, so wasn't sent specifically to more mature testers.

Lip treatments: *our award winners*

For lips and the surrounding skin, a treatment product can be a boon. The winners here are mainly uber-lip balms, which condition lips (and some plump them out). Use them on your lips for daytime hydration and at night on your lips and lip zone to target feathering

Among the many, many lip treatment options out there, these earned the biggest smiles from our panellists – and congrats to Clarins for grabbing the top two slots.

REVIEWS

Clarins Moisture Replenishing Lip Balm

8.35/10 Ingredients in this little tube of lip magic from the Clarins HydraQuench collection include essential rose wax, ceramide 3 (a super-moisturiser), shea butter and rice oil. It's not specifically designed to be 'anti-ageing', but Clarins submitted it for this category and the responses from our testers show it rose to the challenge.
Comments: 'Felt good and really delivered on performance: lips are smoother, softer and look more fulsome' • 'quite sticky to start with but soon absorbed and lips look healthier, plumper and more youthful' • 'healed my son's trumpet-playing sore chapped lips in 24 hours'.

Clarins Extra-Firming Lip & Contour Balm

8.31/10 Unlike the Clarins product above, this comes in a glass jar that's more bathroom- than handbag-friendly. Silky-soft and lightweight, the balm features Clarins's lip-plumping Maxi Lip Complex, to help boost production of collagen and plump and smooth fine lines, plus vitamin E. The fragrance is attractive, with star anise, cardamom, cinnamon and vanilla.
Comments: 'Lip-plumping, moisturising and really hydrating – fab, fab, fab!' • 'my lips look plumper and healthier and there is a slight reduction in feathering around them' • 'a soothing balm with a velvety texture which improved the condition of my lips 100 per cent; lips moister and more kissable!'.

Institut Esthederm Cyclo System Lip Contour Youth Cream

7.86/10 This cream formula – from a French brand with over 30 years of skin research under their belts – incorporates 'plant-based filling spheres' for an instant effect, together with shea butter, centella Asiatica, vitamin C and lipopeptides, plus what they call 'Cyclanol', to 'reactivate vital skin functions and compensate for hormonal deficiencies' (!). Don't just use it on lips: they recommend smoothing into the expression lines that go from nose to mouth, too. The pretty pot comes with its own spatula, which testers liked.
Comments: 'Excellent product. I applied night and morning as directed and it helped to alleviate the vertical lines between my nose and lips; lips are softer and fresher and skin around them softer and less lined' • 'oozes luxury and dermatological care: slight reduction in fine lines around lips'.

Renu Lip and Eye Active Lift

7.81/10 This does double duty: for eyes, as a targeted line treatment for furrows/grooves – and as an age-defying lip treatment. It's for this last purpose that our testers scored it highly. The wheat-free, pump-action formula works to resurface fine lines and 'targets deeper wrinkles with a firming, plumping action', Monu (who make the anti-ageing Renu range) tell us. Testers mostly liked the fact it meant one product for two purposes.
Comments: 'Increased lip plumpness and helped reduce lines; liked the pump action dispenser' • 'went a long way as one pump decanted enough for lips and eyes, very light, smooth and sheer; clever!' • 'lips felt smoother and lipstick seemed to bleed less, saw a distinct change in my eyelids too'.

AT A GLANCE

Clarins Moisture Replenishing Lip Balm

Clarins Extra-Firming Lip & Contour Balm

Institut Esthederm Cyclo System Lip Contour Youth Cream

Renu Lip and Eye Active Lift

♡ WE LOVE...

Ritualised several-times-daily use of a balm (our very own Beauty Bible Lip Balm, a real steal too!) goes a long way towards keeping our lips soft and supple, and Jo also applies Liz Earle Naturally Active Superskin Lip & Eye Treatment around the lip area, which she feels helps with any incipient 'feathering'. She also loves By Terry Or de Rose, a pink-tinted balm shimmering with 24-carat particles of gold (yes, it's a lip luxury). Sarah adores lip balms but isn't yet evolved enough to use another treatment – but she does smear her night facial oil over her lips, so perhaps that counts!

$\mathcal{L}$Moisturising lipsticks: *our award winners*

Don't know about you, but we like our lipsticks dewy, comforting and lip-replenishing. (Since they lack oil glands, lips are prone to dryness.) However, at this stage in life a moisturising lipstick offers more than a mere feel-good factor: its softly sheeny appearance is infinitely more flattering than any matt lip look

Which to choose? You'd do well to start with these top-scorers, from the couple of dozen we dispatched to testers. (NB: the one downside of moisturising lipsticks is they often need more frequent slicking, as the richer and creamier a formulation, the faster it slides off lips. But we think it's worth it, for sheer comfort and flatter-factor.)

REVIEWS

Clinique Colour Surge Butter Shine Lipstick

 Jo's favourite, this: really lip-quenchingly comfortable, with a beautiful glossy finish that lasts longer than most lipsticks, she finds. Its secret: special butters, moisturisers and modern waxes that melt at body temperature for a silky texture, plus high-shine 'gellants'. (A new word in beautyspeak!). Fifteen flattering shades (testers received 426 Perfect Plum, a soft mauve-y nude).
Comments: 'Really liked the glossy sheen; moisturising like a balm but with reasonable coverage and no lip gloss stickiness! Really pretty packaging. Not particularly long-lasting though' • 'very moisturising and creamy with a nice sheen' • 'smooth, velvety texture is absolutely lovely on lips, didn't leave my lips dry at all' • 'tube is gorgeous to whip out at a party and colour goes with almost everything in my wardrobe and I don't feel overdone: *love* it'.

Clarins Perfect Shine Sheer Lipstick

 Another very comfy, sensually-textured lipstick, with 'shine-activator' pigments that deliver the sheen-y, very sheer finish. There's mango butter, too, for a super-smooth,

lip-conditioning reflective surface, and of the ten shades available, we trialled browny-pink Praline.
Comments: 'Keeps lips feeling supple without clogging; slightly thicker than my usual Dior Addict Supershine, and stays on longer: I was impressed, good looks and good staying power' • 'very moisturising, lovely texture and glossy finish from this' • 'lips felt wonderfully soft and moisturised; could build up colour with several layers as texture was not too soft, rather medium-hard' • 'seemed to make my lips look fuller, which might have been down to the shine' • 'loved the gorgeous mirrored tube, beautiful for the summer, very natural colour with high gloss and glittery shimmer which caught the light – my new favourite!'.

YSL Rouge Volupté

 A really interesting texture which 'liquifies' on the lips, and is packed with hyaluronic acid microspheres 'to smooth, plump and beautify' (so YSL tell us). Weightlessly comfy, delivering a satin-smooth finish, and boasting a subtle mango fragrance, Rouge Volupté also shields lips with a protective rice bran compound, plus its SPF15. Our testers trialled Sweet Honey, a soft nude which we love but some of our testers didn't! – and marked it down solely because of that.
Comments: 'Lovely smooth, silky texture, sheer finish and very hydrating, fab packaging' • 'gorgeous glossy finish, smooth buttery texture – just lovely – who can beat YSL? Made me feel like a Hollywood starlet' • 'supremely comfortable, very soft, smooth and moisturising, glides over the lips almost by itself – gave glossy, sheer finish but with a

AT A GLANCE

Clinique Colour Surge Butter Shine Lipstick

Clarins Perfect Shine Sheer Lipstick

YSL Rouge Volupté

Benefit Silky-Finish Lipstick

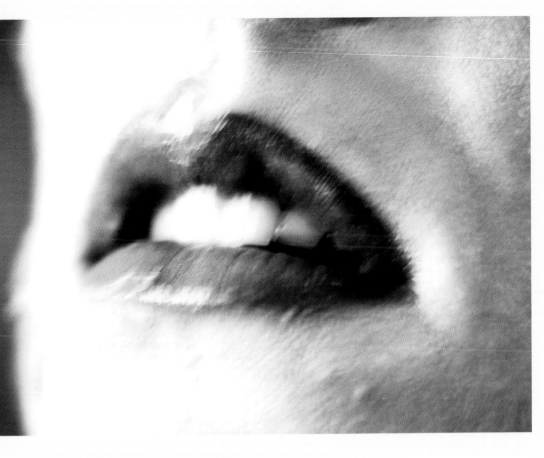

♡ WE LOVE...

The ranges Jo likes best offer a wide shade choice of lush-textured lipsticks: **Clinique Colour Surge Butter Shine Lipstick** (favourite shade Berry Blush, a terrific neutral), **Bobbi Brown Treatment Lip Shine SPF15** in Rosy (a warm pinky-brown) and **L'Oréal Color Riche Shine Gelée**, enriched with royal jelly for a balm-like feel in 303 Sweet Tea. For daytime, lazy Sarah usually wears a tinted lip balm (such as **Lanolips Lip Ointment in Rose**) over a natural-coloured lipliner (**Putty Lipliner by Valerie Beverly Hills**). She's also a big fan of **Clinique's Vitamin C Lip Smoothie Antioxidant Lip Colour** in soft rosy-brown Strawberry Fudge.

good colour; after a few days I thought my lips even looked a little fuller. And the ultimate accolade? It's the lipstick and shade I'll be wearing on my wedding day'.

Benefit Silky-Finish Lipstick

7.87/10 This tied with the YSL lipstick, above, and also offers a fairly light wash of colour that is 'buildable'. (You'd get extra strength of colour by applying with a brush.) There are 24 very wearable and mostly neutral shades and – OK, we own up – we forgot to note which our testers received.

Comments: 'Am loving this absolutely fab lipstick, would buy it for friends but can't bear to give the secret away! Mine all mine…!' • 'lovely silky, creamy texture that gave glossy finish, really moisturised lips, and lasted through three cups of coffee over two hours' • 'yummy, really soft and smoothing, like a duvet for the lips! Leaves my lips soft and kissable' • 'slanted angle made it easy to apply' • 'dream to apply, has a great sheen, very moisturising; wow, it looks so natural and feels so luxurious!'.

FINDING YOUR PERFECT LIP SHADE...

On younger women, paler-than-real-lip colours can look fantastic – but not now! And too dark shades can make an older mouth look harsh. Soft pinks, subtle corals and rosy-browns are the safest bet, subtly putting back the colour that disappears with age (because pigment decreases). Avoid opaque lipsticks: as you get older, solid colours can make the mouth look mean, while the drier matt formulas make lips look tiny and show every line. (That's why we've chosen specifically moisturising lipsticks here.)

Love your life

You can't freeze-frame life. It changes all the time, sometimes slowly, sometimes with chaotic speed. But what you can do is to adopt strategies to help you cope with the rollercoaster. How does that fit in with anti-ageing? A calm mind and taking joy in life make you look beautiful and live well. So laugh as much as you breathe and love as long as you live

Here are some of our favourite strategies, many of which are now used in healthcare.

Be loving to yourself. Sometimes loving and valuing yourself are very hard. That's when we're likely to cause ourselves grief, rely on others for our self-esteem, and make decisions – big and small – based on other people rather than what we really want for ourselves. You could start by just saying to yourself that you are a good person, not perfect – no one is (and please do give yourself permission to get things wrong, make a muddle, be imperfect in everything) – but you try your best. If you believe in spirituality, try thinking of yourself as 'a spark of the divine'. And above all, when you're faced with a decision, ask yourself what you really want to do. (And, of course, extend this loving way of thinking to everyone else too.)

The day starts better after a good night's sleep. We find we sleep soundly when we're glad and grateful. So when you go to bed, write down – or just list in your mind – at least three nice things that have happened. They can be as simple as hearing the birds sing, seeing the sun, or a phone call from a friend. Or praise at work. Or a great cup of coffee. A funny TV show… Then send blessings to the people you love. (And the world in general.)

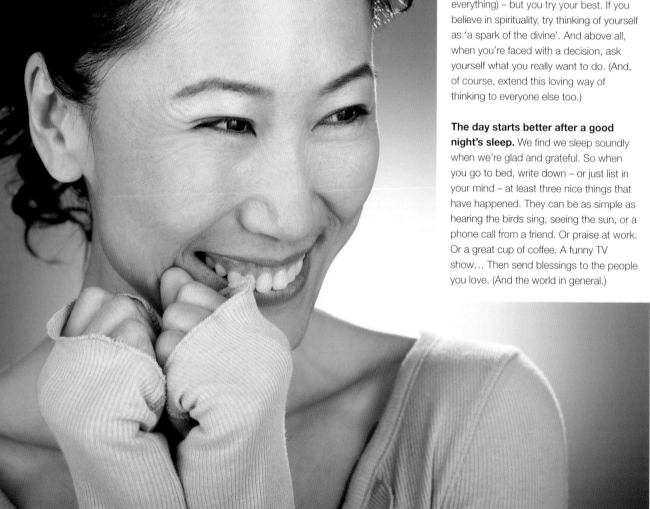

TIPS

Make things fun: wear a tiara when you're hoovering (try accessories or toy stores for gorgeous bargains); brighten tedious chores with your favourite music; trade help with a friend. Reward yourself with flowers, a movie, a good cup of coffee or tea with a friend.

Keep a Happy Box: collect mementoes of joyful times – letters and cards, emails these days! – inspiring photos, tickets from planes, boats, trains and concerts – and leaf through them when you're having a doleful day.

Don't make decisions in the middle of the night. Around 4am (when women tend to wake if there's something on your mind) is the dark hour of the soul, according to psychiatrist Dr David Servan-Schreiber, author of *Healing Without Freud or Prozac*. 'There's a fragile moment at the end of the first long period of deep sleep (about four hours into the sleep cycle) when we cross over into the lighter REM sleep [dreaming time]. Underlying anxiety – especially separation anxiety where we feel a threat to important relationships or a lack of fulfilling ones – manifests then.' Your brain can't process things then, he says, so please don't try: do the breathing exercise right, and if you don't fall asleep read a novel, do the ironing, listen to the radio or even watch a dotty DVD on your laptop.

When you wake up, decide that just for today your intention is that you will be as happy as you can be. Whatever happens. This doesn't mean you won't notice difficulties – of course you will. It does mean you will try to live in the solution, not the problem.

Breathe. Inhale for a count of four, hold for seven, then exhale very slowly to a count of eight. Repeat four to six times, feeling your breath go in and out of your body. If you like, imagine your breath is like a wave coming up a beach, hovering at the top, then ebbing slowly out to sea. Do this whenever you can during the day, but morning and bedtime at least.

Think of someone you love and stretch out your arms to them – literally. (If they're there to hug in person, so much the better.) You will find you're smiling and your heart is warm. Carry that feeling through the day.

Stretch some more. Do some yoga poses if you know them (for more on yoga, see page 204). Or just stretch your arms and legs out, shake your feet and hands – feel the fizz of energy.

Make yourself look as gorgeous as you can. Especially if it's a grey day – weather- or mood-wise. Wear colours, put on make-up, brush your hair.

If you have a wobbly moment of any kind, do the breathing exercise again. Bring your attention to the centre of your chest and widen it – don't cave in. Feel your shoulder blades sinking back, down and together. Then try saying 'yesss!', even 'thank you', and looking forward and up to a hill, a spire, the sky. (To understand why we suggest this, contrast it with looking down and saying 'no'.)

Never lose hope. If it seems to be slipping away, phone a friend but choose one who will support and encourage you – avoid the Eeyores.

Smile. Research has shown it sends feel-good hormones called endorphins rushing through your mind and body. You feel better. So does everyone else. Smiles make friends.

Examine the wobbliness. If you've done something wrong, put it right. Most likely you haven't and it's an old tape replaying in your head and body. Have a few drops of Bach's Rescue Remedy and count up the good healthy positive things in any situation. If the wobbliness persists, repeat again. If it is really troubling you, consider talking therapy of some kind and/or homeopathy.

Reach out to other people. Be nice – it's so much easier. Pay compliments. Listen, really listen.

Notice good things. Even tiny ones: store them up to remember at night and when things are difficult.

Never give up on passion. (We heard novelist Edna O'Brien say that, and she's now in her late seventies.) Yes, we do mean the physical sort of passion! And being passionately interested in people and things of all sorts. Be passionately creative too: paint, sing, play an instrument, garden, take photos – whatever you enjoy, do it!

Cultivate peace. We can't really tell you how – try seeing what makes you feel peaceful and doing more of it. Or it may be a case of 'being' rather than 'doing'.

Make yourself look as GORGEOUS as you can. *Wear colours*, put on make-up, brush your hair

Hang on to your marbles

Fewer lines and a trim waistline are all fine and dandy – but in the bigger scheme of things, nobody would question that keeping your brain sparky and your memory sharp(-ish) is going to do more for your quality of later life than pretty well anything else in this book

'Not fade away' is a BIG theme of *The Anti-Ageing Beauty Bible* – and it applies just as much to our brains, as well as to hair, complexion, eyebrows and so on.

Memory loss is probably the biggest brain-related anxiety we experience, once we hit a certain age. We're not talking about full-blown dementia, such as Alzheimer's disease – though that prospect can be seriously angst-inducing, especially if there's a family history – but about the Craft (Can't Remember a Flipping Thing) moments that strike everyone, usually kicking in around perimenopause. Naturopathic physician Dr Mosaraf Ali explains, 'Anxiety, depression, physical fatigue and anything which causes less blood flow to the brain weakens the ability to store or recall memories.' So: when you bump into someone unbelievably familiar but you can't remember their name (or how you know them), stress or exhaustion are the most likely explanations.

The good news is that, as experts agree, there are many, many lifestyle steps that we can all take to improve our memories.

Eat oily fish. It's rich in omega-3 essential fatty acids (EFAs), which researchers world-wide agree are vital for brain function; they have been shown to help depression and general mental acuity, as well as helping age-related memory loss and just possibly helping to prevent dementia (research is ongoing). These brain-friendly lipids can't be manufactured by the body, and must come from our diet. And the richest source of omega-3 EFAs is oily fish. So if you're vegetarian, like Jo, take them in the form of supplements (see page 180 for our suggestions). Everyone should also consume lots of dark green vegetables such as spinach, watercress, dried seaweed and spirulina (all of which also contain B group vitamins – see box opposite), walnuts, flax and hemp seeds and their oils, try these over vegetables and we like them stirred into baked beans... Phosphorus may also help the brain, and is needed for the body to absorb those vital B vitamins; it's found in oily fish and also in nuts (including walnuts, Brazil, cashew, peanuts, pecans and pine nuts), eggs, lentils, soya, wholegrains and – yay! – chocolate (the darker the better). You can self-test to see whether you are deficient in omega-3 EFAs with a simple at-home blood test (see DIRECTORY).

Do sudoku or quizzes or crosswords. And/or play a lot of Scrabble. All of these help with memory. The general principle is that exercising your brain with any different routines and new

tasks is effective. Learning to play the piano (it's never too late), a new language, even finding your way around a new city – any new skill – gives the memory area of your brain a vital workout.

Train your brain with an App. Every day at 8am, Jo's iPhone reminds her: 'It's time for your brain training.' She spends five minutes doing online games (matching shapes, colours, etc) which improve attention and memory, and speed up thinking time. The App is Brain Trainer by Lumosity (www.lumosity.com) and is available via iTunes. Graphs help you chart your progress – and the alarm is a reminder to do the brain exercises. (Although as your memory improves, the hope is you won't need a prompt.)

Eat ten almonds a day. They contain an incredible array of nutrients and are the richest source of vegetable protein. Soak them in room-temperature water for 24 hours, peel off the skins, crush and eat with a teaspoonful of Manuka honey, to benefit from micro-nutrients essential for brain function. Or add to muesli.

Support your memory with supplements. Ayurvedic practitioner Sebastian Pole prescribes Brahmi Plus, which combines organic herbs including gotu kola and bacopa monnieri, which increase memory and enhance concentration; it also lowers anxiety, clears your mind and revitalises your intellect. (We're sold on it.) We're also considering taking phosphatidylserine (PS), a phospholipid which has been shown to improve memory and mental acuity, due to multiple functions which basically help your brain cells talk to each other. (We're told Memory Lane by Power Health is a good formulation.)

Massage your head, neck and shoulders. This not only helps quell anxiety, but boosts blood flow to the brain. We are particularly keen on scalp massage as stress shortens the muscles in the scalp, making the scalp all but immobile in very frazzled people. Firm pressure with the pads of the fingers is pretty darned miraculous – or better still, book in for an Indian

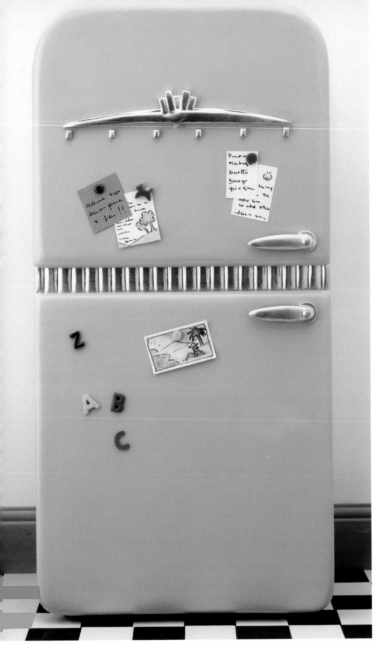

BE ON THE BALL WITH B VITAMINS

Over the past decade, research has increasingly shown that taking high doses of three B vitamins (B6, B12 and folic acid) can help age-related memory loss. These B vitamins help keep homocysteine (an amino acid) at a healthy level. Raised homocysteine may increase the risk of Alzheimer's and heart disease. Taking the vitamins probably won't help if you don't have a mild degree of memory loss but won't harm you and may help other things, eg, stress. If your brain is as sharp as a needle, we think it makes all-round good sense to eat plenty of foods containing these Bs. Find vitamin B12 in meat and fish, with folic acid and B6 in asparagus, lentils, most beans and leafy green vegetables (see our Supergreens Facelift Diet, page 176 – and combine the benefits for face and mind!). For specific supplements of the vitamins, see page 180.

yoga – nature's greatest anti-ageing wonder, in our opinion – see page 204.)

Avoid alcohol, coffee and cola-style drinks. Alcohol in particular is linked with poor memory (and not just in a where-the-hell-did-I-leave-my-keys-after-that-second-bottle-of-champagne way); if you are experiencing regular Craft moments, try cutting down or cutting out alcohol and seeing if that makes a difference, because it does affect the way brain cells communicate. (We're not suggesting that anyone becomes a nun. A special occasion is a special occasion, but for many people a few glasses of wine a day is a habit that's surprisingly easy to give up, once you've made the link with positive improvements.) Caffeine can exacerbate stress – and there's some evidence that, over time, the gradual increase of stress hormone (cortisol) levels in the blood can prevent the brain laying down a new memory, or from accessing existing ones.

Get plenty of sleep. We all know that when we're sleep-deprived, we can hardly remember our own names, let alone phone numbers and the fact we have to pick up our dry-cleaning. Sleep is the brain's way of processing events into memories. For more wisdom on better sleep, see page 208.

Head Massage, which many massage therapists are trained in. Use Google to find someone near you.

Don't multi-task. OK, so for most women this is like telling you to stop breathing. (Men, of course, are another matter…) But studies have shown that memory-related tasks can suffer in the hands of multi-taskers. At the very least, focus on doing – and finishing – one thing at a time. Practise mindfulness (more on page 144). You can sit still to do a waking mindfulness meditation – heck, you can even practise it while washing up. It's all about bringing your consciousness gently back to what you're doing. Whether that's walking, daydreaming – or doing the dishes.

Practise Iyengar yoga. The Cobra pose, which enhances circulation, may be of particular help to your brain. (For more on

And if all else fails, write it down. Whoever said you were meant to remember everything: birthdays, anniversaries, shopping lists, To Do lists, not to mention matching every name in your bulging address book to a face…? Be kind to yourself: the pressure we put our brains under is unprecedented in the history of humanity. Try not to stress out when your memory fails you, or feel it's the start of a slippery slope – it only makes things worse. It happens to us all. Stop, take a deep breath and let your mind rest for a moment. And remember (little joke!) that's what pens, paper, diaries, iPhones and online reminder services were meant for.

Be mindful of life's pleasures

Forget diets. It's time to enjoy your food, eat just the right amount through 'mindful eating' (and lose that middle-age spread effortlessly)

As the years go by, it's ridiculously easy for the pounds to roll on. For most women after the menopause, the evidence is probably lurking around your waistline (we tend to gather fat around our middles due to a shift in the ratio of oestrogen to testosterone). Clothes are tighter. Maybe there's a muffin-top that didn't used to be there. And suddenly, you get as excited over a new pair of Spanx control pants as you once did over frilly, skimpy smalls.

Traditionally, women have turned to extreme diets to combat excess pounds. Trouble is that diets tend not to work long term because they're hard to stick to (and some you shouldn't stick to 'cos they are just plain dangerous).

But there is new thinking that part of the reason we gain weight is that in our busy, stressful world, we're simply not paying attention to what we eat. Think on this. What did you last eat? What did it taste like? Smell of? Did you really enjoy it? Chances are you just don't remember… We're so used to filling our tummies with food like we fill our cars with fuel that we mostly do it on autopilot. Mindlessly. While we do six other things. (Multi-tasking can be a disadvantage sometimes.) The result is that, often, we eat far more than we need because we just don't notice what we're doing. And we pile on the pounds. Because we've eaten too much. Simple!

But it's also quite simple and fun to practise 'mindful eating' – as well as eating well, of course (it won't work if you eat mindfully mashed potato, pasta, cakes and puds for every meal). The bottom line is: it's all about loving your food! 'Mindful eating' is a new (well, old but rediscovered) approach, which is proving very helpful for people who want to lose weight on a permanent basis, not the see-saw of weight loss and gain that's so familiar from so many diets.

So: let's start again…

Go and make yourself something you really enjoy. Needn't be complicated but take enough time to make certain it tastes and looks delicious. Find your favourite place to eat, sitting at a table. Or treat yourself to a coffee or tea and lemon tart at your favourite patisserie.

Now…start by taking a few slow breaths to relax. Look at the food. Notice the colours, texture, smell. Then take the first mouthful. Don't do anything else at all. Just look and taste and smell. Swallow slowly, chewing thoroughly if necessary. Go on to the second mouthful and do the same. Finish your food in the same way, deliberately paying attention to it. That's what mindfulness is – being fully aware of what's happening. With food, it's the sensations and thoughts that occur as we eat. The colours, aromas, textures, flavours, even sounds of the food. And drink – think of the sensation as you taste the chocolate powder on a cappuccino, encounter the cool milky foam, the contrast with the hot, intensely-flavoured coffee.

If your mind wanders, just bring it gently back to what you're consuming. Sometimes it's helpful to say it to yourself, aloud or in your head: 'Now I'm biting into a peach, through the furry skin into the flesh, feeling the juice run down my chin…'

If you like to read or watch TV when you're eating on your own, try to do one thing at a time. So stop reading while you take a mouthful, taste, chew, swallow. Then pick up your book. You will focus on both more completely. (Ideally, ditch the book and switch off the TV.)

If you're eating with friends, it's still possible to be mindful. The key is to do it slowly – and lovingly. So often when you eat out, the food which your host/ess (or the restaurant chef) has cooked and cosseted like a baby is dispatched without anyone really appreciating it. Thinking and talking about each part of the meal is a compliment. So it's win-win!

MORE ON MINDFULNESS

Mindfulness is based on Buddhist philosophy; it's not a religion and you don't need to be religious to practise it. It's the art of staying in the moment and accepting what is – because it is already here. It's a way of slowing thoughts and feelings, keeping the helpful ones, gently discarding any that are foolish and/or harmful without criticising yourself in any way. So that you can access peace of mind at any time. It was developed in the West by Professor Jon Kabat-Zinn, who studied molecular biology and also yoga and Buddhist studies. He developed the concept of mindfulness, and Mindfulness-Based Cognitive Therapy (MBCT) to help people cope with stress, anxiety, pain and illness.

The New Economics Foundation (an independent British think-tank focused on economic wellbeing) says that being mindful is 'noticing'. Look at the number of things we all do mindlessly every day: the article you read without retaining more than 10 per cent, the people you talk to without listening…and the meal you ate without tasting a morsel. You can shift that, suggests the NEF, by bringing your attention to the present: 'Be curious. Catch sight of the beautiful. Remark on the unusual. Notice the changing seasons. Savour the moment. Be aware of the world around you and what you're feeling.' We promise: life tastes sweeter when you're mindful.

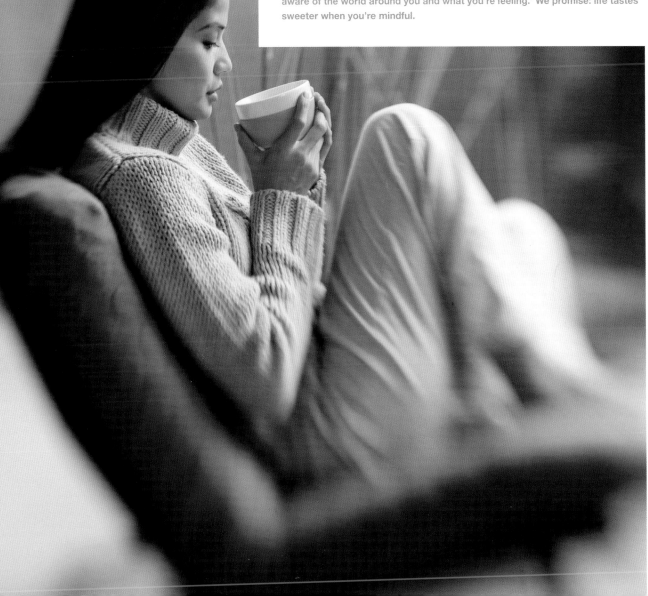

Minimise those bad (facial) hair days

Stop yourself turning into a moustachioe-d lady – here's the lowdown on hair removal

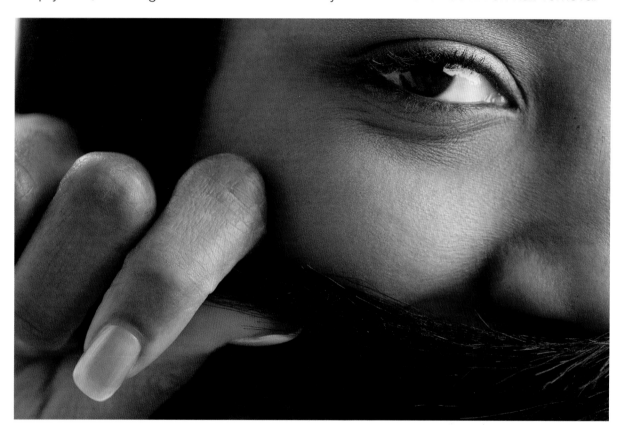

One of the most common questions we're asked is how to get rid of moustaches and, to a lesser extent, other areas of facial hair. We recommend having an appointed 'facial hair buddy' who will tell you when you're sprouting, and you can reciprocate. Mole hairs, in particular, make a break for it after menopause and, as eyesight fades, they can be easily missed.

Now conversely, one of the great blessings of ageing is that elsewhere on the body hair becomes finer and may even disappear altogether (hoorah!). But if you're still fighting excess hair anywhere on the face/body, here's a useful rundown of all the removal techniques you need to know about.

One warning with moustaches: depending on the density of down on the rest of your face (we all have it so don't have conniptions!), completely removing your moustache may leave an obvious hairless patch. In this case, electrolysis is a good option

as the therapist can just take out the coarser, more visible hairs. Alternatively, you could have the whole of your face threaded (but that's quite high-maintenance, so be warned).

Never shave your face. We differ about shaving for legs: Jo does, Sarah doesn't. (If you do, make sure to use a razor dedicated for just this purpose – Jo favours the Gillette Venus range.) But shaving a moustache leads to stubble, and you eventually end up having to do it every day, and fretting over someone feeling a bristly upper lip when they kiss you.

First try bleaching – not so much removal as a disguise. Many of us grew up with crème bleach, and for fine, sparse moustache hairs, it's still an option. However, some testers report that it can sting so much, particularly on your face, that you end up red-skinned, with varying shades of ginger facial hair because you've had to wash it off too soon. Bleach comes in different versions for face and body: get the right one! And please read and follow the instructions to the letter: do a patch test first, every time, don't use with Retin-A, or fruit acids of any kind, and only use on the areas it's listed as safe for.

Experiment with tweezing. Simple, cheap and great for eyebrows, but not recommended for more than the odd stray hair on the rest of your face as it may irritate hair follicles, causing sensitivity and even scarring.

Melt hair clean away with a depilatory cream. These relatively cheap products dissolve hair at the base of the follicle and are useful for legs and underarms (though you'll need to do it often), less so for the face as even dedicated facial versions may irritate sensitive skin, and may not remove all the hairs.

Find a good salon, and try waxing. With waxing, warm/hot wax is applied to skin, then ripped off with a muslin strip bringing the hairs with it. It's usually effective for upper lip and fine hair on the sides of your face, but not suitable for coarser hair on the chin. Never let the therapist use a metal knife for this: it may burn your skin – they should only ever use a wooden implement, and we like salons best which provide a hygienic pack in which every single spatula is used once only, rather than repeatedly dipped.

Get sweet on sugaring. Sugaring uses the same procedure as waxing except that the sugar tends to stick only to the hairs not the skin – so it can be more comfortable. It does need a skilled practitioner to be effective.

Or try threading. (We love threading.) This is an ancient method of hair removal practised in Asian countries. A pure, thin twisted cotton thread is rolled rapidly over untidy areas. As well as shaping brows, skilled practitioners can remove hair anywhere on the face, all over if desired. It's not painful in our experience, but not comfy (it 'pings'). Again it's temporary and needs upkeep.

For permanent hair removal, look at electrolysis. A fine needle conducting an electric current is inserted into the hair follicle, destroying it. You may need several sessions with some maintenance later, but it's an ideal option for a small number of coarse facial hairs, although it is impractical for larger areas, according to consultant dermatologist Dr Nick Lowe of the Cranley Clinic, London.

Laser hair removal is another option. Here, the hair follicle is effectively cauterised with a laser. It's a perfect choice for upper lip hair, says Dr Lowe. Advances in technology mean that any hair with pigment in it can be lasered. (Which usually precludes

treatment of white or grey hair.) There used to be a problem treating coloured skin but new lasers protect tanned, Asian or black skin from losing pigment. These newer modified lasers incorporate cooling technology, says Dr Lowe, who uses the Alexandrite 755 nanometre laser, which cools the skin with a high-flow jet of cold air.

Be aware: laser hair removal won't give you results overnight. (And it's expensive.) It will take between three and six sessions to get the optimum reduction of hair growth, depending on the thickness. And please note: reduction not permanent removal. 'None of the lasers will totally and permanently remove all hair, but this method will achieve up to 70 or 80 per cent in a lot of patients, and patients can come back for maintenance sessions,' advises Dr Lowe. To help extend the time between maintenance (and minimise regrowth), he recommends a prescription cream called Vaniqa, which interferes with some of the proteins that form hair. On the positive side, Dr Lowe says laser hair removal usually works extremely well, and is also useful for ingrowing hair.

Appoint a facial hair buddy who will tell you when you're sprouting

Don't go near lasers if you have pigmentation problems. Laser hair removal is not suitable for anyone with vitiligo (patches of de-pigmented skin) as it may stimulate new areas. Anyone with eczema, psoriasis, hives or urticaria should have a patch test first.

Beware of IPL. Many beauty salons offer treatment with IPL (Intense Pulsed Light), as do some cosmetic surgery clinics. However, Dr Lowe advises caution: 'I've seen so many patients that have had burns and blisters, loss of pigment and scars.' (Dr Lowe uses IPL systems for removal of thread veins, sun spots and for rejuvenating skin.)

And be very careful where you have any laser or IPL treatment. Dr Lowe cautions against booking laser hair removal at beauty salons: you should go to an experienced trained physician at a reputable clinic. We recommend you follow the same guidelines for this as any 'cosmetic tweak' such as Botox, etc, to optimise your chances of the best outcome – see page 46.

A final caution: very occasionally with these high-tech methods of hair removal, hair growth may be stimulated instead of reduced, due to the technology not delivering enough energy to the hair follicle; usually the problem can be overcome by switching to a different laser system. But it's another big argument for going to someone who is trained properly and experienced.

'The only real
ELEGANCE
is in the mind;
if you've got that,
the rest *really*
comes from it'

Diana Vreeland

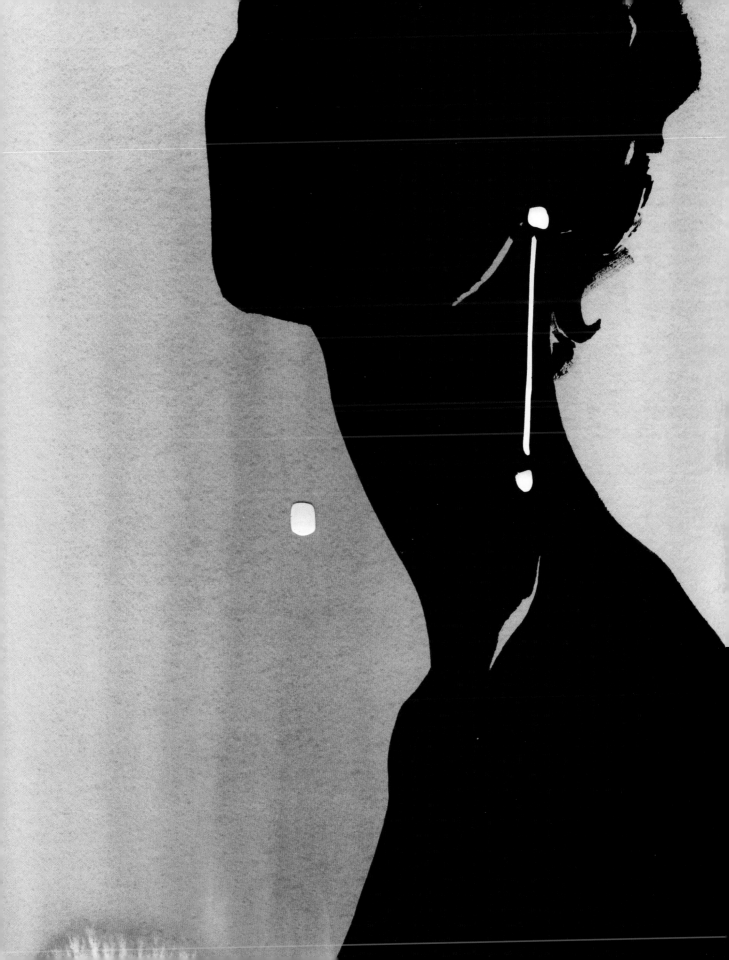

Nourish your neck
(and keep it swan-like)

As our necks start to sag and the texture looks crêpey, our hearts begin to sink. The reality is that the skin is much thinner on the neck than on our faces, and thus more easily damaged. (And we do tend to overlook it.) So, no more neglect – just lavish it with loving care

To misquote Nora Ephron, don't feel bad about your neck.
We love Nora Ephron (screenwriter for *Heartburn*, *Julie & Julia*, etc), and author of the hilarious collection of essays, *I Feel Bad about My Neck*, in which she writes: 'One of my biggest regrets – bigger even than not buying the apartment on East Seventy-fifth Street, bigger even than my worst romantic catastrophe – is that I didn't spend my youth staring lovingly at my neck. It never crossed my mind to be grateful for it… Of course now I am older, I'm wise and sage and mellow. And it's also true that I honestly do understand just what matters in life. But guess what? It's my neck.'

We agree with Nora that necks can be angst-inducing. But we say: any neck – even 'turkey neck' (that unpicturesque term for a sagging neck) – can be improved, with targeted and diligent TLC.

Make like a Frenchwoman and 'double-moisturise'. One of the key issues with the neck is crêpiness, as the skin on the neck has relatively few oil glands and without moisture and lipids, it can start to look papery super-fast. Get into the habit of applying everything you put on your face right down to the bra-line. At the same time, sweep any body lotion up to your chin, so it gets twice the nourishment. Your neck and chest should be part of your 'cleansing zone', but avoid using a scrub on the neck, although a muslin cloth (used with cleanser) is fine.

And consider a targeted neck product. For our testers' favourites, and ours too, see overleaf.

Protect your neck with an SPF15 plus. As dermatologist Dr Nick Lowe tells us, 'The neck is easily damaged by sun exposure as the skin is much thinner than it is on other parts of the face, and its support structure is not as effective.' So the ceaseless battering of UV light breaks down collagen and elastin, leading to sagging. Any SPF you apply to your face – your first line of defence against ageing – should be applied to the neck, the chest and the décolletage, religiously. End… Of… Story. If you tend to 'miss' the sides of the neck because your hair's in the way, scoop it off your face pre-application. If you do have 'age spots' on your neck and chest, see our recommendations for treating these on page 190.

Avoid wearing perfume in the sun. Many a woman's list of neck woes includes pigmented areas either side of the neck. Certain fragrance ingredients – generally citrus-derived – contain psoralens, components which over-stimulate the pigment-producing cells. This produces localised brown patches (medically called Berloque dermatitis), that look like a streak of brown pigment rather like a raindrop running down a window pane. (Plus the alcohol in the scent dries out the skin.) The solution? If you want to enjoy a summer fragrance in the sun, try spritzing it on your clothing rather than your skin. (Check first, of course, that it doesn't discolour the fabric: you can try it on a tissue.) Or wear a ribbon around a wrist or your neck, drenched in scent, à la Marie Antoinette and her mob. Spritz a hankie with scent and tuck it in your bra – or your swimsuit, as long as you're not planning to get wet. And, of course, enjoy liberally after dark. Just be certain to cleanse away the fragrance the next morning with a wet flannel, before you go anywhere near the sun.

Take up yoga. One of the key reasons women develop 'turkey neck', double chins and those 'necklace rings' on the neck is because underlying muscles are weak. So neck firming is yet another reason to add to the list of why embracing yoga is a good idea (more on page 204). It's fantastic, fantastic, fantastic for strengthening the neck and the jaw and – as we've observed in previous books – we know seventy-something yoga devotees who have sharp jaw-lines and smooth, swan-like necks. And we want to be like them. It's not just us. Esteemed dermatologist Dr Karen Burke observes: 'If you do yoga you can postpone facelifts for years. People have those sharp jawlines because they're doing a total stretch.'

Raise the height of your computer screen.
Whether you use a laptop or a full-size screen on your desk, you should make sure that it's high enough for you to look straight at it, rather than looking down.

Embrace polo-necks, pashminas, scarves and pearl chokers. If you really still feel Nora Ephron-ish about your neck, short of surgery/lasers (we'll come on to that), camouflage is your best option. These all hide a multitude of sins. Not everyone suits a polo-neck, but if you generally look better with a scoop- or a v-neckline, you can create a flattering optical illuson that draws attention downwards by hanging a necklace or rope of pearls over the top. Wear earrings, too, which distract the eye from your neck. But you have to trust us: nobody looks as unforgivingly on your neck as you do.

As a last resort, there's surgery. And fillers. And Intense Pulsed Light (IPL) treatments. We are going to point you in the direction (not for the first time in this book) of Wendy Lewis, who is the fount of all cosmetic surgery wisdom. In her book *Plastic Makes Perfect* (see ANTI-AGEING BOOKSHELF), she devotes several pages to all the options, which range from 'plastysmaplasty' (to tackle 'turkey wattle') to liposuction and the fillers Restylane and Perlane. But any procedure to do with the neck is A Big Deal (remember: your main artery and all the important nerves go through the neck); botched neck treatments happen. If you can afford any of these procedures, you can afford to talk to Wendy first: she is completely independent and not affiliated with any doctor, but knows better than anyone on the planet who's best at what.

And if you still feel bad about your neck, read Nora Ephron. Because at least there's someone who feels worse about hers than you do.

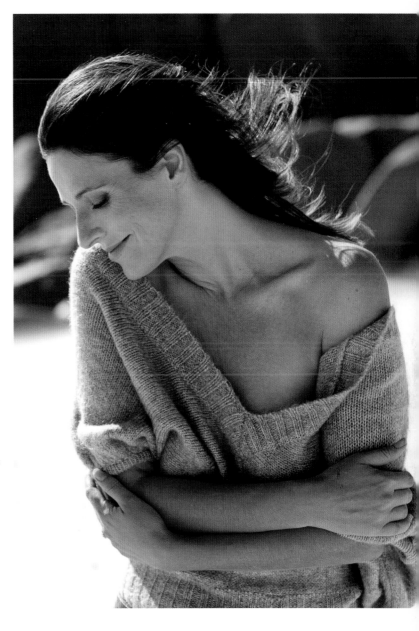

'I look forward to getting older when looks should become less of an issue, and when who you are is the point' Susan Sarandon

N

Neck treatments: *our award winners*

Why do so many women buy neck creams, only to leave them languishing on the bathroom shelf? Is it a belief that nothing can make a difference to this notoriously hard-to-treat area? Certainly, the key with any neck treatment is ritualistic use – preferably twice a day (and it does no harm to shield the area with an SPF15 during daylight) – and a high pleasure factor helps to encourage that ritual. If you follow our testers' recommendations and are religious with any of the following creams (the victors from among more than 40 trialled just for this book), you may be as pleased as they were

AT A GLANCE

Clarins Super Restorative Décolleté and Neck Concentrate

Liz Earle Superskin Concentrate

RéVive Fermitif Neck Renewal Cream SPF15

Liz Earle Skin Repair Moisturiser Dry/ Sensitive

This Works Perfect Cleavage for Neck & Chest

Lulu's Time Bomb Trouble Shooter Neck, Jaw & Chest Firming Cream

REVIEWS

Clarins Super Restorative Décolleté and Neck Concentrate

 This fluid treatment is instantly skin-firming, moisturising – and features a combination of plant extracts for its age-defying power (we really don't think you need the complicated, Linnaean list of specific botanicals!). It is also said to lighten pigmentation spots, used over time, through a vitamin C derivative. Clarins recommend a specific one-minute massage technique to enhance the effects (you'll find it slipped inside the box).

Comments: 'Such a treat – can't emphasise how much I loved the silky texture and beautiful smell: you're advised to massage it in so it's a treat that way too: neck and décolletage appreciably smoother and softer, less fragile and with a slight gleam – lovely, lovely, lovely!' • 'fine lines have much improved, some disappeared, and deeper ones less noticeable; texture and sink-in-ability faultless' • 'very definite improvement in neck area especially, much smoother, less crêpey, necklace lines much less visible, looks younger and smoother – am so pleased and impressed!'.

Liz Earle Superskin Concentrate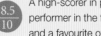

 A high-scorer in previous books, a stellar performer in the facial oil category here, and a favourite of Jo's… Well, Liz Earle sent another ten bottles of this to be trialled as a

neck treatment, and they obviously knew what they were doing: the argan- and rosehip-rich oil, turbo-charged by vitamin E, came up trumps here too. (NB: the aromatic essential oils are said to aid restful sleep, as a bonus.)

Comments: 'Very noticeable difference immediately; greatly improved smoothness, which continued with use; skin feels softer and smoother, the biggest difference is to fine lines which are far less noticeable – a fantastic product' • 'neck felt and looked plump and smooth; healthier, fresher skin' • 'skin looks and feels beautiful, and younger because smoother' • 'I love, love, love this product! Smells great, feels great and makes my skin look great! Neck is certainly less craggy, has eliminated all signs of crêpiness and dryness, lines finer and less visible, skin moisturised and supple'.

RéVive Fermitif Neck Renewal Cream SPF15

 We often wonder why more neck creams don't incorporate an SPF, since the neck's so vulnerable to sun damage. Hallelujah: this one does (a chemical sunscreen, note), in a luxurious, softly rose-scented cream with special firming agents from wheat protein and barley extract, plus what RéVive call their 'youth molecule'.

Comments: 'Skin immediately lovely and velvety to touch, supple and plumped up; with regular use, everything is smoothed out and fine lines much

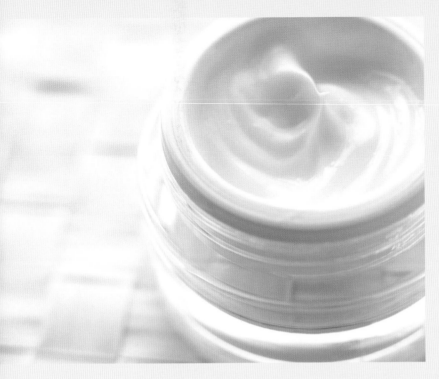

more faded, neck looking much younger' • 'skin on neck and décolletage feels much firmer, softer and looks better – more supple, wouldn't have believed that this product could make such a change' • 'skin looks glossier and firmer – just loved this product and think it does an amazing job'.

Liz Earle Skin Repair Moisturiser Dry/Sensitive

8.41/10 Interesting! This everyday moisturiser from Liz Earle did well in previous books as a neck treatment, even though it's not specifically labelled as such. Once again, they sent us ten pots to be specifically trialled for this book. And guess what? Once again, Skin Repair got a great score from this entirely new bunch of neck-conscious testers. Packed with plant avocado and borage oil, echinacea, pro-vitamin B5, antioxidants – all the botanicals which are the signature of Liz's so-successful range, in fact.

Comments: 'Fantastic: the skin on my neck drank up this product like it had been stranded in the desert, immediately became plumper, smoother and felt more comfy; neck looks much younger and healthier – you absolutely must try it!' • 'gave a kind of "soft focus" effect to lines' • 'skin felt instantly nourished by this rich, light cream, absorbs like magic, have never used a cream that made my skin feel so soft, supple and moisturised – would like to score it 12/10!'.

♡ WE LOVE...

From being too lazy to use anything at all on her neck, full-on neck panic now has Jo veering between two favourites. The serum-like Liz Earle Superskin Bust Treatment is now (at Jo's own suggestion!) going to be rebranded as Neck & Bust Treatment, because it's also fantastic for this purpose. But the incense-y smell of Neal's Yard Remedies Rejuvenating Frankincense Firming Neck Cream also inspires Jo's slavish devotion. Sarah has always slathered moisturiser on her (long) neck and chest and now slops on facial oil too (any, all!), which is very effective.

This Works Perfect Cleavage for Neck & Chest

8.28/10 We're personally delighted that this product from our beauty editor friend Kathy Phillips's range did so well here, having previously had so many anecdotal good reports. With larch extract, yellow algae and pomegranate, rose oil, patchouli and tonka bean, it's sensually-scented, the packaging's chic – and Kathy's own smoothly swan-like neck is Perfect Cleavage's own best advertisement. (Though the yoga – which she's practised daily for decades – may help…!) Testers particularly liked its effect on the décolletage.

Comments: 'Nice texture that's easy to spread, sinks in very quickly and smells absolutely lovely; the wrinkles on my neck look much better and I have had less spots since using' • 'less crêpiness with this lovely serum – I have gone and bought a couple more, which says it all' • 'dryness and texture improved, encouraged me to put cream much lower down than just my neck – lives up to its promise of being tightening, nourishing and shimmering!' • 'loved this product, which improved fine lines, crêpiness and made neck look younger and smoother'.

Lulu's Time Bomb Trouble Shooter Neck, Jaw & Chest Firming Cream

8.25/10 This formula from the ever-youthful singer's age-defying range was created to firm skin and lighten age spots, blending 'chrysanthellum extract' (to target jaw-droop), vitamin E, pea extract, shea and sunflower seed butters, plus white truffle extract. Happily, it smells gorgeously of Lulu's favourite lavender oil, rather than a risotto…!

Comments: 'Loved this thick cream that absorbed like a lotion and felt incredibly hydrating; definite improvement in fine lines and sagging under chin, jaw contour looks more pronounced, neck looked considerably younger and smoother' • 'really liked this product, nice texture, smells lovely, did improve my neck – made it very soft and smooth' • 'neck did feel very smooth and tightened, soft and supple'.

'Lift' your face – without surgery...

(Yes, it's possible.) Maybe you want to look your best for a special occasion. Or perhaps your face would love a boost after a stressful time. But you're not up for surgery, fillers, dermabrasion or lasers – so what's to do…? Here are the (non-surgical) fixes that we know really work

Try CACI. Over the years we've been in the beauty business, we've pretty much tried out all the non-surgical facelift systems. These mostly involve probes carrying low-voltage electric currents which are moved over your face to make the muscles jump around and work harder, giving a temporary lift – sometimes versions of these are used in tandem with facials. Of the many that have been launched over the past two decades, the one that has stood the test of time world-wide is CACI, which stands for Computer Aided Cosmetology Instrument. From the one original option (CACI Classic), there's now an almost bewildering range – which extend to microdermabrasion and ultrasonic peeling, and beyond the face to include CACI for bust enhancement, stretch

marks and cellulite. We honestly don't know how well all that works – but we do know that for a temporary (24 to 48 hours) boost, a CACI treatment can be rejuvenating. (And just lying still for an hour or so is a big bonus for many busy women.) For longer-term results, CACI recommend ten to 15 treatments and then maintenance sessions every four to six weeks. (Worth considering, we'd say, if you enjoy it, like the results and your budget permits.)

Find a great facialist. For our money, a good facial with massage by skilled hands can give some gorgeous instant results. (On page 79 you'll find our favourite facialists, but talk to girlfriends and investigate local talent – you might find a hidden magic-worker just around the corner. (Tell us if you do, at www.beautybible.com!) Some facialists undoubtedly have healing hands; indeed one of our fave raves Emma Hardie (who now has a lovely skincare line with products that regularly feature in our award winners) started out in the early 1990s with her own natural lifting and sculpting facial. Sarah wrote about it for *YOU magazine*, other beauty editors (including *Harper's Bazaar*'s Newby Hands) endorsed it – and Emma has become a legend in natural rejuvenation.

Get the needle! We swear by facial acupuncture. And believe us, the needles truly aren't scary. (The only version we did find too much to take was electro-acupuncture, where the needles carry a current which is progressively increased. You need to be made of sterner stuff than we are for that.) Sarah really loves a treatment from Annee de Mamiel, formerly a successful banker who studied acupuncture after recovering from cancer. Annee treats your whole body, explaining: 'Beauty is about being balanced on the inside, in every way – physically and psychologically. If you feel good about yourself, it reflects in the way you look. Dry, wrinkled, saggy skin mirrors what is happening in your body, so I look at the roots of the problems and treat those too.' For instance, the common problem of vertical lines between your eyebrows can relate to liver energy not flowing properly (frowning too much is a factor too!), so as well as needling the lines themselves, Annee treats the liver. As well as acupuncture, she makes up specially blended oils for each client plus a herbal tea to take home. Annee incorporates stimulating Tui Na Chinese massage (to invigorate the skin) and lymph draining massage and acupressure to relax you from top to toe. An increasing number of acupuncturists now offer facial acupuncture; ask friends for recommendations. (Jo sees a fab Hove-based therapist called Steve Mason for this.)

Just say 'ouch'. Much the most painful treatment Sarah has endured is having the muscles inside the mouth at the base of the tongue released by osteopath Vicky Vlachonis in London (who learned it from French obstetrician Michel Odent). As she wrote at the time, 'The results are extraordinary: any downward drift perks up and the contours of your face seem redefined – truly a non-surgical facelift moment.' And the pain is definitely worth the

TIP

If there's one low-tech gizmo we'd recommend for ironing out your face at home it's Sarah Chapman's Facialift, an odd-looking contraption with eight small knobbly cogs on a handle which rotate as you push them up and down your face. Good for massaging in product, or simply for stimulating the skin tissue and encouraging lymph drainage.

'BEAUTY is about being balanced on the inside. If you feel *good* about yourself, it reflects in the way you LOOK'

gain, according to Carine Roitfeld, editor of French *Vogue*, who recently revealed that this internal facial massage is her secret for looking younger. 'They put on gloves and massage inside because all your stress is in your jaws. It hurts very much, but is my beauty secret,' she says. NB: if you want to try this do make sure you go to a practitioner who has really learnt this technique: you don't want to be a guinea pig.

Do it yourself. If you haven't got the time, budget or opportunity to have a treatment, you really can achieve wonders by yourself. Start by sipping some still room-temperature water, then spend a moment or two focusing on your breathing, as Annee suggests:

● Do this breathing exercise throughout the day: inhale through your nose to a count of three, exhale through your mouth for five, then pause for a second or two and let your body and mind go still and release tension.

● If possible, apply an instant face reviver (see page 212 for our testers' top-scoring products).

● Massage your face to relax muscles, allowing oxygenated blood to flow freely and toxins to be released, leaving you with a fresher, brighter complexion, less puffiness and fewer wrinkles. (See page 78 for guidelines.)

● Practise some yoga, or lie flat on your back for five minutes (more if you have it), knees bent, eyes closed (with damp teabags over them if possible). In your mind's eye, see blue sky – and as stray thoughts pop into your brain, convert them into clouds and let them float away.

Think nice thoughts. Your skin and face reflect your state of mind. If you're stressed, you run the risk of looking pinched and peaky. Try thinking of a couple of nice things that have happened to you today – remember someone you love and, if you're having an iffy day, that you never know what delicious thing might be around the next corner. Even if life is really tough (and it happens to everyone), there's almost always something positive. Gratitude and hope are great beautifiers.

Night treatments: *our award winners*

On this page you'll find the 'miracle' products which – according to our testers – really do transform mere slumber into beauty sleep. Because of the body's repairing rhythms, most cellular patching-up happens while we're slumbering, so that many 'miracle' treatments are specifically designed to be used overnight. And because we don't need to slap on make-up over the top, night creams tend to be richer. Here are the night-time products our testers loved – out of over 90! – with some truly spectacular scores. (For day-time miracle treatments, turn to page 16 – also see Korres's entry, right…)

AT A GLANCE

Elemis Pro-Collagen Oxygenating Night Cream

La Prairie Anti-Aging Night Cream

Korres Thyme Honey 24-Hour Moisturising Cream

REN Omega 3 Night Repair Serum

Crème de la Mer Moisturizing Cream

Caudalie Vinexpert Night Infusion Cream

REVIEWS

Elemis Pro-Collagen Oxygenating Night Cream

 9.37/10 This outstandingly high-scorer is the night-time 'sister' product to a cream that's excelled in previous Beauty Bible books. Said to increase oxygen levels in the skin by 'up to 41 per cent', it combines an anti-ageing hexapeptide, marine extracts, antioxidants and *padina pavonica*, a potent algae to boost firmness and elasticity. Luxuriously priced too.

Comments: 'My skin just drunk it in, skin was plumped up and very soft, helps with wrinkles because it's so hydrating; skin looks much better and someone I hadn't seen in a while complimented me on a healthy glow' • 'a little goes a long way, so probably quite good value' • 'skin looks much fresher and plumper in the morning, smooth and calm; does enhance radiance, dehydrated areas have improved dramatically and wrinkles appear greatly reduced' • 'skin looks better in every way, clear, soft and glowing, skintone more even and calmer' • '*padina pavonica* seems to be a magic ingredient – this is the best night cream I have ever found, my hormonal skin has never looked better'.

La Prairie Anti-Aging Night Cream

 9.08/10 Again, a luxe-priced winner – though not as pricey as some La Prairie supercreams. We wondered how some of the key luxury names in skincare would perform in our trials – but our testers' comments show this sensuously-fragranced cream earned its high-scoring place purely on merit. Rich in peptides, it also features an extract of green micro-algae (again, to help production of collagen and elastin), plus La Prairie's signature Exclusive Cellular Complex. Allow a month to see a real difference, they advise.

Comments: 'LOVED it! Inside the silver box is a silver jar with a spatula and when you apply the cream skin feels nourished and has a radiance, makes you feel as if you have done something really, really good for your skin' • 'my skin is glowing and silken, more toned, lines beside eyes less visible, and two rather large frown lines between my eyebrows have lessened; I'm its biggest fan' • 'my mature fair skin looks younger, definitely addressed fine lines particularly around my mouth – I've had compliments – and my husband has bought me some more of their range' • 'skin greatly improved, softer and plumper, most fine lines reduced, some bigger wrinkles too, and I am told I look younger'.

Korres Thyme Honey 24-Hour Moisturising Cream

9.03/10 Just behind La Prairie, an impressive, lusciously honey-scented entry from Korres, a fast-growing Greek natural brand. Thyme honey is rich in antioxidants, as well as helping to maintain skin's ideal moisture level. Oops: our testers were asked to put it through its paces as a night treatment but it's designed to be used in the morning too.

Comments: 'Skin felt softer and silky smooth with a glow but not greasy; I absolutely love the honey smell, so good you could almost eat it! Left a soft, velvety feel to my skin, hydrates well for 24 hours; people say my skin is glowing' • 'skin felt instantly nourished, smooth and renewed when I used it for the first time; sinks in within a few seconds, my skin is in a lot better condition and plumper, so fine lines not so apparent; my two daughters say my skin certainly looks better' • 'a little goes a long way' • 'skin plumped up the first morning after I applied it, had a pretty immediate effect with less obvious lines and much fresher – a little sticky but it does seem to get results and the smell is addictive!'.

REN Omega 3 Night Repair Serum

8.93/10 A rich, unctuous night serum, certainly not something for applying under make-up. Blended with rosehip seed oil, gold of pleasure oil, coconut oil and wheatgerm oil, plus soothing chamomile, it has generous levels of omega-3 fatty acids. To be honest, we could have categorised this as a facial oil, or a serum, but went by REN's stated purpose for their product: 'To ensure skin gets its beauty sleep'.

Comments: 'Skin looked more luminous after 48 hours; liked the rich but light texture which was very quickly absorbed into skin, definitely enhanced radiance; very pleasant smell – like honeysuckle – would definitely buy' • 'I am impressed, skin softer, more rested-looking, brighter and healthier – I look like I've had more sleep than I have, even my husband said I looked young and fresh-faced – does it come in industrial-sized vats?' • 'my skin looks finer and smoother so younger!' • 'it makes a real difference to my skin, more so than many products that claim anti-ageing benefits'.

Crème de la Mer Moisturizing Cream

8.85/10 Aha! We knew it! Any doubting Thomasinas who are cynical about Crème de la Mer's anti-ageing powers can please be silenced now. In our totally independent trial, this legendary rich cream – created by a NASA scientist to deal with severe chemical burns, based on a 'Miracle Broth' including marine ingredients – has put on a stellar performance. Our experience is that it's suitable for even the most sensitive complexions, but it's rich and best applied with a special 'pressing' technique (explained inside the box).

Comments: 'Can I give this 11 out of 10? The difference is unbelievable, skin much plumper and "rested", softer and more alive, sank in quickly and I felt a slight tightening and toning effect; definitely has anti-ageing benefits, lots of friends have commented how well my skin is looking – bring it on!' • 'amazing! My skin looks wonderful, so smooth, soft and with an extra brightness; I look years young and fresher, as if I've slept well for a month' • 'I loved this product: I've always been against paying so much – but it's worth it' • 'absolutely fantastic; it saw me through a very nasty chest infection when I would usually have looked corpse-like, and even looked good after insufficient sleep too – a real bonus'.

Caudalie Vinexpert Night Infusion Cream

8.71/10 Grapes – grape-seed oil, grape-seed extract, grape-seed polyphenols or the uber-antioxidant resveratrol – are the signature of every skincare creation within the Caudalie range, which was born on a vineyard near Bordeaux. This nourishing night cream also features shea butter, with a pretty, fresh scent from lime and orange blossoms, verbena and aromatic herbs.

Comments: 'Sank in like a dream leaving my skin feeling silky smooth; after regular use skin brighter, much, much softer, crêpiness in jaw and neck area reduced, small reduction in fine lines around mouth and in frown line above nose on forehead – for me a must-have product' • 'main benefit is in the softness and a slight reduction in fine lines' • 'skin felt softer, smoother, much brighter and plumper – looks younger – a wonderful product'.

♡ WE LOVE...

After Jo declared Liz Earle Naturally Active Superskin Moisturiser 'the best moisturiser ever, ever, ever', what else could she use before bedtime? And it's now three years on. 'It's rich, nourishing and the "plumping" action is amazing,' she says. When Jo had her facial moisture levels checked at a recent launch for a skin cream, she scored the highest percentage for moisturisation of any beauty editor. Sarah is very happy with her night cream (which can also be used for daytime) Temple Spa Skin Truffle, with a rejuvenating formula including truffles, diamonds and pure gold (gosh!).

TIP

Many people we know swear by a silk pillowcase to sleep on, insisting that they wake up without the 'sleep creases' that can develop in skin as we slumber. Also a silk pillowcase – unlike cotton – doesn't absorb either your skin's natural moisture or the cream you put on, so you're giving your skin the benefit of any anti-ageing ingredients – not your pillowcase...

Give aches and pains plenty of TLC

We're not talking here about the sort of pain that comes with acute illness or injury. This is the general wear and tear that we're all prey to and which can make us look and feel older – so here's our prescription for kissing it better!

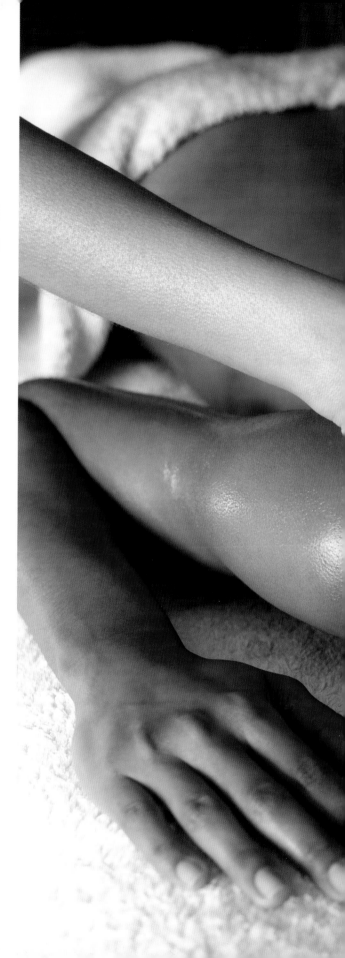

Two out of three people suffer neck and shoulder pain in their lives. Back ache is endemic, affecting eight to ten of us, the majority aged between 35 and 55. Then there are the usual headaches, not to mention sore feet (for more about them, see page 96). And none of them are beautifiers: we furrow our brows, the light goes out of our eyes, we stoop or slouch. (And left untended our joints may suffer irreparable damage.) So it's worth having strategies to deal with aches and pains. First of all, prevention – below you'll find the most useful tips we know for everyday stuff. And if despite your best endeavours you do end up in agony, see overleaf for advice.

Stand up straight. Improving your posture reaps heaps of benefits – preventing aches and pains, making you look slimmer, and even keeping you happier. Ears, shoulders, hips, knees and ankles should be in a straight line; pull your tummy button towards your spine. Breathe slowly. (See the box overleaf for more.)

Make sure you can see clearly. Having the right specs will help prevent that tortoise-poke-forward as you peer at a book, the

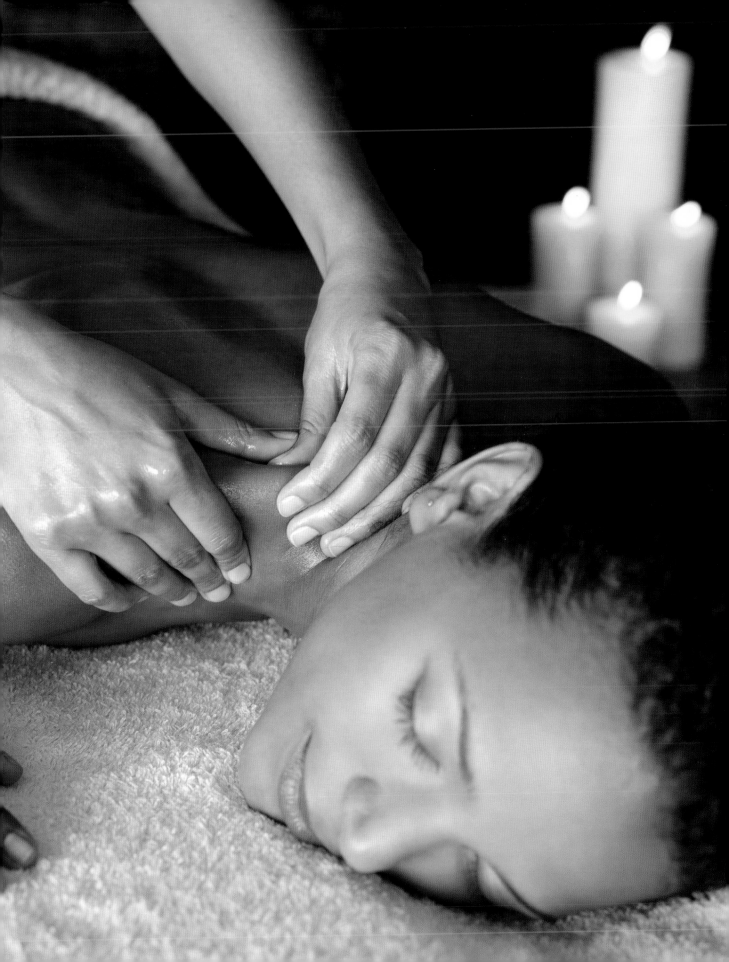

screen – or the road ahead (as well as stopping you frowning, which should save a few pounds on face creams). Have your eyes tested at least every two years, annually after the age of forty if you have glaucoma in the family (it can result in blindness, so this is vital). Check your lighting: if you're working at a screen, the main source should come from behind it to avoid reflections on the screen. If you're reading, the light source should preferably come from over your left shoulder; in the darker winter months, you will need stronger light than on a bright summer's day. (We like Serious Readers dedicated lamps.)

Keep moving. Our bodies were not designed to sit still for long periods. Neck, shoulder and back aches often come from sitting in a fixed position at screens (laptops are worst of all, see right) and also driving, lifting, etc. The golden rule is: get up and walk around every 30-40 minutes – more if possible. Sip a glass of water as you amble, and you'll be doing double beauty duty.

Position your head correctly. It's very heavy (about 12 pounds) and needs to sit directly on top of your spine rather than poking forward, straining muscles and causing injury. Aim to have your ears, shoulders and hips in a straight vertical line. Lifting your chest and letting your shoulders roll back and down helps; gently push your shoulder blades together (see exercises below).

Have your knees slightly lower than your pelvis when sitting. This helps put the spine into neutral position. If you don't have a chair with an adjustable seat, try putting a couple of folded towels under your bottom, and sit into the back of the chair.

Your screen should be at eye level. Have your forearms at right angles to your body and in a straight line to your fingertips. An arm rest may help. Your mouse should be easily accessible by swinging your hand round, to say 45 degrees maximum. You shouldn't have to lift your elbow or make a claw. RSI sufferers should choose a big 'elephant's foot' mouse or trackball.

Keep the documents you are working on at eye height to avoid squinnying at the bottom of the screen.

Do simple, gentle exercises to keep your circulation moving. A counter-stretch will reverse the hunched position, particularly after using a laptop; imagine you're 'opening like a flower', says Tim Hutchful of the British Chiropractic Association. Reach your arms out to the side, palms up, then open your fingers and turn your palms down to the floor; look gently up to the ceiling, push your shoulder blades together and hold for ten seconds. Follow with a 'chin tuck': pull your chin into your throat as if you are trying to make a double chin and hold for ten seconds. Also shrug your shoulders up to your ears and circle them back and forwards. (For a quick exercise programme for all ages, visit www.youtube.com and put Straighten Up UK! in Search – fantastic if you're feeling tired and/or looking peaky.)

POSTURE

Bad posture is to blame for all sorts of aches and pains. But here's an interesting thing: good posture can actually help to change your mood. If you feel low, you tend to look down, which keeps you feeling, well, low and down. Matters get worse if you hunch your shoulders and clasp your arms or hands in front. 'You're closing off your chest, which means you don't get as much oxygen in your lungs and your brain,' explains body language expert Robert Phipps. 'If you straighten up, open your chest and shoulders, look ahead and around keeping your eye movements horizontal, you start to feel better. Looking down connects with the emotional part of your brain whereas looking up and to the right engages with your future. You will notice your breathing changes, and your whole body lifts.'

Posture is also a vital component of social signalling: 'If you adopt a confident body posture, you project confidence. Barriers and defensive postures signal fear; uncrossing your arms and lifting your chin signals "I'm not afraid". Our minds and bodies are in a constant feedback loop, conveying information. Animals respond purely to body language; humans put a social veneer on behaviour but we always revert to animal instincts,' says Phipps.

A tip: on a first meeting or at an interview, mirror the person's body language for three or four movements, match their rate of talking and breathing, then sit back in your chair. 'At an interesting moment in the conversation, pause, lean forward and drop your voice slightly so they have to come forward to you. They are then mirroring you – through your confident strategy,' says Phipps.

Of course, posture isn't just about your social life. 'Good posture keeps your bones and joints in alignment so you can use your muscles properly and keep them fairly relaxed to avoid painful tension,' explains chiropractor Tim Hutchful. 'It should also prevent your spine being distorted into an abnormal position, which can lead to

LAPTOP KNOW-HOW

Laptop computers have liberated us in many ways but, according to chiropractor Tim Hutchful, the downside is that they can cause considerable damage to your neck and spine, resulting in lots of aches and pains including headaches. 'Because the laptop keyboard and screen are integrated, you risk compromising your neck, shoulders, arms and/or back when using one, so there's potential for problems in all these areas,' he says.

● Taking a small keyboard with you (pack everything in a rucksack so the weight is even) may seem like trouble but it can really help you avoid it.

● Try to work with your arms supported (on a train or plane table, or even on cushions if you're in the back of a car), to avoid neck pain from the muscles that hold up your arms.

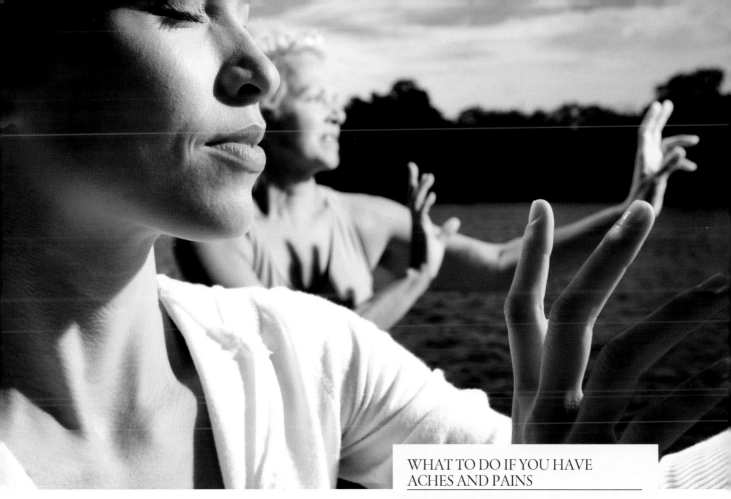

T'ai chi helps many aches and pains, including knee osteoarthritis and fibromyalgia, as well as quality of sleep. It may also benefit bone density, and increase musculoskeletal strength.

pain in different parts of your body. Additionally, if you're evenly balanced, it helps to reduce abnormal wear and tear of joints. Remember that good posture is just as important when you're moving as when you're still,' he adds.

To support your spine, it's vital to strengthen the corset of abdominal muscles between the lower margin of your ribs and your waist, all round. Simply contract those muscles as you sit at your desk or stand at the bus stop. To create a 'cross bracing effect', try the Superman exercise: go down on all fours like a coffee table, arms and upper legs at right angles to your body. Raise your right arm and left leg to the horizontal, hold for five to ten seconds, then swap sides. Repeat five times. (Don't do this if it's uncomfortable.)

WHAT TO DO IF YOU HAVE ACHES AND PAINS

Spray on magnesium oil: it will relax the muscles in that area and should provide quick relief. You can use it several times a day, and before bed. Genius! (Try Magnesium Oil by Better You.)

Take an anti-inflammatory: we don't get on with conventional versions, so took the advice of integrated medicine guru Dr Andrew Weil and keep a stock of Zyflamend by New Chapter, a combination of plants that help reduce pain and inflammation in the joints (can also be used for skin).

Try Bromelain, an enzyme with remarkable painkilling properties, that's been extensively studied for use in digestive disorders (eg, heartburn, reflux and food allergies), also inflammatory conditions (arthritis, sports injuries and skin conditions such as eczema and psoriasis). (Bromelain by LifeTime Vitamins.)

Explore complementary therapies such as acupuncture, chiropractic (try McTimoney chiropractic if you don't like too much clunk-click stuff), Bowen technique, osteopathy and/or cranial osteopathy. Practise (gently) yoga, Pilates or t'ai chi.

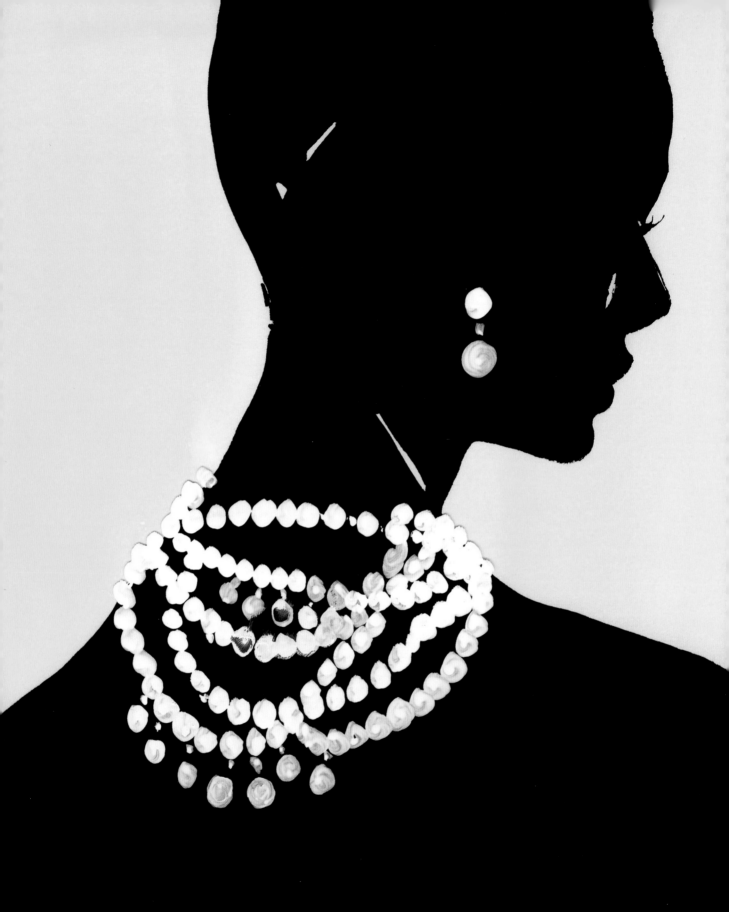

'Beautiful
YOUNG
people are
accidents of nature,
but beautiful
OLD people are
works of art'

Eleanor Roosevelt

Embrace pearls (it worked for Grace Kelly)

We love pearls. Ropes and swags of them. As necklaces, chokers, bracelets and don't forget earrings. Real, cultured or plain fake. Sea or freshwater. Vintage or just-strung. Oversized and multi-stranded or neat, demure singles. White, pink, grey or black. With denim or satin, T-shirt, woolly or your most glam glad rags

Forget diamonds – we say: pearls are a girl's best friend. Why?

Because these lustrous baubles are just about the most fabulously flattering accessory for any mature complexion – whether your skin has warm or cool tones. (Michelle Obama looks amazing in pearls. So do Hillary Clinton, Oprah Winfrey and Elizabeth Taylor, which tells you everything you need to know about how they work for every complexion. Think of Coco Chanel, Audrey Hepburn, Jackie Kennedy Onassis, Princess Diana – all draped in them. And not for nothing have English and North American women traditionally been given a pearl necklace and earrings when they came of age.)

Pearls may swing in and out of fashion, but they are always miraculously flattering. Pearls distract the eye. They're lambent like moonlight, creating a sort of 'halo' effect when close to the face – bouncing light on to your skin and making it appear softer and more radiant.

A pearl collar or choker can disguise a less-than-fabulous neck. Dowager duchesses have always known that, but frankly it's a tip that many of us could make use of if neck-angst kicks in. You don't need a title or family jewels for this: Jo, in particular, is constantly on the lookout for great costume jewellery pearls, but also likes real baroque Indian pearls: she first found them in Anjuna Market in Goa, and while a practised eye might be able to tell them apart from much, much pricier versions, we're just not that snooty about our jewels. We just pile 'em on. Timeless. Classic. Minor-miracle-working.

And add a touch of pearl to your skin, too. Pearl is also a word – or rather, a texture – to bear in mind when it comes to creating a finish for your make-up. Applied judiciously – a touch on the browbone, for instance, or even on the eyelid – pearlised eyeshadow helps create a sculpting light-and-shade effect. Fact: too matt isn't good, after forty, because a face looks dry and dusty. You need a little sheen. But use 'the pearl test' when you're buying glimmering shades of any product, ie, does this have more shimmer than a real pearl? In which case it's probably too shimmery, whether you're looking at a lipstick or an eyeshadow.

LUST FOR THE LUSTRE

Pearlised pigments and, in some cases, real crushed pearl (aka 'nacre') are also being incorporated into skin creams for instant radiance – great in a make-up primer, as it gives skin that 'halo' effect when foundation's applied on top. In make-up, these pearl-esque, light-reflective pigments really can create the illusion of softening fine lines, and minimising under-eye shadows or visible pigmentation.

> 'There is one piece of jewellery that is equally becoming to everybody, lovely with almost every ensemble, appropriate for almost every occasion and indispensable in every woman's wardrobe... Long live the pearl necklace, from our first date to our last breath!'
>
> GENEVIÈVE ANTOINE DARIAUX, *Elégance*

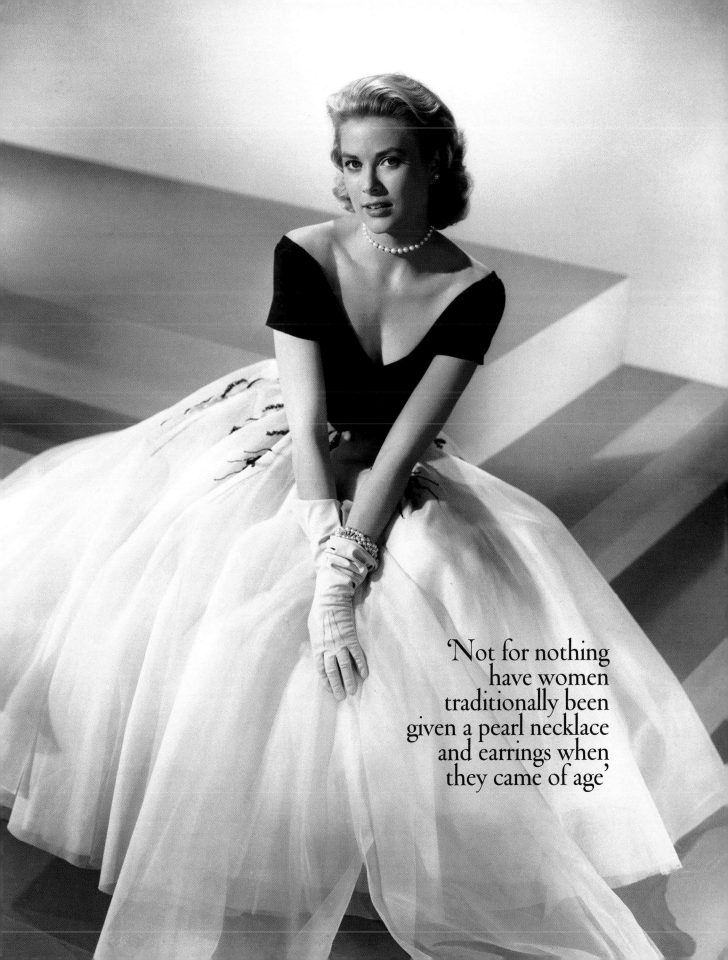

'Not for nothing
have women
traditionally been
given a pearl necklace
and earrings when
they came of age'

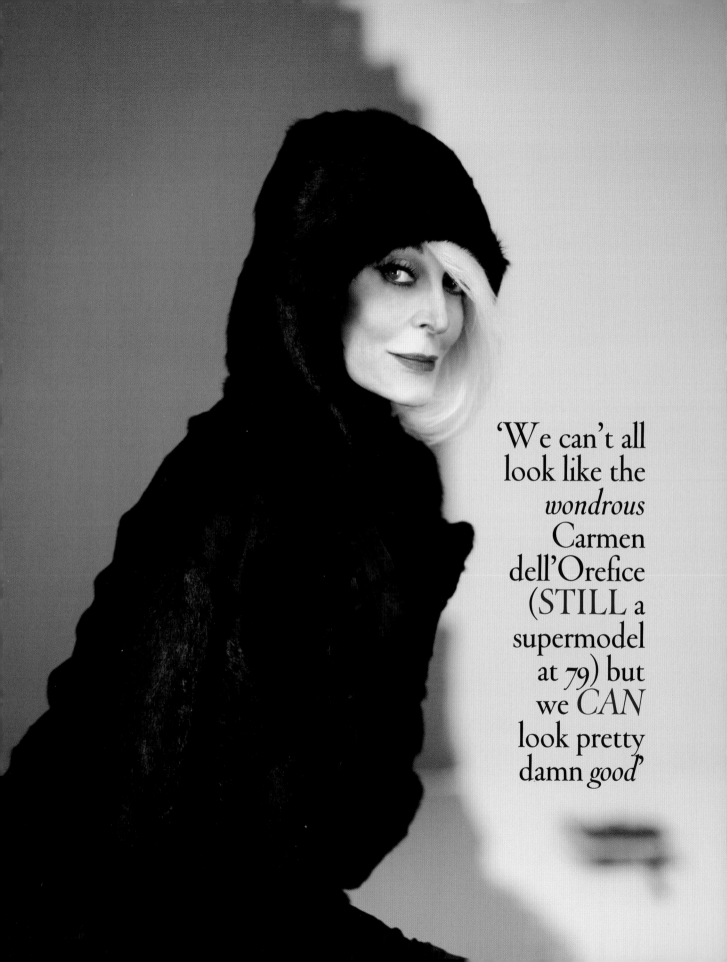

'We can't all look like the *wondrous* Carmen dell'Orefice (STILL a supermodel at 79) but we CAN look pretty damn *good*'

Look good in photos

(And feel better about yourself)

We used to think that a friend of ours – then editor of *Tatler* – was being so grand when she refused to be photographed before lunchtime. Now we absolutely understand what she meant. One of the commonest causes of those 'oh, damn!' moments – when we really feel like we've fast-forwarded a decade or two – is seeing ourselves in a hideous snap. 'Do I really look like that…?' Well, the answer is not really: in real life, people take in all of you (voice, smile, twinkling eyes) – whereas in a snapshot, it's so easy to see only your flaws.

So: we believe in positive reinforcement. It's possible to take a hideous picture of anyone (think of those 'drunken' celebrity shots which caught them mid-blink). But it makes all of us feel better if we can glimpse a photo and go, 'Actually, not looking so bad…'

This may be a cheat, but in the same way that famous people control 'official' images of themselves, we suggest that you only surround yourself with photos of yourself that you really like: from the photos on the mantelpiece to the pix you send to friends. And the photos on your Facebook 'wall', or in your online albums.

There's also a great deal more you can do to look your absolute best in photos than just simply say 'cheese'… We can't all look like the wondrous Carmen dell'Orefice (still a supermodel at 79 as we go to press) but we can look pretty damn good.

Don't be photographed before lunchtime. No, we really mean it: most of the early morning puffiness will have diminished by then – and eyes will appear more awake. (And it also gives time to get to the hairdresser, if required. You think we ever have our official pictures taken without hitting John Frieda first? No. Way.)

Remember: this is no time to go bare-faced. Make-up artist Bobbi Brown recommends a yellow-toned foundation and concealer (rather than anything with a hint of pink), as these look better on film. Use a mattifying foundation, rather than a dewy finish; apply with a sponge sparingly, and use concealer to even out any flaws such as broken veins, under-eye circles. Be aware, though, that pen-style light-reflecting concealers – designed to work on dark circles – can bounce back so much light if used with flash photography, they create a 'reverse-panda' effect. Brush translucent powder over the face and exposed skin on the neckline. Avoid shimmer, as any flash will exaggerate shine.

Use matt eyeshadows. Browns and greys look best in photos, with black or brown eyeliner, close to your lashes on top (and, if you like, bottom) lid. Use black or brown waterproof mascara, as any flash can lead to 'tear-ing', thus smudging your lashes.

Go for an enhanced lip-coloured lipstick. Something mid-rose, or a bit deeper – the colour of your lips only a bit more so. These are the shades we generally recommend anyway, but in pictures bright reds, corals and oranges look super-garish.

Stay out of strong sunlight. This creates major nose shadows and makes you squint. Outdoors, open shade is best – daylight under an awning or a tree. As model Lisa Snowdon says, 'Midday sun is the equivalent of looking at yourself in the mirror under an incredibly harsh spotlight, and is very ageing.'

Try 'the golden hour' instead. As Lisa adds, 'This is the first or last hour of sunlight of the day. This is the optimum time for photographs, when you cannot fail to look your absolute best.'

Pretend the photographer is your best friend. You'll be more yourself and your face will take on a more normal expression.

Relax your mouth. Make-up artist Tricia Sawyer recommends saying A-E-I-O-U to achieve this; to give the face a better shape and diminish a double chin, push your tongue against the back of your top teeth. Try not to crinkle your face into a big grin, as this will exaggerate lines around the eyes, but 'twinkle' with them.

Stand slightly sideways – and follow the beauty queens' advice. Angling the body slightly will make you look slimmer. Then put one foot in front of the other, which miraculously narrows the silhouette of the leg.

Never be photographed from below. This is the fastest-track to double chins and awful photographs. Instead, it helps if the photographer is positioned slightly above you: tilting your face up into the camera is hugely flattering (unless you have a long nose). Shots taken full-on can make a wide face look wider; try tilting your head slightly if the photographer is directly in front of you.

B-r-e-a-t-h-e. Many of us find it stressful having our photo taken, but if you hold your breath you'll look 'frozen'. Breathing out relaxes the face and body; inhaling raises shoulders and can give you a look of panic. So first take a few long, deep breaths.

And if all else fails, retouch. You think Hollywood stars REALLY look the way we see them? Online and on the high street you can get photos retouched. Or change to the more forgiving hues of black and white. Whatever it takes to get a photo you love is fine.

Don't let rosacea give you the blues

It used to be blushing that was embarrassing. Well, nowadays for getting-older women there seems to be an increasing problem with redness and rosacea. If you don't quite love your rosy cheeks (yet), here are some ideas

Although a fiery skin can sometimes affect young women, for others the problem starts as they get older. The causes of redness and rosacea are still pretty mysterious – basically something in the bloodstream triggers the swelling of blood vessels in the skin, causing inflammation (redness and soreness).

The triggers are notoriously individual, including food, alcohol, stress, pollution and perimenopause. There may also be inherited components which predispose people to redness: also it shows up much more on people with thin, fair skins.

However, there are some general guidelines which may help, as we learnt from Marie-Véronique Nadeau, the Californian former chemistry teacher who – after 'struggling' with rosacea from her early thirties – started her own skincare company (Marie Veronique Organics) to help people with problem skins. Here's her advice for dealing with inflammatory skin conditions:

Take turmeric faithfully. This Indian spice is a lifesaver for minimising flare-ups: take a 400mg capsule morning and night. It's hard to get enough by sprinkling it on your food, but do that too!

Use products with zinc oxide. As well as providing sun protection and helping wound-healing, this mineral is anti-inflammatory, so helps with most skin conditions including rosacea and also acne. Apply products which contain it (such as Marie Veronique Organics Moisturizing Face Screen SPF30). Other helpful anti-inflammatory ingredients include emu oil, red raspberry oil and aloe.

Take specific supplements. In addition to a good anti-inflammatory diet (plenty of nuts and seeds, vegetables and fruit, oily fish if you're not vegetarian), Marie-Véronique says it's 'an absolute must' to supplement with vitamin C, vitamin D3 and omega-3 essential fatty acids. (See page 180 for more on supplements.) Rosacea patients may also need more of a specific and powerful antioxidant called SOD (superoxide dismutase), so add that in too. NB: Marie-Véronique advises avoiding iron supplements, particularly if you have severe rosacea, as iron may aggravate it.

Monitor your reaction to 'heating' foods. Caffeine, red wine, curries and so on affect redness-prone people differently (see Maggie Alderson's experience opposite). The only advice is to turn detective and track your own personal response.

Beware the sun (and sunbeds). Ultraviolet light and particularly UVA – the longer-wavelength rays that are linked to skin damage and also now to skin cancers – seem to affect some rosacea sufferers severely. Everyone should take care in the sun – ie, always wear sun protection and never fry your skin. But for anyone with skin sensitivity of any kind, it's wise to avoid sunscreens with a chemical sunblock since they are known to be more likely to cause irritation. Opt instead for sunblocks using minerals, preferably zinc oxide (see left). Additionally, avoid anything with citrus essential oils and any product at all with alcohol.

ROSACEA – WHAT WORKS FOR ME

Novelist Maggie Alderson developed rosacea in 2002, when she was in her early forties. Here, she describes her strategies for making the best of what can be a lifelong condition.

'Tucked away at the top of my bathroom cupboard I keep an insurance policy, in the form of a pack of antibiotics my doctor prescribed for my rosacea. I hate the idea of taking oral antibiotics for anything short of a life-threatening infection, but I keep them there just in case the day comes when I really can't live with the raised and angry red blotches on my face any longer.

'I came close to it last summer after using cheap chemical sunblock on holiday and ending up with cheeks and chin almost as red and sore as the worst sunburn, but I managed to get through it by binning the block in favour of hats and beach umbrellas – and giving up wine with dinner. After eight years with this progressively worsening condition, I have found that what you swallow makes as big a difference – if not more – than what you slap on. Coffee, white wine and spicy food are my worst triggers, but apart from sunblock, the other most aggravating factor is stress. Which is ironic, as having a face like an overcooked pepperoni pizza is pretty stressful itself.

'I have tried legion topical products over the eight years or so I've had the condition, from prescribed antibiotic creams to exotic blue potions from imported beauty companies. Some of them worked for a bit, but none of them will cure rosacea. There isn't a cure but one effective temporary treatment I've found is acupuncture, which can settle down a really bad episode – although I know it will always come back.

'So rather than wasting more time and money searching for the miracle, I've come to accept it and, like someone with a port wine mark, put my energy into concealment. You simply have to wear make-up every day.

'The best conventional base I've found is Giorgio Armani Designer Shaping Cream Foundation SPF20, used with Laura Mercier concealer, but more recently I've been exploring mineral

SUPPLEMENTARY BENEFITS

As well as increasing omega-3 essential fatty acids both in the diet and as a supplement, pharmacist Shabir Daya advises taking a probiotic supplement: 'These beneficial bacteria will help to rid the gut of potential toxins that inflame the skin but more importantly they may ensure that specific "bad" bacteria do not proliferate.' Also try anti-inflammatory herbs such as red clover and echinacea, plus yellow dock and dandelion, which have mild diuretic properties to help eliminate the troublesome toxins. A topical serum with pycnogenol (a powerful antioxidant and anti-inflammatory) may also help, he says: 'It immediately reduces redness and inflammation and also strengthens the collagen matrix and in doing so reduces the capability of these toxins to inflame the skin.'

'I've come to accept it and put my energy into concealment. You simply have to wear make-up every day'

make-up. It takes a bit of getting used to but once you get the hang of layering on the fine dust, the coverage is extraordinary, with a lovely dewy finish which doesn't look – or feel – too make-up-y.

'I'm also seeing signs of improvement to my skin. Bare Minerals claim their products can help rosacea and mine has certainly calmed down significantly since I've been using it. The marks are still there, but they aren't nearly so raised and crusty.

'Most importantly, I know I now have a tool I can rely on to get me out of the house without embarrassment, even if I have the worst flare-up.

'One other tip: as well as the red weals and flaking spots, rosacea makes your facial skin as dry as a crocodile handbag. After sampling every miracle moisturiser on the market, the one that really makes the difference is Superskin Moisturiser by Liz Earle.'

Redness treatments: our award winners

We'll be frank: we didn't have incredibly high hopes for these. However, the products here – all of them trialled by panellists who put themselves forward because they have redness or mild rosacea – out-performed our expectations. We are seeing rapid growth in this category of products: redness has suddenly been identified as a 'boom' area by the beauty industry. So we'll be trialling new products as they appear, for future updates. However, inflamed conditions are notoriously individual, so what works for some may not work for all

AT A GLANCE

Marks & Spencer Advanced Formula Solutions Anti-Redness Serum

Murad Redness Therapy Recovery Treatment Gel

Darphin Intral Redness Relief Soothing Serum

Ole Henriksen Nurture Me

NB **These products are (mostly) not designed as moisturisers, and many women will need to use them with, not instead of, day and/or night creams.**

REVIEWS

Marks & Spencer Advanced Formula Solutions Anti-Redness Serum

 Good old M&S! We have to admit we were a little surprised that the least expensive product we trialled in this category triumphed (with a truly impressive score, when you consider the challenge...). It contains, so they tell us, 'a unique bio-functional complex derived from vitamin E, proven to reduce redness and inflammation'. Suitable for rosacea, thread veins, hormonal blushing and skins challenged by environmental stress.

Comments: 'I have early stages of rosacea and am prone to blushing, and also suffer from hyperhidrosis, so this light product was particularly good as I'll sweat off heavy ones within minutes; I've definitely seen a difference – redness not so fiery and less visible; skin slightly mattified and tone improved, fine lines improved too; I also use a facial oil and together with this, my skin looks much better' • 'I have some permanent redness also heat sensitivity: skin turned red immediately for a few seconds in the first week only, but was then less red; this worked as well as my more expensive brand' • 'very cooling and soothing, sank in quickly, felt less sensitive, looked a bit clearer and less red' • 'very refreshing serum that soothed skin and made it feel less angry with slight reduction in redness'.

Murad Redness Therapy Recovery Treatment Gel

 Uber-antioxidant goji berry is the key anti-inflammatory agent in this gel (goji has 500 times the vitamin C of oranges, and more beta-carotene than carrots, FYI!). It accelerates the healing of dry, flaky skin, and the light gel also features soothing zinc oxide, azaleic acid, vitamin K and peppermint leaf extract, to reduce sensitivity. Dr Howard Murad helped pioneer the whole category of dermatologist skincare, and this is one of a capsule range within his brand specifically to target redness.

Comments: 'Sank in so quickly and left no residue, and I can't tell you how happy I am with this: my redness has demised, and my acne-enraged nose is a distant memory; my skin looks how it used to before all this started. I had become so self-conscious I hated going out even for the school run; I have spent a lot of money on creams before finding this – it's cleared up a lot of the problem with only the odd blip which is gone really quickly and without stress' • 'nice almost milk-like texture and it worked!' • 'left my face a lot less red than it was before – I now use every morning and will buy more' • 'lovely to use and very good results' • 'rosacea is definitely calmed, the broken veins are the same but I flush much more mildly, less red and less often – the only product I have really seen a difference with'.

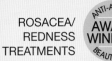

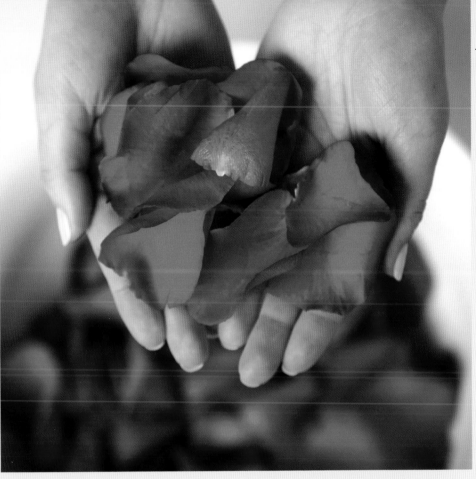

Darphin Intral Redness Relief Soothing Serum

 This is part of a recently introduced range from Darphin for sensitive skins, created to help strengthen skin while diminishing the appearance of redness. Calming botanicals include grape extract, antioxidant resveratrol, chamomile, hawthorn and peony extracts, in a gentle baby-pink serum.

Comments: 'After two minutes, my very red sensitive cheeks with thread veins felt soothed, and smoothed; moisturiser glided on; I looked forward to applying this every morning as it cooled my skin and took the extreme redness from my cheeks; skin more even and hydrated and I didn't have to use so much make-up to cover. Colleagues and family have noticed the improvement, which is lovely • 'finally found something that's gentle and effective, will be investing in the accompanying products. Very, very pleased!' • 'skin looks healthy and not as red' • 'I loved this product, it worked brilliantly – 10/10!' • 'after two weeks my skin was less prone to redness'.

Ole Henriksen Nurture Me

 This lags a little behind the others score-wise because one tester gave it a big, fat zero – which brought down the average considerably. (As we said above, responses are notoriously individual.) This soothing cream features nourishing oils to shield skin (including evening primrose and wheatgerm), plus chamomile extract, calendula and allantoin, and LA-based facialist Ole created it especially for rosacea sufferers. As with the other products, some testers found they needed extra moisturisation.

Comments: 'Lovely cooling and calming effect that is very soothing for my sensitive, redness-prone skin, which tends to flush; definitely lessened redness and skin feels very nice, clear and smooth; I really love this as a daily moisturiser, and will continue using it' • 'I have areas of redness on nose and chin, with a couple of broken veins: really nice cream which sinks in straight away to leave skin matt, feels lovely; a small but noticeable improvement in redness, skin definitely looks better and I use less make-up – really love using this; it's very economical and I will buy more when I run out'.

TIP

A friend with flaming cheeks divulged that her secret soother is a spray of organic Pukka Rosewater which she takes everywhere. (It's in a glass bottle but not too big or heavy for most handbags; at home do keep it in the fridge for maximum effect.)

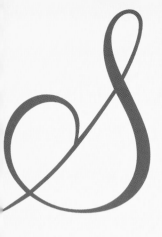

Serums:
our award winners

Serums are hot anti-ageing beauty news. While writing this book, we went to no less than three serum launches from Big-Name Brands in one week alone, so this really is a booming area of 'miracle' treatments. The reason is that it's possible to concentrate higher levels of active ingredients in a serum – so potentially they can deliver impressive results. And you don't have to give up favourite day or night creams because serums are usually designed to be layered with them

AT A GLANCE

La Clarée Oliv' Radiance Elixir

Pinks Boutique Anti-Aging Serum

Sarah Chapman London Skinesis Age-Repair Serum

Guerlain Orchidée Impériale Exceptional Complete Care Serum

TIP

Allow serum to absorb for a few minutes before applying your moisturiser. Pay attention to areas where skin is thin and easily damaged, such as your neck and décolletage.

So: do the benefits live up to the serum hype? Or are serums just another way to get us to part with more hard-earned cash? They can be very pricey – right up to a heart-stopping £1,500, though these winners were significantly less expensive. Our testers were certainly impressed with the following… And remember, more is not more with these products – like facial oils, you just need a very few drops.

REVIEWS

La Clarée Oliv' Radiance Elixir ❀❀❀

 From an organically-certified fave range of Sarah's, the texture of this is more akin to a dry oil than a conventional serum (though 'serums' was the category the brand submitted it for). It's suitable for all skintypes. The key anti-ageing ingredient is an olive leaf extract to fight skin stress and deliver radiance. To be applied morning and evening, massaged into skin with little circular movements. Sarah adores this product – which really does boost radiance – and isn't at all surprised that testers feel the same.

Comments: 'My favourite of all the products I tested: smells gorgeous, and while skin was nicer from first use, after two weeks my eye area has definitely improved with fewer fine lines, not so puffy and congested-looking – youthful and firmer; face appears brighter and fine lines are disappearing!'
• 'just give me more! I'll bathe in it…' • 'within 24 hours, skin was velvety smooth, after two weeks I am a convert, skin is less crêpey, brighter and the smell is divine: a single drop on my granddaughter's eczema made it less dry and itchy immediately!'
• 'my skin beamed at me – dewy, alive – and when I woke the next morning it was plumper, amazingly soft and there were fewer creases, crow's feet softened over time and small crease between my brows definitely softened; stubborn crêpiness improved massively, and skin has a glow about it – I have even been out without foundation on!'.

Pinks Boutique Anti-Aging Serum ❀❀❀

 Intended ideally for use under night cream or balm, a Soil Association-certified blend of rosehip, avocado, camellia and jojoba that's packed with antioxidants and sun-damage-repairing botanicals. British-born Pinks Boutique is one of the few organic 'spa' brands around and if you're a wannabe-natural beauty, their website is worth checking out for salon locations.

Comments: 'Skin immediately looked a bit more radiant, with a bit more colour in my cheeks, and

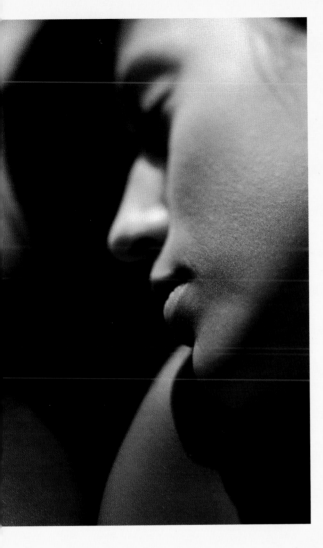

in this book from her elegant seven-product range. Loads of peptides, vitamin E, aloe vera juice and mushroom extract are delicately and prettily fragranced with jasmine, hyacinth and rose essential oils. Stylish pump-action packaging protects the contents.

Comments: 'Immediate and *big* difference in tone, skin brighter and smoother with no tightness; after two weeks, people mentioned I looked great and younger – fine lines disappeared and skin looked vibrant, really bright and smooth with no dark tones, crêpiness lessened – amazing!' • 'my fine lines have almost gone away! A lot of compliments…' • 'really a wow product, you only need a small amount for a great difference in the texture of the skin, which really did appear softer, brighter and more rested; definitely reduced marionette lines near nose and mouth, definitely buying – I look as if I've had a good holiday; colleagues say I look refreshed' • 'after two weeks, skin is 80 per cent brighter, and fine lines reduced'.

Guerlain Orchidée Impériale Exceptional Complete Care Serum

 8.31/10

We have been blown away by the results from Guerlain's ultra-luxe Orchidée Impériale range throughout this book, which has excelled against really, really tough competition in many categories. (Guerlain may be best-known for sublime fragrances, but we've always known their skincare is also exceptional.) A 'Biofilm mesh' offers an instantly firming action, comprised of proteins, sugars and skin-compatible lipids, in a satin-smooth veil. You will definitely need another cream on top.

Comments: 'Beautiful product and my skin felt lovely from the first time I applied it; definitely brighter and smoother, so soft and looks less tired; make-up went on well too; my daughter noticed a real difference' • 'Marks? One million… wow, I can't believe it, my husband noticed a difference in ten minutes…and after two weeks, my face is so much more lifted, fine lines and crêpiness visibly reduced, skin so much brighter and clearer, smoother and more even-toned; it's as if I've been French-polished – and it smells just like my grandmother's rose garden' • 'made my skin very fresh-looking and young, and lifted my spirits too; should be named the fab-feeling-face cream; texture like silk and sunk into my skin like a spoonful of honey slipping down my throat'.

Three, for Jo, who likes to give her skin a boost every few months with a four-week serum treatment programme. There's REN Keep Young and Beautiful SH²C Serum, which she layers under moisturiser (it's light but effectively cell-plumping). There's Neal's Yard Remedies Rejuvenating Frankincense Facial Serum, 'because I'm addicted to the smell of frankincense, and I figure that anything which was used to preserve skin for mummification – as this resin was in ancient Egypt – has to be good for anti-ageing.' And most recently, she's a major convert to Korres Quercetin & Oak Anti-Ageing Anti-Wrinkle & Firming Face Serum, 'as it really does live up to the firming promise'. As you can see from the top-scoring product, Sarah relies on La Clarée's Oliv' Radiance Elixir, and the result elicited big compliments from no less a face expert than make-up artist Barbara Daly.

after two weeks, crow's feet less noticeable, with overall plumpness and healthy glow. I love, love, love it, definitely improves my complexion and makes it looks less tired; plus my big frown line has magically reduced! I've become slightly obsessed with it…' • 'bottle goes a very long way as you only use a few drops, skin looks brighter and healthier' • 'noticeable difference with the side I applied it to – softer, smoother and plumper – and the other side of my face!' • 'skin looked much more nourished, brighter and younger after just two weeks – woo hoo! Lots of fab comments, thank you!!!'.

Sarah Chapman London Skinesis Age-Repair Serum

 8.5/10

A facial with superfacialist Sarah Chapman is definitely worth the waiting list. More readily available, though, is her skincare line – and this silky serum is one of two winners

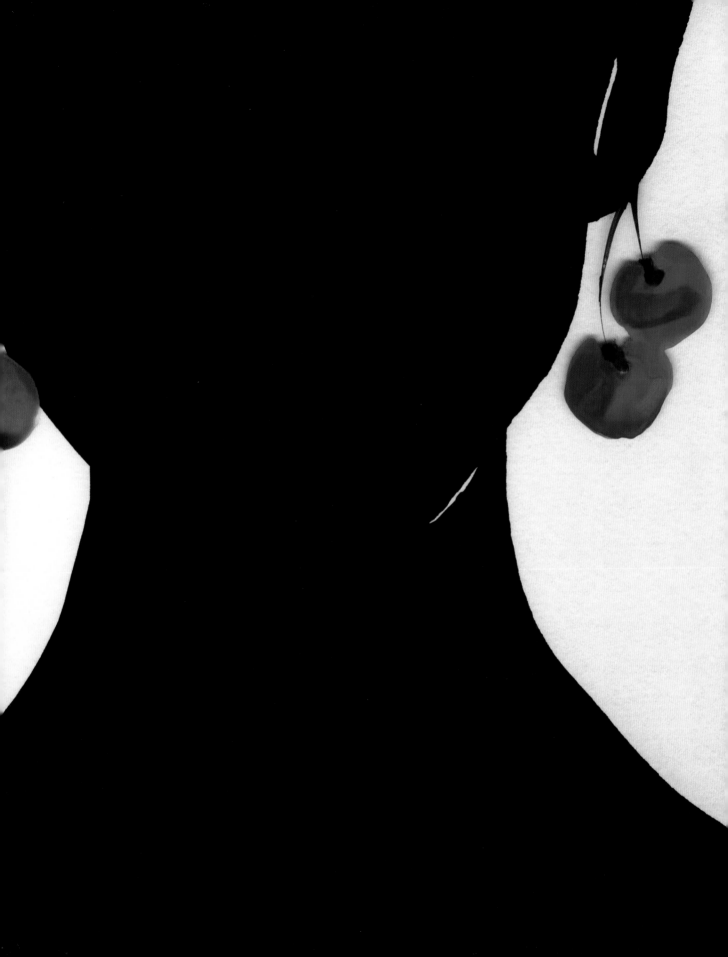

'Don't hold on to *anger*, or *regrets* – it's AGEING. Kindness is GOOD for the skin'

Marie Helvin

Supergreens Facelift Diet

Give yourself a natural face (and body) lift with this plant-loving diet

We could write a whole book about healthy eating (maybe one day we will). And by now you probably know the basics of what you should and shouldn't be munching for general health maintenance. (And if weight has become an issue, you can read all about a different approach to help you shed pounds in our section on middle-age spread and mindful eating on page 144.)

But here's something wonderful. We truly believe that you have it in your power to slow down the process of ageing (or speed it up, of course, if you do the wrong things). We're not talking about delaying the ravages of time with cosmetic surgery but by what you eat. (As well as other lifestyle steps such as sleep and exercise.)

There are two big processes that cause our skin (and indeed all the cells in our body) to age: dehydration and inflammation. You know the culprits! A poor diet, smoking (you don't, do you?), sun and alcohol, plus late nights, psychological stress, a polluted environment and not enough exercise. But eating plants – mostly fresh greens (mostly raw) – helps to hydrate every cell in your body. And that keeps your skin plump and moist. Add in lifestyle shifts such as more sleep, sun protection and exercise, and your skin will 'bounce-back' – as they call its suppleness capacity – like a Duracell bunny!

Chlorophyll-rich greens are packed with amino acids, which are the building blocks of all protein. Unlike animal protein (where the body has to work to break apart the protein into the separate amino acids), green plants offer you instantly absorbable amino acids to transform into protein.

We learned about this concept by trying a green food supplement called Sun Chlorella from Japan. This superfood settles your gut into a state of delicious calm and efficiency. And when that happens, it helps to 'lift' your face and peachify your skin (Sarah couldn't believe it when she first noticed the transformation after taking Sun Chlorella for a month or so).

The reason? Your skin is the mirror of your digestion and, according to Traditional Chinese Medicine practitioner and nutritionist Nadia Brydon, there are two pairs of energy (Qi) lines called meridians running down your face. If your gut is unhappy, the lines droop and so does your face. Stabilise your digestion and whoosh! The energy is replenished and everything goes upwards.

It's not just your face that sags, says Nadia, because the same meridian runs down through your breasts and stomach. 'When we eat too many foods high in calories and refined carbohydrates and low in micronutrients, we're hastening the sagging in these areas too; eat foods high in micronutrients and low in calories – such as fresh greens – and we help to tone, contract, firm and pull up the droops from the inside.'

The Supergreens Facelift Diet (see overleaf) cleanses the skin from the inside, toning, feeding, hydrating, lifting, moisturising, reducing puffiness and wrinkles – and putting back your glow from top to toe! In fact, the very best face and body lift we can give ourselves is to eat more greens in our diet every day, starting with an anti-ageing supergreen smoothie (see box overleaf). Then do the Supergreens Facelift Diet for two to three days once every three months (minimum).

Try following this diet for two days to start with, preferably over a weekend when you can rest as much as you want to. Do some gentle cardiovascular exercise for at least half an hour a day: walking is fine – dancing if you prefer, or jogging, swimming, hockey. Whatever pleases you.

Do remember this is not meant to be a penance. Make sure you have lovely clean fresh bedlinen, bath towels and nightie; your favourite music and DVDs, a stack of glossy magazines and whatever else you enjoy! Go out if you want to – lead your normal life, just stick to the diet.

It's often fun to do these things with a partner, so ask a girlfriend – or lover/spouse if they're game. But choose someone where there's no tension attached.

> 'If you starve yourself to the point where your brain cells shrivel, you will never do good work' Cate Blanchett

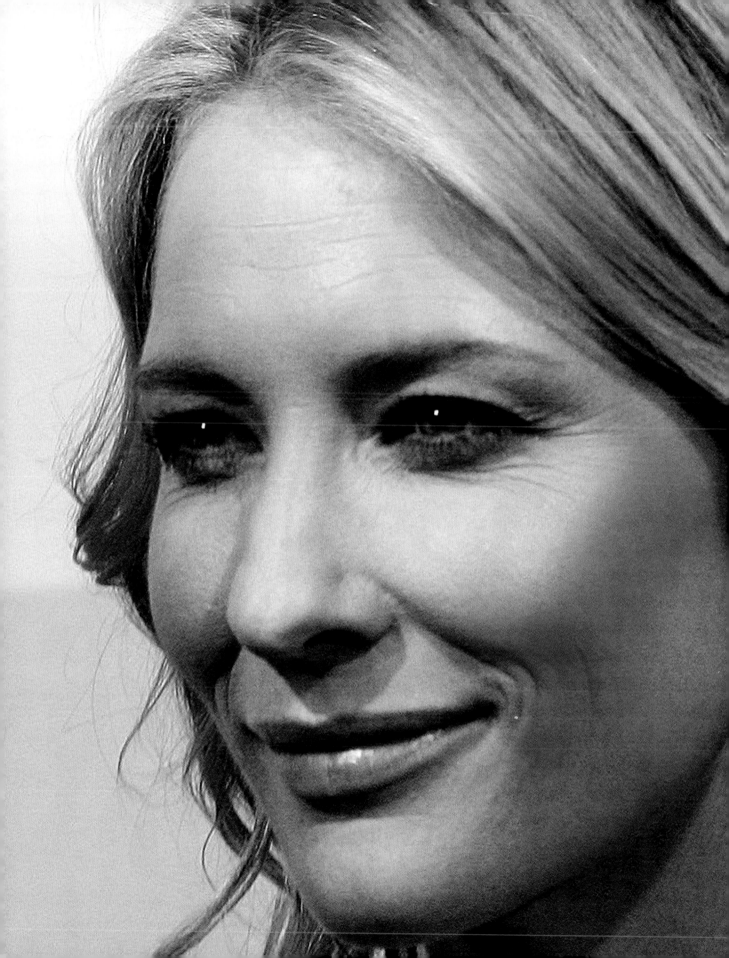

FRIDAY NIGHT

Prep for your weekend by eating a light evening meal between 6pm and 7.30pm. Always leave at least two hours between eating and going to bed. And do plan for an early night.

SATURDAY/SUNDAY

● First thing, drink a large glass of room-temperature water, with a slice of lemon if liked.
● Follow with half an hour of yoga stretching and meditation, or a walk. Salute to the Sun will start your day beautifully whatever age/fitness you are; for easy-to-follow instructions see www.yogasite.com/sunsalute.htm.
● Apply a hair mask before starting, if you wish.
● Brush teeth and tongue, gargle with slightly salted room-temperature water and splash face with cold water to wake up and contract facial skin cells.
● Before showering, body-brush your whole body with a soft, natural brush or mitten to help stimulate and detox the skin and lymph system. Brush from extremities towards the heart.
● Take a shower, ending with hot and cold hydrotherapy water treatment: alternate hot and cold water for half a minute each, repeat seven times in all. End with hot water before bed, cold water in the morning or before a night out. This contracts and relaxes every cell and moves the circulation, so helping to eliminate toxins.
● Shampoo and condition your hair in the shower.
● Moisturise from top to toe.
● Fill 2 x 1 litre bottles with natural spring (or filtered) water, and sip through the day.

THE DIET

Breakfast
Drink half your Supergreen Smoothie (see recipe right)

Mid-morning snack
● Sip half your remaining Supergreen Smoothie
● 50g soaked almonds and 100g white grapes or raw peas, carrots/cucumber sticks

Lunch
● 100–175g steamed or grilled fresh fish of any sort (just not tinned or frozen)
OR 100–175g fresh tofu
OR half an avocado
● 200–400g mixed salad: make a big salad with some or all of the following: torn leaves of lettuce, rocket (arugula), watercress, basil and spinach; chopped red pepper and cucumber; grated carrot and beetroot, radishes, spring onion; 110g living sprouting seeds, eg, alfalfa, pulses, mung bean shoots; 1 teaspoon pumpkin and sunflower seeds. Dress with 1 tablespoon extra virgin cold pressed olive oil and lemon juice, with salt and freshly ground black pepper to taste
● Pudding: 200g mixed berries
OR 100g papaya
OR 100g apple/pear/grapes
● Sip 350ml natural spring water (more if wished)

Mid-afternoon snack
● Drink remainder of anti-ageing/anti-inflammatory Supergreen Smoothie
● Apple or pear or 100g grapes
● 350ml natural spring water (more if you wish)

Evening meal
● 100–175g fresh organic chicken
OR fresh tofu
OR avocado
OR roasted/steamed vegetable medley seasoned with fresh herbs
● Mixed salad and pudding, as above
● 350ml natural spring water or more if desired

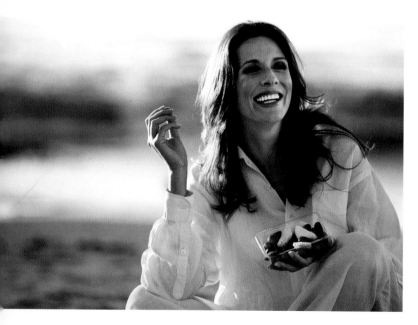

SUPERGREEN SMOOTHIE

Pure rocket fuel! This will help reduce your appetite, rejuvenate your skin and whole body, plus give you endless energy. Drinking it in the morning reduces your appetite for sweet tastes so it helps balance blood-sugar levels. Always store in the fridge in a screw-top jar (or wide-necked vacuum flask) and make fresh daily.

Makes about 1 litre in all. All measurements are approximate, so don't fret about being exact.

Blend together
- 600ml still mineral water
- $^1/_2$ chopped cucumber with skin and pips
- $^1/_4$ peeled avocado
- 1 chopped celery stick
- juice of $^1/_2$ lemon or lime
- $^1/_4$ teaspoon unrefined salt
- small double handful of mixed green leaves (60–80g) from the following: spinach, chicory, watercress, rocket (arugula), Savoy cabbage, chard, lettuce, kale, bok choy (Chinese cabbage), sprigs of mint, parsley, coriander, basil, etc (you can often buy bags of organic mixed green leaves)

- 5–15 pillules Sun Chlorella A (if not used to greens in diet, use 5 tablets for the first 3 days, then build up to 15 over the week)

Plus, optionally
- 1 clove garlic
- 1-2 slices of fresh ginger (5-10g)
- 1 small chopped spring onion
- $^1/_2$ apple or $^1/_2$ pear or 100g papaya, mango or melon to sweeten slightly

If you are constipated
- 1 tablespoon fresh flax oil or ground flax seeds

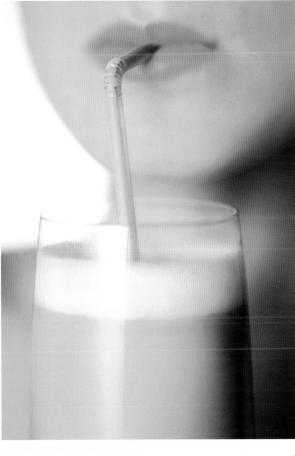

'Eat food. Not too much. Mainly plants'

Michael Pollan's 'Food Rules'

LOVE THESE FOODS

Organic where possible
- Fresh vegetables, freshly made veggie soups and juices
- Fresh salads
- Sprouted seeds and pulses
- Fresh fruit
- Nuts and seeds (soak nuts for 12 hours at room temperature)
- Fresh fish including sushi
- Tofu
- Lean meat/game
- Hot water with slice of lemon
- Spring water
- Herb teas eg, ginger, fennel, peppermint

REDUCE THESE FOODS

- All processed sugar and sweeteners
- Processed and tinned foods
- Junk foods
- Dairy products
- Wheat products (especially 'industrialised' bread; if you want to eat bread, look for long-fermented sourdoughs from artisan bakeries)
- Red meat
- Crisps and peanuts
- Pasta and pizza
- Any foods with E numbers and additives
- Sweets/chocolate
- Tap water
- Coffee
- Fizzy drinks
- Alcohol

Discover the supplements you really need

You could spend a fortune on supplements. Or you could miss them out altogether. Neither are good options for optimal health and beauty, we feel…

Consider investing in these basics. Leading experts worldwide consider these the ones you really should include.

● **Multivitamins and minerals:** research shows that even people eating the best diet possible nowadays are deficient in some essential nutrients. Result: you feel and look under par, you're more likely to get ill and you have less energy all round. Invest in a good product, food state if possible for maximum absorption (and value).
Try: All Natural Perfectly Balanced Multinutrients, which contains vitamins, minerals, antioxidants, green foods (including blue green algae, chlorophyll and spirulina), plus liver-cleansing herbs and probiotics (to keep your gut in great order).

● **Omega-3 essential fatty acid:** our bodies don't make essential fatty acids, of which omega-3 is the most important. We need it for pretty well everything in our bodies, including keeping our skin plump, soft and supple. It fortifies hair and nails too. If not veggie try to eat two portions of omega-3 rich oily fish a week, and consider a supplement. Look for a product with EPA and DHA, either based on fish oil, krill or the plant echium.

Try: Ideal Omega 3 by Ideal Omega, a particularly pure form of fish oil, but for those who don't like fish, or are veggie, try Echiomega from the plant *Echium plantagineum*.

> ## 50 per cent of adults are deficient in 'sunshine' vitamin D, particularly as we get older

● **Vitamin D:** research suggests that at least 50 per cent of adults are deficient in this 'sunshine' vitamin, particularly as we get older. It's vital for your bones, muscles and the immune system, among other functions. It also helps to ward off low mood and depression. Scientists now suggest taking 1,000-2,000 IU daily.
Try: D Lux 1000 spray by Better You – it tastes of lemon and is absorbed rapidly.

We think it's worth adding in these too: you probably won't need or want to take all of them, so read through and see which seem most relevant to you.

● **Phyto-oestrogens:** we don't take HRT (though we're totally sympathetic to women who've tried everything else and feel it's worth the risks), but we do like plant oestrogens which help to mimic our natural hormones and help with hot flushes, night sweats and vaginal dryness.
Try: Sage Complex by Food Science of Vermont, which contains sage, wild yam, dong quai, red clover and a bunch of other herbs including Siberian ginseng, hops, pomegranate extract, fenugreek seeds and kudzu.

● **Digestive enzymes:** as the years pass, our natural supply of digestive enzymes to process food declines, leading to bloating, wind, bad breath – oh dear!
Try: Extrazyme-13 by LifeTime vitamins – a capsule before a meal should do the trick.

● **Hyaluronic acid:** the latest compound to be dubbed the 'fountain of youth' – and with some justice. A protein that can hold 1,000 times its own weight in water, it plumps up skin cells, so helping to erase fine lines and wrinkles. Levels decline with

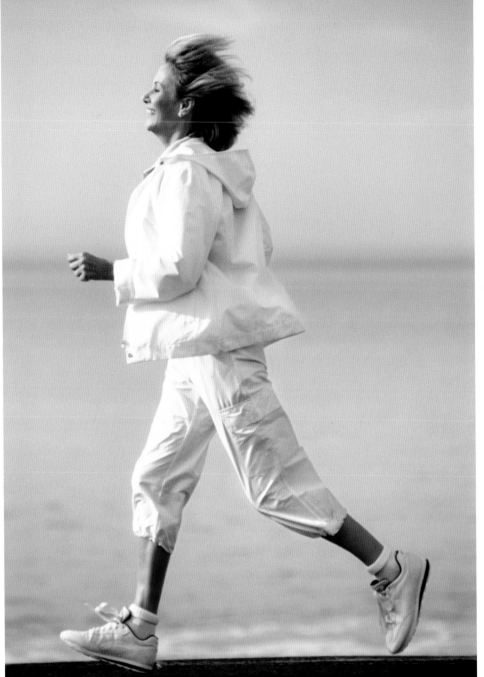

age: as much as 50 per cent by the age of forty. It's also a key factor in keeping joints lubricated and working smoothly. And another thing (or two): it may help dry eye syndrome and also vaginal dryness.

Try: Hyaluronic Acid Capsules High Strength by LifeTime Vitamins, one to two capsules daily.

● **Co-enzyme Q10 (aka Co-Q10):** this vitamin-like compound, which also declines with age, is essential for keeping your muscles (including your heart), gums and immune system in good shape,

and it's vital for anti-ageing in all ways, as well as helping with energy generally. NB: if you take a statin (to lower cholesterol), it's important to take Co-Q10 too as the statin can block production of Co-Q10 and this may create problems in itself.

Try: Super Ubiquinol by Life Extension – ubiquinol is the active form of Co-Q10. Most products are formulated as ubiquinone which is then converted into ubiquinol; taking this supplement as ubiquinol tends to suit people with any sort of digestive problem such as IBS (irritable bowel syndrome) or sluggishness. Take one daily with food.

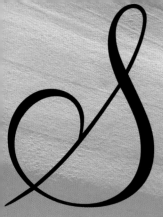

How to fade your stretch marks

Most women have looked down their body at some point and gasped as they saw the zigzag lines embellishing their skin. We can't really pretend they're gorgeous, so if you can't learn to love them (or at least live with them), we have ways of making them less…

Stretch marks shouldn't be called stretch marks at all – they're really 'hormone' marks. They may happen at puberty (when hormones kick in), pregnancy (ditto) and even sometimes at menopause (which seems especially cruel, if you ask us, considering all the other stuff we have to deal with). It's a bit of a hormonal lottery as to whether you'll get them, but women (and some men) do also get them after weight loss and weight gain (that was Sarah). And the bottom line is that however stretch marks appear on your body, they can cause some distress. So: what to do? Below you will find some general tips – and overleaf, the products our ten women tester panels voted the most effective (and somewhat to our surprise, some really were).

Do as they do in the Mediterranean. Oil yourself. Liberally. Regularly. Olive oil, cocoa butter, shea butter, rosehip oil (which has shown great skin-healing results): all manner of rich and lavish oils will lubricate and nourish the skin. So: anoint your stretch marks at bedtime with oils. When skin is well-nourished, the marks are less obvious. It will also feel smoother and sexier, and more strokeable generally. We're all for that.

Eat foods rich in vitamin K, and plenty of essential fatty acids (EFAs). Vitamin K is a fantastic 'skin-healing' vitamin, found in leafy green vegetables (Brussels sprouts, broccoli, spinach, parsley, okra, mustard greens, peas, artichokes), lentils, kidney beans, plums, liver (if you're not vegetarian) and dairy products. To preserve the vitamin K, all the vegetables should

ideally be consumed raw, or very lightly cooked (save the water for a soup or stock, to reclaim its nutritional value). See page 180 for more about EFAs and their sources.

Live a more holistic lifestyle. This is pretty much the advice that you'll find scattered through this book (because when it comes to looking and feeling fabulous IT WORKS), but eating a good diet, exercising regularly and maintaining a stable weight may have another benefit: it may just help fade your stretch marks. OK, so this is just us speaking (not some doctor with a string of initials after his name), but Sarah used to have shiny stretch marks zigzagging up her hips on either side of her belly. After several years of healthy living – and oiling her body (see left) – she realised the marks had literally vanished. When Jo read this in the answer to a reader's question to www.beautybible.com, she decided to check out her own ancient stretch marks and discovered – to her astonishment – that they had faded too. Not a sign. We can only attribute this to consistent healthy living, and a diet that incorporates plenty of EFAs (plus supplements) and literally mountains of the types of veggies mentioned left.

Try Heal Gel. Anecdotally, Heal Gel has had remarkable results on many different types of scarring (including tough-to-treat keloid scarring). Developed by leading plastic surgeons with a biochemist, this treatment – which also works on sprains, sunburn and bruising – can be worth a shot. You need to apply it two or three times daily, and although you only need a titchy bit, that could prove an expensive option. For other options, trialled by our tester panels, see overleaf.

Buy a tankini. It's tummy stretch marks that really seem to upset the women we know. (Despite the fact that the marks are usually a proud badge of motherhood.) If the one thing standing between you and baring your stomach in public is a network of stretch marks, consider a tankini: the vest top of this style of two-piece swimsuit can be rolled up when nobody's looking, so you get the glorious feeling of air on your skin (and a touch of sun) in the privacy of your back deck/garden, or rolled down in company. Your bikini days may be over, but your tankini days needn't be.

If they really distress you, consider laser or IPL treatment. This works best with pigmented stretch marks; pale or flesh-toned marks don't respond so well to treatment – although there are now re-pigmenting lasers that can help with this. The Lux1540 laser has been approved by the FDA in the US for the treatment of stretch marks, but is only available in a handful of locations. We would certainly suggest only going to a 'master' of laser surgery (local clinics may promise the earth to get your bucks, but as with all high-tech treatments we advise major caution). Be sure you are armed with all the right questions, as per Wendy Lewis's advice on page 46. You may want to consider a pre-treatment consultation with Wendy herself (Wendy works in the US but you can contact her via email and she does consultations on Skype – see DIRECTORY). Beware: this will be expensive, and at this stage in life it's unrealistic to expect to go back to your smooth-skinned former self.

STRETCH MARKS: THE SCIENCE BIT

Stretch marks – as many of us know – start as fine red or brown lines (sometimes raised) and can deepen to purple on some people. But it's the legacy of stretch marks that causes so much heartache: they fade to a white or silver colour (usually lighter than your natural skintone), but the skin can be much (much) slacker – so it folds and, yes, hangs differently. They're most common on the abdomen, breasts, thighs and buttocks. As well as reproductive hormonal changes, why are stretch marks also linked with gaining and losing weight? According to Dr Eric F Bernstein (Clinical Associate Professor of Dermatology at the University of Pennsylvania School of Medicine, and head of the Scientific Advisory Board of www.stretchmarks.org), 'When people gain weight, our hormones are metabolised by fat cells. Hormones resemble fat and cholesterol, so when we gain and lose weight it affects the hormones in our body – and also the hormones in our skin.' Normal skin is 80 per cent collagen and just 4 per cent elastin, but that elastin is oh-so-important for skin resilience – and stretch marks are basically damaged elastin fibres. According to Dr Bernstein, 'Elastin fibres are the single hardest thing to repair in skin.'

SCAR GAZING

Beat-generation poet Fran Landesman, who's still writing and doing readings in her eighties, wrote a poem called 'Scars' – and it applies just as much to stretch marks (except that wouldn't sound so poetic...). Fran has had grateful fanmail from women who she's helped to come to terms with their scars. You can find the whole thing on www.franlandesman. com – do look. Here's a snippet we love:

Don't be ashamed
Everybody's got scars
From our various wars
On the way to the
　stars
So I'll show you my
　scars
If you show me yours
In the streets and the
　bars
Everybody's got scars
On their way to the
　stars
Everybody's got scars

SKIN TAGS

Skin tags: these tiny little growths, which may be flesh-colour, or sometimes look brown or purple-ish, are not harmful but are often unsightly and can be irritating if they are near or on your eyes, or where clothes rub. An old-fashioned DIY method was to tie a piece of cotton tightly round the base, blocking the blood supply so they eventually dropped off (ligation). However, this carries a risk of infection, so do consult your family doctor or dermatologist who can remove it with a minor surgical procedure. The most common options are cryotherapy (where very cold liquid nitrogen is applied directly to the area), cauterisation (heat is used to burn off the tag, called electrolysis), and excision (the tag is cut off with a scalpel). Your doctor will use local anaesthetic if necessary and provide an antibiotic ointment to prevent infection. If the tag is very close to the eyelid, the procedure may need to be done by an ophthalmologist.

Stretch mark treatments: our award winners

Stretch marks are a concern for expectant mothers but as the collagen and elastin in skin break down with ageing, they can be even more anxiety-inducing later in life. (As we say, for some women, stretch marks make an unwelcome appearance at menopause, since they're linked with hormonal upheaval rather than 'stretching'.) With an increasing number of treatments on the market, this was one of the toughest challenges in the book: can anything lessen or reverse stretch marks? Our testers were rather pleasantly surprised (and so, to be honest, are we!)

AT A GLANCE

Aromatherapy Associates Renew Rose Massage & Body Oil

Bio-Oil

This Works Stretch Mark Oil

Erbaviva Stretch Mark Cream

TIP

One tester trialling the top-scoring cellulite product Thalgo Crème Thalgomince (page 38) noticed that it had a double-whammy effect, not only greatly improving cellulite but also helping to fade her silvery stretch marks. Result!

REVIEWS

Aromatherapy Associates Renew Rose Massage & Body Oil

 8.75/10 As regular readers know, Aromatherapy Associates' oils are long-standing favourites of ours. They submitted this rose, orange blossom and evening primrose-based oil for this tough stretch-mark category, with recommendations to apply daily. A light oil, it's easily absorbed. In fact, this oil's effect on stretch marks was not as crucial to testers as its knockout effect on skin generally and the fact they adored using it so much.

Comments: 'Absolutely divine smell, stretch marks less unsightly after using, also helped fresh scarring, I am completely hooked on this and will be buying copious bottles regardless of price; the bonus is that it keeps your whole skin glowing and moisturised all day long' • 'skin took on youthful bloom and was very soft' • 'my worst stretch mark is much paler, skin much smoother but to be honest, I wasn't bothered: too busy loving my skin. I am a convert – my skin is so happy and so am I' • 'my daughter watched me changing and after a few minutes said, 'Mum, your skin looks lovely!' • 'vast improvement in skintone and I think stretch marks also improved – I certainly felt much happier wearing a swimming costume than I have in years' • 'the silver of my marks didn't change but they are much smoother, and I loved everything about this product'.

Bio-Oil

 8.21/10 Bio-Oil is something of a beauty legend, with many women we know swearing by its effect on scars and stretch marks, as well as an everyday (or rather, everynight) facial oil. We'd never managed to put it through its paces till the trials for this book, and it performed very well in this challenging category. We do need to knock one myth on the head, though: there's a common misconception (echoed in their marketing) that Bio-Oil is 100 per cent botanical, when the key ingredient is mineral oil. (That does happen to be amazing for helping to maintain skin's moisture levels, FYI.)

Comments: 'Lovely fresh smell and after a few weeks, old scars have begun to fade considerably, some gone completely, skin is smoother and less crêpey and in time I think even my older stretch marks will fade: excellent product' • 'also very good on eczema on hands and boobs' • 'absorbs easily and no residue on clothes, have lots of quite deep stretch marks on tummy, skin now looks smoother and improvement in general texture; stretch marks still visible but on the plus side my C-section scars have nearly vanished!' • 'I've used this as a preventative long term during my pregnancies and through diets and had very few stretch marks, which have faded by now; I've used other products that don't work. This is great'.

This Works Stretch Mark Oil

7.8/10 Our friend, beauty editor and This Works founder Kathy Phillips truly believes in the power of massage to prevent stretch marks (she had a massage every two weeks while expecting her son Oscar). In her range, then, she made sure to include a rich blend designed to counteract the appearance of stretch marks, blending oils of passionfruit seed, gold of pleasure, rosehip seed, alongside coconut and soothing chamomile. This product had the most positive comments about actual effect on stretch marks of all we tested, as well as a high pleasure factor.

Comments: 'Over one month of use, dark stretch marks faded considerably and some of the new ones had disappeared; skin very hydrated; what a shock that a stretch mark product actually works! Wonderful!' • 'just perfect for its job – getting rid of those awful stretch marks; love the fact it's natural too' • 'This Works actually WORKS – what a little miracle' • 'sank in immediately, very attracted to the smell, my skin drank it in and the overall look was improved, as well as helping stretch marks – a marked improvement: treat to use' • 'a joy to use; divine smell, very nourishing product that leaves skin looking and feeling wonderful, with stretch marks much improved; has definitely made my 17-year-old-marks much less noticeable and I would highly recommend it to any mums-to-be'.

Erbaviva Stretch Mark Cream

7.25/10 This USDA-certified organic cream – rather than an oil – is packed with shea butter, sea buckthorn, algae extract, allantoin and feverfew extracts, deliciously scented with organic lavender, mandarin, rose and sandalwood. Erbaviva – a natural brand with a particular focus on motherhood and babies – recommend using this in tandem with their Stretch Mark Oil, but our testers got good results from this alone.

Comments: 'Stretch marks became less noticeable and slightly faded, very easy to use and I think marks would greatly improve with time' • 'light pink and silvery marks on lower tummy from weight gain/loss have really improved; I wasn't that bothered but seeing the difference has made me committed to using this product' • 'skin softer and more supple, does look better' • 'marks started to fade a little after a week's use'.

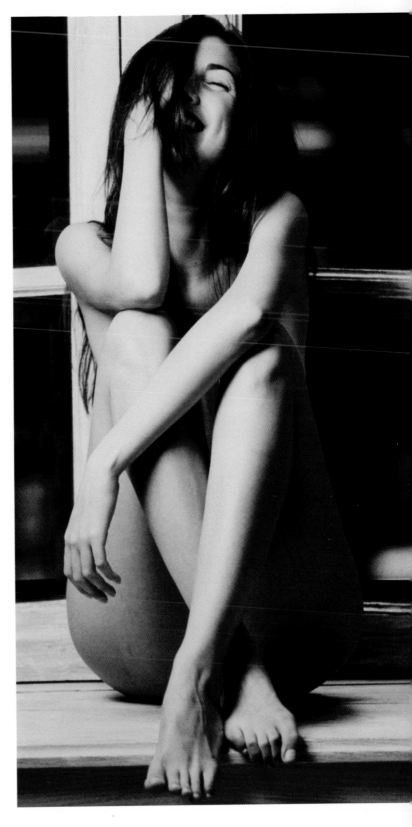

Put sun spots in the shade

Age spots. Liver spots. Whatever you like to call them, they're something we can all live without

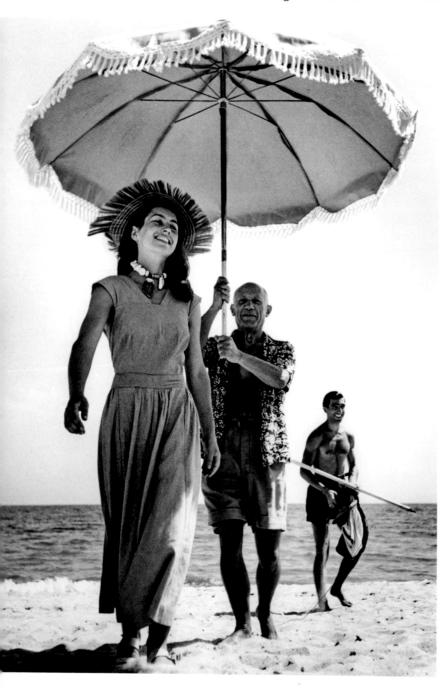

Lines we can live with. (Just.) But according to research carried out for Clinique, the problem of uneven pigmentation can be more distressing than wrinkles. The research also identified that from the perspective of a stranger looking at your skin, pigmentation issues ('dark spots', 'sun spots', 'age spots' – or to give them their formal name, 'solar lentigines') can increase your perceived age. Ironically, according to Dr Daniel Yarosh (who's Senior Vice President, Research and Development Basic Science at Estée Lauder), 'Today, these spots are appearing in people decades before their first senior moment. That is a dangerous sign that sun worship is out of control.'

It's fair to say that tackling the problem is one of The Big Beauty Challenges Of All Time (which is one reason we're so tub-thump-y about sun protection everywhere in this book) – but on the upbeat side there are steps you can take if you're troubled by uneven pigmentation.

Never venture out without an SPF30 or over. And please Start Right Now! This is non-negotiable; it should prevent the spots you have from getting any worse, and may actually go some way towards slightly fading them. If you aren't affected by age spots so far? A daily SPF15 (or higher) will go a long way to preventing their future appearance; for a rundown of the daily sun-protective moisturisers which our testers liked best, see page 188. Hand creams with a built-in SPF can be super-useful on the backs of hand/forearms. If you tend to spend a lot of time outdoors, apply regular sunscreen to these vulnerable zones, and remember to repeat after hand-washing (advice which we echo in our HANDS section, page 122).

Wear a hat. If you have sun spots, or seek to avoid their appearance, we also advise: get yourself a fabulous, stylish collection of fairly tightly-woven straw hats, and keep on a peg near your door/s, for easy grabbing when you go out on a summer day (not a baseball cap because the brims aren't big enough, plus they miss your ears which are very vulnerable). Sometimes anti-ageing solutions can be wonderfully low-tech. Wide-armed, large-lensed sunspecs also help.

Try a specific 'age spot' treatment. A vast amount of cosmetic research dollars is currently being channelled into this area of skincare. Dermatologists in some countries can still prescribe hydroquinone for the problem, but in others this skin-lightener has been banned (research showed that it caused mutations in DNA in animal lab tests – though we totally disapprove of those). And even in the US, where its use is popular, treatment with prescription 4 per cent hydroquinone is restricted to a maximum of 12 weeks. We would suggest one of the alternative over-the-counter cosmetic options – and for a shortcut to the most effective, see what really works on page 190.

Apply the product very carefully – don't slap it on before reading the directions. Be aware: most of these treatments take some time to kick in, and there are no overnight miracles here. (You're probably looking at three months minimum, which is longer than most 'miracle' wrinkle treatments take.) Be aware, too, that some are for all-over skin application, and others are literally 'spot-targeted', requiring the use of a cotton bud to apply precisely. Get out your magnifying glasses and read the instructions before throwing out (preferably recycling) the box. Another tip is to apply a thin amount to dark areas at least one

THE SCIENCE BIT

Sun spots, explains Dr Daniel Yarosh, are a direct result of accumulated sun damage, which triggers melanin-producing cells in the skin to lose control and produce too much pigment as a defence mechanism – on the face and chest, in particular, but also the arms and backs of the hands, where they're harder to conceal. Fairer skins are more susceptible – and against a paler background, age spots show up more, too. Jo had one of those 'oh s**t' moments when a dermatologist told her that the dark patches on the side of her face were sun spots, not – as she'd thought/hoped – beauty marks. Which goes to show how easy it is to miss the edges of the face and the outer jaw-line when applying sunscreen. So be sure to smooth your morning SPF into the whole face. Many botanicals have proven pigment-lightening actions, including azaleic acid (from barley and wheat), kojic acid (from fermented mushrooms), retinoic acid and retinols (vitamin A derivatives which are also famously effective against lines), magnesium ascorbyl phosphate (a stabilised form of vitamin C) and liquorice. They all work by inhibiting the melanin-producing enzyme tyrosinase.

KEEP AN EYE ON YOUR MOLES

Most people have ten to forty moles, some many more. Most moles are benign but it's always worth doing a mole check every month or so from top to toe, including your back. If you notice changes in colour (especially if moles are bi-coloured), size, height or shape, or they bleed, ooze, itch, appear scaly, or become tender and/or painful, consult your doctor or dermatologist.

hour before bedtime; this will let it fully absorb into the skin so it won't slide into your eyes when you press your face into the pillow. (Although the products are mild, skin-lightening ingredients can still sting eyes.)

Use make-up to conceal the spot. Once you've got an age spot, what's to do? For a quick fix, turn to make-up. As we explain on page 88, after your primer, dot on a matt, yellow- or peach-based corrector or concealer (deeper peach for women of colour), with a little brush,

then press it in with your finger – don't sweep it on. If needed, top with cream or liquid foundation or brush on a mineral powder base.

Be careful with fragrance. Certain perfume ingredients – particularly some derived from citrus (such as bergamot) – can interact with sunlight to cause permanent pigmentation problems, in the form of 'staining' of the skin, with dark streaks or patches – typically on the neck and chest, where perfume is spritzed or splashed. We counsel: in summer, it's safest to apply perfume to skin for evening only rather than daytime, or put it where the sun won't strike directly. (So long as there's no risk of staining your clothes, fabric is a wonderful 'carrier' for scent, too; more on page 102.)

Zap 'em. The super-high-tech solution is laser treatment, which can disperse these patches of pigmentation, literally 'zapping' the melanin into oblivion. It's painful. It's expensive. If you really decide to go down this route, turn to page 46 and arm yourself with all the advice that you need to shop around to optimise your chances of a safe, effective treatment.

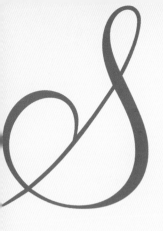

Sun protective day creams: *our award winners*

Repeat after us, please: 'The very best way to stop my face from ageing is to protect it from the sun.' It is never too late to add an SPF day cream into your skincare regime – but it's never too early, either. This goes for all skin colours and types, dermatologists insist, to prevent the signs of ageing. And for anyone already suffering age/sun spots, sun protection is essential to prevent further damage and give any targeted pigmentation treatment the best chance of working. (More about those overleaf)

A good SPF day cream, though, doesn't just offer protection: it sinks in sufficiently well NOT to leave skin either greasy or with a white film of sun-protective ingredients on the surface. The following creams – each with an SPF15 or above – fit the bill beautifully, according to our panellists. Optimum protection starts here.

REVIEWS

Clinique Superdefense SPF25

 8.88/10 Another impressively high score for Clinique, who've done very well in this book. Their thinking is that 'stress ages skin, making it dull and lifeless' (we agree!), so alongside the SPF25 (higher than most daily creams), there are 'skin de-stressing' ingredients, including a rare red microalgae extract. It's lightweight and – being Clinique – hypoallergenic and fragrance-free.

Comments: '10 out of 10: sank in easily, gave dewy effect and kept skin moisturised all day; good base for make-up and skin doesn't dry out after foundation/powder are applied' • 'skin felt soft and moisturised all day, looks radiant' • 'love it! Moisturises very effectively, absorbs very well with no residue, I thought it would be far too heavy and make my skin shiny but it didn't aggravate my acne and was a very nice base for foundation' • 'you use

very little so it lasts a long time' • 'moisturised really well, the best I have tried; sank in well leaving dewy glow and was rich enough for the dry parts of my face – would like it in a tube rather than a pot though'.

Sarah Chapman London Skinesis Dynamic Defence Anti-ageing Day Cream SPF15

 8.64/10 Sarah Chapman has become one of our favourite facialists (we're lucky enough to be fast-tracked up her waiting list), offering treatments from a tiny Chelsea clinic for which women fly from around the globe. We're fans of her signature skincare products, including this rich, subtly jasmine/hyacinth/rose-scented daily moisturiser, which is packed with vitamins, antioxidants, omega-rich oils and a broad-spectrum SPF15. A fave of Jo's (see We Love…).

Comments: 'Fantastic! Left skin dewy and well-balanced' • 'easily absorbed rich cream which leaves my very dry skin supple, silky, dewy and clear; I have fallen in love with this product and would buy it again' • 'superb packaging with integral pump, although possibly a bit rich for my shiny skin, which is prone to spots' • 'brilliant product which moisturised well so my skin kept a lovely glow; make-up went on very well after' • 'very rich cream which felt divine and smelt really nice but subtle' • 'lovely matt finish once it sunk in'.

♡ WE LOVE...

For day, Jo alternates between three SPF moisturisers (switching when she gets to the end of the product, so there's no risk of the SPF degrading): Dior Hydra Life Pro-Youth Protective Fluid SPF15 is great for summer (it's super-skin-quenching but not greasy), while Sarah Chapman London Skinesis Dynamic Defence Anti-ageing Day Cream SPF15 and Vaishaly Anti-Ageing Day Moisturiser (Dry/Sensitive) are more suited for the chillier seasons. Sarah too has several favourites, including all-natural Kimberly Sayer Anti-Oxidant Daily Moisturizing Cream SPF25 (for summer) and our award winner Clinique Superdefense SPF25 (for winter).

Estée Lauder Time Zone Line and Wrinkle Reducing Crème SPF15

8.42/10

With a light, fresh scent, this rich, skin-plumping cream harnesses two of the breakthrough technologies from their super-boffins: replenishing Tri-Hyaluronic Complex and Sirtuin EX-1 Technology, 'to help skin naturally stimulate its proteins'. What you'll really want to hear, though, are these real-life tester comments on its peformance.

Comments: 'Very, very effective – great moisturiser but feels lightweight; sank in fast, and not at all greasy; skin felt much smoother and even, make-up much easier to apply; loved this and saw a huge difference to my combination skin – more moisturised, fewer breakouts, even colour, it ticks all the boxes' • 'keeps skin feeling moist, lovely fresh smell, shiny at first but sinks in nicely, and keeps skin settled during the day' • 'left a great dewy/healthy glow, and make-up sits on top very well' • 'perfect moisturiser which I've been using for months, makes my skin look more radiant and feel completely moisturised – one of my Holy Grail products to fight the signs of ageing!'.

Eve Lom Moisturiser + SPF15

8.25/10

Legendary facialist Eve Lom has now added an SPF day cream to her range, which moisturises while delivering a matt finish. There are antioxidant red, green and white teas to protect against environmental damage, soothing bisabolol and yarrow, firming chestnut, plus shea butter for moisture power. There's a teensy bit of lactic acid to brighten skin, but Jo (who's sensitive to alpha-hydroxy/fruit acids) gets on fine with this. No fragrance that we can discern!

Comments: 'The best moisturiser I have used, my skin feels great! Heaven in a pot – like putting whipped cream on your skin; melts in skin quickly leaving it soft and hydrated and make-up went on beautifully after' • 'loved the fact it had SPF15 but left no white residue' • 'I've been using it twice daily for six weeks and am about halfway through the pot so it goes quite a long way' • 'quenched my thirsty skin, left it glowing and bright from within but not shiny or weighed down; looks thick and gloopy but very light texture and immediately absorbed' • 'doesn't clog up skin which is very important for sensitive complexions like mine'.

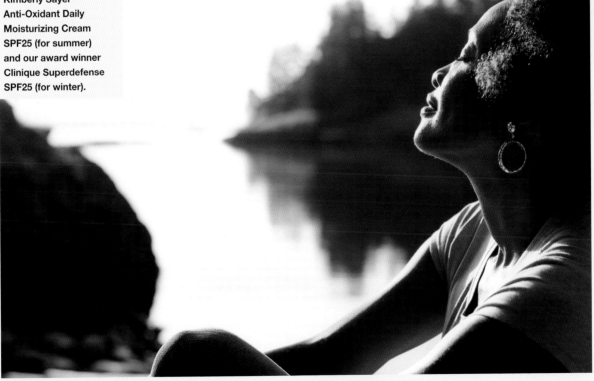

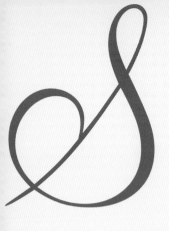

Sun spot treatments: *our award winners*

In recent years, the beauty industry has declared sun spots (aka brown, liver or age spots) Public Enemy Number One, with lots of launches targeting hyperpigmentation. Bold claims are made but we weren't sure whether any would demonstrate a real and visible impact on pigmentation marks

Our testers were asked to trial products on specific, affected spots on their faces, and monitor very carefully the improvements (if any). The scores varied widely so the averages aren't that high. And the results were mixed. For the products below, an average of just under half the testers saw some visible improvement (usually slight) in sun spots BUT they loved these products for their skin-brightening, decongesting, rejuvenating, skintone-evening effects – and would buy them just for that. (Our testers of miracle creams also noted that Melvita Naturalift Anti-Ageing Cream lessened hyperpigmentation, see page 18.)

REVIEWS

Dior Capture Totale Radiance Enhancer

 This luxurious pale pink serum/cream (at an accordingly luxe price) is instantly luminous, so the appearance of pigmentation and redness are toned down straight away. (Think of it as a bit like an all-over light-reflecting concealer.) Over and above the instant concealing effect, two testers felt it improved the sun spots on their faces somewhat, a third said it helped those on her hands; the rest saw no long-term difference in pigmentation but voted it a 'miracle' cream for improving vibrancy, tone and clarity.
Comments: 'Some improvement in sun spots after two weeks but my skin generally just looked so much better; fantastic product that made my skin appear younger and more vibrant' • 'when I finished the product, age spots weren't as noticeable, skin

more even, with pigmentation faded and so looked slightly younger' • 'after two weeks sun spots began to fade slightly and weren't as noticeable; by the end of the product, they were much less visible though not completely gone, but I can't see them after I put on make-up' • 'I have quite a few tiny sun spots on my cheeks and this evened out the tone immediately, though didn't really make a difference long term: but skin was smoother and brighter and clearer so I love it and don't want to stop using it!' • 'no difference to age spots but my skin is much brighter; I am hooked on this gorgeous cream'.

Origins Brighter By Nature High-potency Brightening Peel with Fruit Acids

This is a brightening solution based on AHA/fruit acids impregnated into (wet) pads to swipe over the face, with high-potency skin-brightening botanicals derived from coconut and salicylic acid (willow bark), balanced by soothing cucumber extract, aloe, Japanese basil leaf and caffeine, plus a mega-antioxidant complex. In their own clinical tests, Origins observed results comparable to a 30 per cent glycolic peel.
Comments: 'I have areas of pigmentation on cheek bones and upper lip; after two weeks using these slightly abrasive pads there was a slight fading of age spots, overall skin felt smoother and brighter immediately, less congested; by the end, the pigmentation had faded slightly but no dramatic improvement, however the overall skintone and clarity has improved' • 'after two weeks, the spots on my forehead going into my hairline became

AT A GLANCE

Dior Capture Totale Radiance Enhancer

Origins Brighter By Nature High-potency Brightening Peel with Fruit Acids

L'Occitane Immortelle Very Precious Brightening Concentrate

Origins Brighter By Nature Skin Tone Correcting Serum

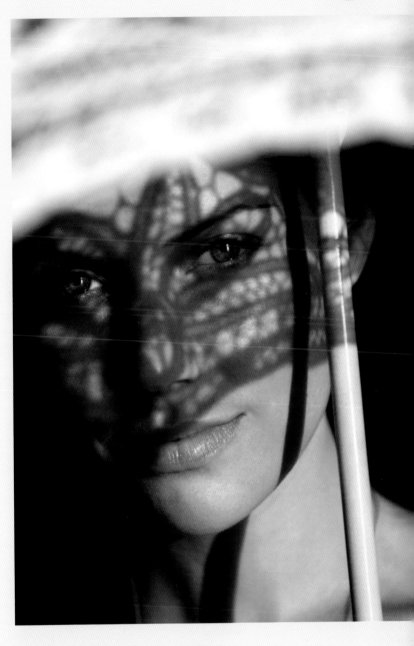

micro-sized, and are now unnoticeable, plus my skin looks a lot younger' • 'no difference in age spots but the product is definitely peeling away redness and fellow book clubbers noticed improved clarity, brightness and more even tone' • 'I do believe my age spots and pigmentation have faded a little, so I do look younger and people say I look healthy'.

L'Occitane Immortelle Very Precious Brightening Concentrate ❀ ❀

 7.28/10

Immortelle is a 'wild and mysterious flower from Corsica which yields a miraculous essential oil' and the signature ingredient in this Provençal brand's eponymous anti-ageing skincare. Over 3,000 Immortelle flowers are concentrated into a single bottle of Brightening Concentrate (essentially a facial oil), with a vitamin C derivative, combined with orange and grapefruit oils (mmmm, lovely smell) to even out the complexion.

Comments: 'Sun spots reduced drastically by the end of testing, and skin was toned, brighter, fresher and younger-looking – despite being off work for long-term sick leave, colleagues said I looked well and my skin healthy' • 'skin looked and felt much fresher and "alive"' • 'sun/age spots slightly improved but tone much better and skin looks younger' • 'truly gorgeous product but don't think it's made a difference to the targeted sun spots' • 'tried this on two sun spots, one on my nose, another on my forehead, which have both faded though still quite visible – initial results impressive but little difference after first few days' • 'helped to fade pigmentation and skin brighter and smoother'.

Origins Brighter By Nature Skin Tone Correcting Serum ❀

 7.25/10

This time a lightweight serum from Origins, which showed a 42 per cent reduction in age spots in their own eight-week trials, with participants using it twice daily. The secret is a potent blend of Japanese basil leaf, salicylic acid, vitamin C and yeast extract, plus complexion-nurturing sunflower seed cake (truly!) and barley extract, with cucumber.

Comments: 'My very small sun/age spots on my forehead are slightly reduced with this light serum; skintone improved, smoother and brighter: my husband said I looked radiant!' • 'tried this on the spots on the back of one hand and they're now definitely lighter than those on the other, clear difference!' • 'really liked the product but no change to my long-term sun spots' • 'definitely evened out my skintone, sun spots faded and age-related redness – my whole face is more uniform in colour'.

Brush up on tooth wisdom

The thing the majority of people remember most vividly from a first meeting is your smile. (Why do you think Julia Roberts became galactic?) OK, as the years go by, flashing a Californian-babe beam may look out of place but long term, caring for your teeth (and gums) is vital for your appearance, confidence – and your general health

We've become a bit obsessed about our teeth and gums. We're both lucky in that we have quite strong teeth and, partly because we eat well, they aren't discoloured or stained. (Though Sarah had veneers applied in her thirties because of brown stains and shortened teeth due to tetracycline antibiotics as a child.) But we want to keep them that way, and also keep our gums in good shape so that teeth don't get loose. (The thought of putting them in a glass at night is a powerful incentive.) Plus, your whole mouth structure is so important for literally holding up your face – if that gets slack and/or you lose teeth, your cheeks cave in, and that really does age you in a trice. So we're going to spend a bit of time in this section of the book giving you expert advice from London-based holistic dentist Dr David Cook, who has transformed the mouths (and in some cases lives) of several people we know.

So, what ages your smile?
● Stained, discoloured or mismatched teeth.
● Gum disease, which causes gums to recede so teeth look long and horsey; gaps like black triangles often appear at the gum line; loose gums mean teeth may fall out.
● Tooth loss (also grinding, see below) can lead to the lower part of your face looking 'caved in', appearing pinched and shorter with more lines and folds, as well as having gaps (obviously).
● Grinding your teeth at night (bruxism) wears them down, making them shorter and squarer, which distorts the proportions and makes them look less attractive when you're smiling.
● Grinding also causes jaw muscles to bulk up so you get a square-jawed look (not very feminine).

Can the state of your teeth affect your health? In a word, yes…
● Gum disease (aka gingivitis) increases the risk of heart disease, stroke and, in women of child-bearing age, low-birthweight babies. There is also increasing evidence of a link with osteoporosis, type 2 diabetes, Alzheimer's disease and other inflammatory conditions.
● The bacteria that cause gum disease can be passed to others, so partners, children and grandchildren are at increased risk. (Kissing babies is a bad idea if you have gum disease.)
● Poor oral hygiene and gum disease are the primary causes of chronic bad breath (halitosis) and the sufferer is often unaware of the problem.
● Tooth wear and loss can lead to the collapse of your ability to bite down on food – this means your jaw muscles and joints have to work harder, putting strain on them and causing pain and further bite problems.
● Grinding your teeth at night can cause poor sleep patterns, with all its related problems.

WE LOVE…

Dental Miracle, an all-natural green powder with orris root, juniper berry, peppermint, calendula and acacia gum, which leaves your breath fragrant and has a gently abrasive action to leave teeth sparkling clean. It also claims to help 'reinforce' gums, as well as preventing and getting rid of plaque.

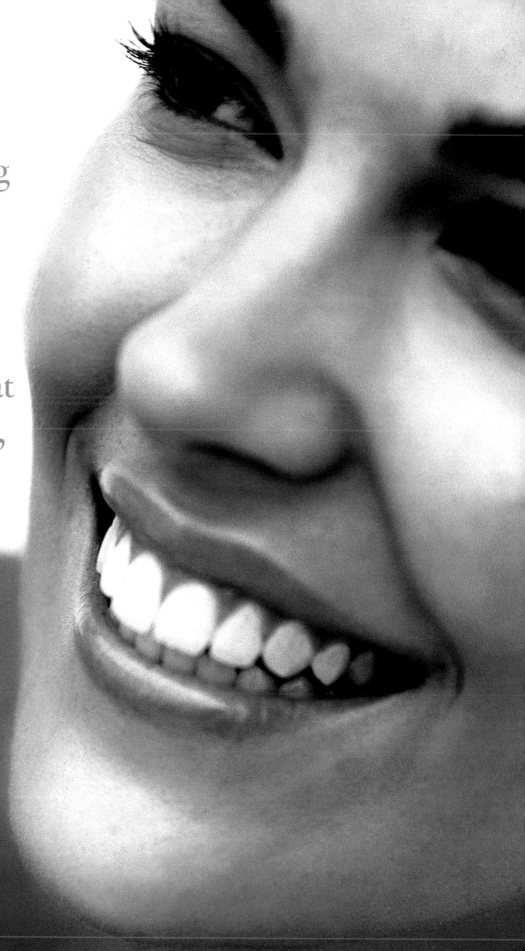

'Nothing makes a woman more beautiful than the belief that she is beautiful'

Sophia Loren

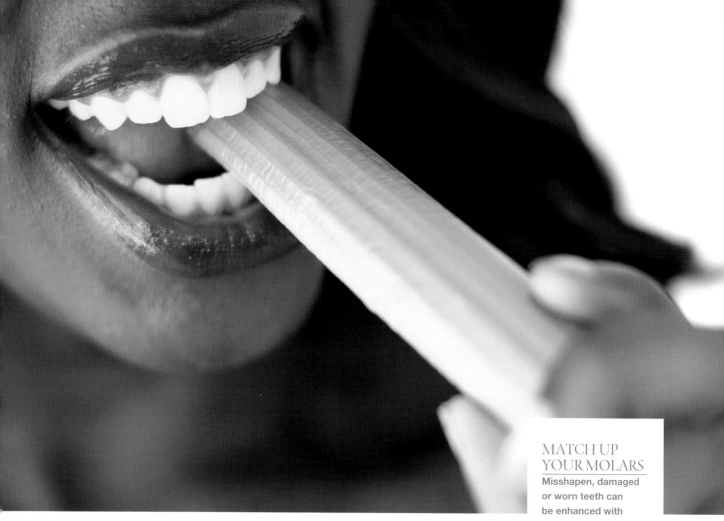

So what exactly is going on?

Read Dr Cook's advice on common problems and how you can treat them.

Brighten stained and discoloured teeth

As teeth age they tend to get darker, due to stains building up on the surface of the teeth and also penetrating the surface through micro cracks and porosities. Tea, coffee, red wine and tobacco are the main culprits here, and surprisingly herbal and fruit teas are notable culprits too.

A twice-yearly professional clean by a hygienist can work wonders. Once all stain and surface discolouration is polished away you may be surprised at how good your teeth look. After that, using whitening toothpaste with a sonic toothbrush can be very effective at reducing the rate of further stain build-up. (You may need advice from your hygienist on how best to use a

sonic toothbrush; also see box page 198.)

Teeth that are badly discoloured or have lost their sparkle and vitality can be rejuvenated with whitening (aka bleaching), using hydrogen peroxide gels which work all the way through the teeth and actually change the colour. Gel concentration and safe application time varies widely, so this should definitely be done under the supervision of a dentist. Provided that tooth whitening/bleaching is done professionally, it is safe, very effective and has few side effects apart from temporary sensitivity. Over-the-counter (or internet) whitening products are usually ineffective and may be damaging due to high acidity, so they should be avoided.

MATCH UP YOUR MOLARS

Misshapen, damaged or worn teeth can be enhanced with porcelain veneers, crowns or onlays to give a beautiful and functional appearance. These techniques can also be used to restore a severely worn or damaged bite, which returns facial balance and gives support to cheeks and lips – (that's why it's sometimes known as the 'dental facelift').

FIX CROOKED TEETH/ BAD BITE

A crooked smile or bad bite can be corrected with braces, and modern techniques are quick, comfortable and can be virtually invisible.

Love your gums

Gum (periodontal) disease is a chronic bacterial infection of the supporting tissue of the tooth (gums and bone). As the body tries to ward off the infection, inflammation develops; over time this leads to bone loss around the teeth. Often this happens with few external signs and little or no discomfort until quite advanced, which is why regular dental visits are so important. If the reversible early stage of gum disease (gingivitis) is allowed to continue into periodontitis, the bacteria and inflammatory cells can leak into the bloodstream and be carried around the whole body contributing to the problems highlighted on page 192.

What you can do:

● Brush your teeth! The first line of defence is hygiene – meticulous, thorough, regular cleaning with a toothbrush and floss will remove bacteria, reducing inflammation and aiding healing. Aim for twice a day at least.

● Regular visits (usually twice-yearly) to your dentist to monitor disease progress, and to the hygienist to clean the mouth thoroughly and advise on effective homecare – every mouth and person is different, so homecare needs to be tailored to individuals.

● Don't smoke – smokers are more prone to gum disease and once established it will progress much faster than in a non-smoker.

● Eat well: a diet low in all forms of sugar with healthy levels of antioxidants is beneficial. There is growing evidence that supplements of vitamin C, coenzyme Q10 and zinc (antioxidants which also act against inflammation) are also helpful. Natural live yoghurt which has both calcium and lactose bacteria appears to help prevent gum problems.

● Take exercise – it can help to reduce inflammation.

● Try to avoid stress as this leads to a higher risk of disease.

● Drink lots of still water (but not fizzy! See page 197).

● Gum disease runs in families, so be extra vigilant if there's a family history. Women are more likely to suffer, which is probably related to reproductive hormones.

● If you have another inflammatory disease, such as diabetes, keep tight control on blood-sugar levels.

● Brush your teeth! Again!

MAKE UP FOR LOST TEETH

Losing teeth at an early age affects your appearance as well as the way they function (or don't…), plus other teeth can drift around the jaw, leading to bite imbalances. Replacing lost teeth as soon as possible helps prevent more complex problems. There are three basic options to replace missing teeth, all of which can work well.

1 Implant: screwed into the bone, this is effectively a like-for-like replacement which can last a lifetime and is considered the gold standard.

2 Bridge: this uses adjacent teeth to support a replacement unit but can involve damage to the supporting teeth and commonly needs replacing after several years.

3 Denture: this is removable and allows easy cleaning, but can be uncomfortable.

Deal with tooth grinding and bite problems

The wear caused by teeth grinding at night and/or from a 'bad bite' (where your teeth are misaligned so they don't meet correctly when you bite) can cause the structure of your teeth to be badly affected. This can lead to problems such as sensitive teeth, receding gums, and broken teeth or fillings.

Grinding your teeth can actually lead to bite problems because of the damage to tooth structure. The whole thing can become a vicious cycle, causing pain in addition to the other problems above.

Additionally, persistent grinding at night prevents the jaw muscles from relaxing and can lead on to muscle spasm, cramps, head and neck pain, even migraines. Night grinding also disturbs sleep patterns, which can lead to tiredness, stress and so more grinding…

What you can do:

● Have your bite, jaw muscles and joints assessed regularly to catch any problems early, before too much damage occurs.

● Many people with a problem will benefit from a night splint – a custom-made appliance worn over the teeth when sleeping to position the jaws so as to allow muscle relaxation and better-quality sleep, and to help prevent further damage.

● If the damage is more advanced or symptoms are severe, your dentist may advise some form of bite reconstruction (potentially surgical); when done correctly this can not only restore appearance but prevent future problems. NB: this needs an expert practitioner.

● Tension in the head and neck due to a bad bite can be relieved by skilful use of complementary therapies such as physiotherapy, osteopathy and chiropractic. Simple exercises and home massage of the jaw can help greatly (as Sarah knows from personal experience).

A colleague who was prescribed a 'bite splint' says:

'From the first night, I slept more deeply than I had in years. I felt better, looked better and people started asking whether I'd had a holiday'

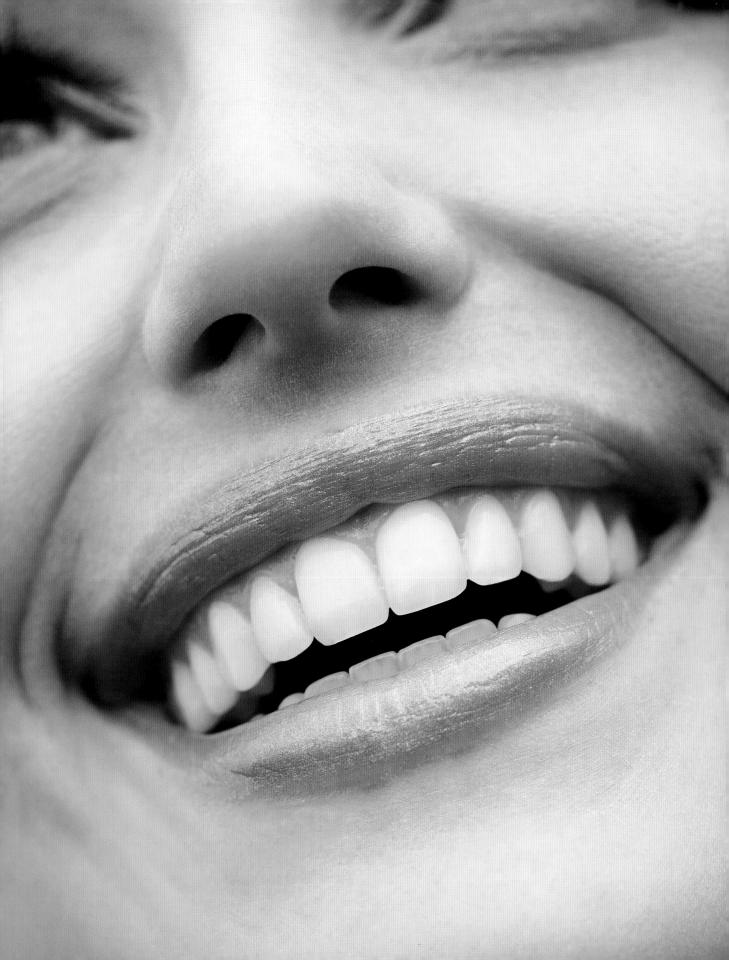

Learn about dental decay – the great enemy for teeth

We all know that sugar is a big problem food in tooth decay. But it's not just eating candy and cake, modern processed foodstuffs often contain hidden sugar, which is tricky to detect. What's more, from a dentist's perspective, natural sugar sources such as fruit and honey are just as problematic. And don't let's even mention fizzy drinks – yet…

To understand what's happening, the all-important link between sugar, acid and tooth decay and what to do about it, we need to know a little bit about the science. (It's riveting, promise!)

Here's Dr Cook's explanation: 'The human mouth is full of bacteria, happily living in the microscopic nooks and crannies and most of them causing no harm – in fact, some give us protection from more dangerous organisms. But certain types love to feast on sugar and the more sugar they eat, the more they multiply. The problem for your teeth is that as the bugs consume sugar, they produce acid (as a waste product) – and that's the agent which attacks and weakens teeth. The acid environment in your mouth also encourages more bacteria, so more acid is produced, and so on…and on…

'The body's defence against each sugar dose is saliva, which neutralises the acid. But this process takes about 45 minutes, during which the acid launches an attack on your teeth, dissolving some of the hard mineral coating of the tooth [demineralisation of the enamel]. Once the saliva has neutralised the acid, the minerals it contains begin to repair some of the acid-damaged enamel [remineralisation]. But if another dose of sugar comes along too soon – continuously sucking sweets, say, through the day, rather than in separate "hits" – effective repair is impossible and the weakened enamel begins to break down and dissolve again. This creates a protected home for more bacteria which can't be completely cleaned off – and a cavity becomes established. The sugar also forms a gungy residue called plaque, which sticks to the tooth.

'But there's an extra threat to your teeth in the shape of acidic foods and drinks, notably carbonated drinks, tea – including fruit teas, coffee, vinegar, alcohol, salad dressing and ketchup.'

What you can do:

● Clean away as much of the bacteria and plaque as possible – brushing and flossing thoroughly, ideally after every meal but at least twice a day.

● If you have snacked on something sugary or acidic (see next point), wait 30 minutes before brushing to allow the acidity in your mouth to become more neutral.

● Remember: the main offenders are sugary foods (including most fruits and fruit juices) and acidic ones (including fizzy drinks, tea, coffee, alcohol, vinegar, ketchup and most salad dressings).

● It is the repeated frequent acid attacks that cause the major damage, so if you want something sugary/acidic, eat it all in one go. Best of all, go for nuts or unsweetened natural yoghurt as a snack.

● Help the naturally protective saliva by chewing sugar-free gum after a meal, preferably one sweetened with xylitol (eg, Trident sugarless gum). This speeds up the neutralisation of acids and the xylitol – a natural sweetener and proven tooth (and bone) strengthener – helps stop the plaque from sticking to teeth.

● Drink plenty of water – this helps flush away acid and keeps saliva flow high.

● End a meal with a little cheese or unsweetened yoghurt: this helps speed up acid neutralisation.

● If you've had a lot of fillings in the past or some of the enamel has been demineralised, you can use a remineralising paste, smeared over the affected areas and left overnight or held in a custom-made tray. This can significantly increase the chance of reversing very early decay (water-based, sugar-free GC Tooth Mousse from your dentist is the most effective).

Know your fillings

Amalgam is a mixture of mercury with silver, copper and tin, which forms a strong, relatively stable material when set. It's been in use as a filling material for over 150 years and continues to be used today, largely because it's inexpensive and requires little skill to place quickly and successfully. So why the fuss? Because mercury is a known poison and extremely toxic. While the majority of the mercury in a dental filling is stable within the amalgam, small amounts are continuously released. If this were anywhere other than inside someone's mouth, it would be classified as an environmentally contaminated zone… Over the past decade, concern about toxicity from mercury in amalgam has increased and many countries restrict the use of mercury-based products.

As a patient, potentially the biggest exposure to mercury is when you are having old amalgam fillings removed. This can be accomplished safely. Check that your dentist understands the risks (you can afford to be blunt). Ensure that a rubber dam will be placed around the tooth to isolate it from the rest of your mouth. Dr Cook normally advises swallowing two activated charcoal tablets before treatment (these mop up any debris that slips past the dam). For more sensitive patients, a clean air supply during the procedure may be advisable, plus specific nutritional supplements afterwards. Once the amalgam is removed, there's a range of options as replacements:

● **Porcelain:** this is very aesthetic, strong and can be used anywhere.

● **Gold:** very noticeable (so unaesthetic), but the strongest and can be used anywhere.

● **Composite resin:** this looks very good and is durable in small- to medium-size cavities, but it is not suitable for back teeth unless they are small.

In Dr Cook's opinion, 'The aesthetics of porcelain outweigh the slightly better strength of gold – particularly "Emax", the latest generation material which is incredibly strong and looks fantastic. But any of the options above can perform very well. However, to get the best out of them requires meticulous technique and is time-consuming, so the procedure will be more expensive than amalgam.'

KEEP YOUR TEETH BEAUTIFULLY CLEAN

The reality is that it's less about what you use and more about how. The basic equipment of a toothbrush with a small to medium head and dental floss is all most people need – if they use it correctly. Having said that, electric brushes, particularly sonic ones, are very effective and there's a wide selection of different brushes specially developed for cleaning between and around teeth and gums.

Every mouth is different, and the correct tools and technique need to be tailored to each individual, so the best advice is to ask your dentist or preferably your hygienist to advise and demonstrate a personalised cleaning routine. Also have it checked after a couple of months to make sure you are managing it correctly. This is probably the best investment of time and money you can make and could save you many times the investment in the future. (For general guidelines, see box left.)

Mainstream toothpastes are all effective (although specific smokers' pastes and powders can be very abrasive and damaging). Fluoride is a naturally occurring element which is incorporated into tooth enamel, making it harder and more resistant to decay. Fluoride toothpaste has been shown to reduce the level of dental decay, so unless your diet and hygiene are perfect, not using a fluoride toothpaste may mean you need more dental work.

The evidence for a protective effect when fluoride is swallowed (in the water supply or as a supplement) is less clear and it can have toxic side effects, so using fluoride like that is controversial. However, if fluoride is applied as a toothpaste in the correct and tiny amount – a pea-size for an adult and half a pea of an appropriate product for a child – and not swallowed, the benefits can be great and the risk is probably negligible. (This is Dr Cook's opinion, which we respect – though we prefer to use natural fluoride-free toothpastes ourselves.)

Another controversial toothpaste additive is sodium lauryl sulphate (SLS): this is a chemical foaming agent common in many household products – shampoo, bubble baths, detergents, etc. It has been shown to cause skin reactions and ulceration. SLS-free toothpastes are available: Dr Cook's favourites are Tom's of Maine Clean & Gentle Care, and Sensodyne Total Care Gel. (We like the Green People and Weleda ranges, which have peppermint-free options suitable for people taking homeopathic remedies.) If you suffer from mouth ulcers, it's worth trying an SLS-free toothpaste.

TEETH-CLEANING TECHNIQUE

Brush your teeth outside and inside for two to three minutes twice daily (at a minimum), after meals, and follow with flossing. If you use a sonic toothbrush, all you need to do is hold the head steady against each tooth where it meets the gum – counting to six on each side. If you're using a manual brush (choose a soft one), hold the brush like a pencil and go round and round gently in little circles on the chewing surfaces of each tooth. The brush should be at a 45 degree angle towards your gum so that the tufts are pressed into it.

TIP

Toothbrush heads harbour bugs, so do change them regularly and particularly after you recover from any infections.

Brightening toothpastes: *our award winners*

A first, for us: we've never trialled toothpastes before. But since a brighter smile can be instantly 'de-ageing', we figured: why not trial brightening, whitening toothpastes alongside all the beauty lotions and potions? With tooth-bleaching procedures more popular than ever, these are the low-tech, daily-use alternative. So: is it possible to brush your way to a brighter smile...? The averages here aren't spectacular but tend to reflect the fact that for some testers they worked really well, while others didn't see much difference. Still, if you're looking for a shortlist of where to head first when looking for a whitening toothpaste, we suggest you start here.

Aquafresh Iso-Active Whitening

A unique 'foaming-gel' – featuring a special ingredient that activates the gel as you brush – this 'directly targets bacteria to fight a key source of oral malodour'(!), and within the Iso-Active range this is the tooth-brightening option. In a pump-action dispenser (which testers mostly disliked, on the score there was too much packaging and the nozzle didn't work that well).

Comments: 'You apply this just like ordinary toothpaste but thinner, rather like Pearl Drops; teeth feel extra clean and mouth very fresh, better than a normal product, so I would buy though not certain if teeth actually whiter' • 'thick paste that really foamed up when applied, very minty but not so much that it stung, teeth felt really fresh and clean after, my slightly stained teeth look much brighter: did get compliments! I love this and won't be without it from now on, lasts a long time and my mouth feels so much cleaner as well' • 'after ten days of using this, two people in two days asked whether I had had my teeth whitened, so they obviously noticed a difference – though to start with I didn't...' • 'I was very sceptical but I have to say my teeth did look much whiter – I was impressed!'.

Beverly Hills Formula Total Breath Whitening

Beverly Hills Formula were pioneers in whitening toothpastes, and promise 'whiter teeth in one minute' from what is now a wide range of formulations. This particular toothpaste features an antibacterial formula to help fight plaque (and bad breath) – leaving breath fresher for up to five times longer than a regular toothpaste, so they say.

Comments: 'Nice light toothpaste with minty aftertaste and I definitely saw a difference, my teeth were much whiter and my family noticed; I tried the tip about leaving it on the tongue for a bit before brushing for freshness and this worked well' • 'my teeth do look good and don't feel rough to the touch as they did at first' • 'I have started drinking green tea without milk and noticed how much it stains the cup: I think it would have stained my teeth but this has kept them looking clean and bright' • 'I enjoyed using this and my teeth did look a little bit better'.

AloeDent Triple Action Toothpaste

AloeDent takes its name from the soothing aloe plant, a key ingredient in this natural toothpaste range, which also combines tea tree oil and green tea extract to fight against bacteria, plus Co-Q10 for healthy gums. The naturally whitening mineral silica is significantly less abrasive, they promise, than conventional stain-removing ingredients.

Comments: 'Really nice taste, no difference in amount of foaming, my teeth felt really clean after' • 'definitely makes my slightly yellow teeth whiter, difference showed up pretty much the first time of use; teeth feel very clean after using too' • 'I thought aloe vera would be horrid but I'm a convert! Teeth feel really clean and mouth fresh' • 'loved the taste – teeth and mouth felt clean and invigorated; though I didn't notice any difference in whiteness, I love this product: it may cost a few pence more but it's really worth it'.

AT A GLANCE

Aquafresh Iso-Active Whitening

Beverly Hills Formula Total Breath Whitening

AloeDent Triple Action Toothpaste

♡ WE LOVE...

Jo uses a natural toothpaste with no specific brightening promises... Sarah particularly likes natural brands with xylitol, a compound that helps prevent bacteria sticking to teeth: these include Xyliwhite Toothpaste, which is fluoride-free, as is Tom's of Maine Tartar Control Plus Whitening Toothpaste, which contains xylitol, zinc citrate and silica (though they appear to contain forms of sodium lauryl sulphate which we don't like so much...).

TIP

Once you've brightened your teeth, keep stain-causing liquids from reversing the improvement by using a straw. (You can do this for hot drinks but it takes a bit of getting used to!)

Tinted moisturisers: *our award winners*

Tinted moisturisers are absolutely brilliant for evening out skintone without making a face look over-made-up. Some, though, are just too moisturising (and so shine-inducing), while others aren't quite dewy enough, so they go on patchily (and so need a moisturiser underneath). With a couple of dozen products to trial, we asked our panellists to help us identify which really are 'the business'

NB: a plea to brands – most women wanting to use a tinted moisturiser are also concerned about sun damage, so could you please start incorporating an SPF in more of these creams? Or is it just a conspiracy to get us to layer on yet another product, come summer…? Most of the winners here do feature an SPF, but that wasn't the case with many contenders.

REVIEWS

RéVive Tinted Moisturizer SPF15

 A sheer, featherlight moisturiser that adds a healthy hint of colour, this is from an advanced skincare range 'infused with Nobel-prize-winning technology' (so RéVive tell us!). A true treatment product, it's packed with antioxidants and vitamins, marine extracts and EGF (Epidermal Growth Factor), to increase cell renewal. It also has an SPF15. (As we say, we wish all tinted moisturisers did.)

Comments: 'I like this; nicely moisturising, with an SPF, covers quite well but not heavy-looking, evens out skintone so it just looks better but not made up' • 'skin feels slightly greasy initially but soon settles to feeling soft, smooth and full of moisture; product has slight luminosity which makes skin more alive and full of bounce' • 'maybe not for oily skin but suits my drier skin beautifully' • 'great velvety texture, not too thick or liquid, blended well to look completely even; covered thread veins, small

spots and dark marks completely, didn't sit in lines and wrinkles'.

Marie Veronique Organics Moisturizing Face Screen SPF30

 From a bijou American natural and organic brand with the highest ethics, this is a non-nanoparticle zinc-oxide-based sunscreen (so no synthetic chemicals here), in a glass jar with a pump action. It comes in two shades of tint (light and medium), and features sea buckthorn, red raspberry and emu oils to moisturise and heal skin, plus a heftier-than-most SPF30.

Comments: 'Did enhance radiance, skin looks better after using this, small blemishes covered; I like it a lot, particularly with the SPF30; not exceedingly moisturising but went on well after a serum' • 'barely there colour, but skin looks bright from the light-reflecting particles; lovely subtle, slightly luminous pearly look; minimises open pores but too sheer to cover other blemishes' • 'made my skin look lovely and good alternative to facial sunscreen'.

Philosophy The Supernatural Poreless Flawless Tinted SPF15

 Oil-free and peachy-toned (very flattering, actually), this also features an SPF (hallelujah), and can be used on its own to even out complexion or as a pore-minimising primer under foundation.

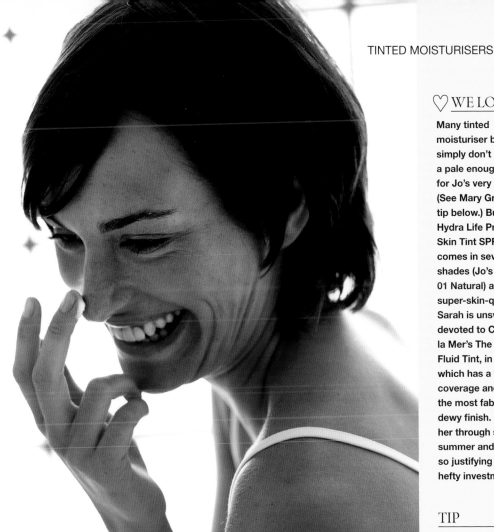

♡ WE LOVE...

Many tinted moisturiser brands simply don't come in a pale enough shade for Jo's very pale skin. (See Mary Greenwell's tip below.) But Dior Hydra Life Pro-Youth Skin Tint SPF20 comes in several shades (Jo's is 01 Natural) and is super-skin-quenching. Sarah is unswervingly devoted to Crème de la Mer's The SPF18 Fluid Tint, in medium, which has a bit of coverage and gives the most fabulous dewy finish. It lasts her through spring, summer and autumn – so justifying a hefty investment.

TIP

Mary Greenwell insists that tinted moisturiser should be viewed more like a lightweight foundation than as something to change the underlying tone of your skin. She prescribes the same colour-matching technique as for foundation: apply to just below your jaw to find the shade that will blend in seamlessly. If you're very pale, you'll need to check out one of the ranges which now offers a selection of shades – many tinted moisturisers are one-shade-fits-all options, and one shade DOESN'T fit all.

Comments: '10/10! Went on smoothly, felt moisturising, and blended easily; skin looked clearer and brighter; preferred it for daytime to my usual Chanel foundation as it felt so light' • 'perfect for a day look' • 'needed to go over a moisturiser but felt like silk velvet – lovely! Skin felt and looked smoother' • 'loved this product, skin looks smoother and more radiant; would definitely buy for the summer' • 'good creamy consistency but no greasy feeling or shine; easy to blend in' • 'smoothed out skintone and filled in fine lines, disguises open pores better than anything I've found so far; if my skin looked like this all the time I would be very happy!'.

Mádara Moon Flower Tinting Fluid ❊ ❊ ❊

Organically-certified by Ecocert, Mádara is an award-winning range from Latvia – and the range features characteristic Baltic herbs and plants (calendula, plantain, rosehip, etc). This tinting fluid is part of a small make-up collection, for a natural, sun-kissed look – and it comes in two shades, Moon Flower, for paler skins (our testers had this) and Sun Flower, which is slightly warmer in tone. Mádara recommends using over a moisturiser for maximum effect, though some testers didn't need it.

Comments: 'Very easy to apply with fingertips, and very effective on me; usually I apply these products on top of a moisturiser but didn't need one; skin looks glowing; reduces the look of fine lines and doesn't settle in bigger ones; disguises flaws quite well' • 'husband commented favourably, which is a miracle in itself' • 'lasted all day on holiday in very hot weather without sliding off' • 'for something that feels so light it covers really well, especially at my age (55)' • 'skin looks clearer since I've been using this product'.

Say goodbye to spider veins!

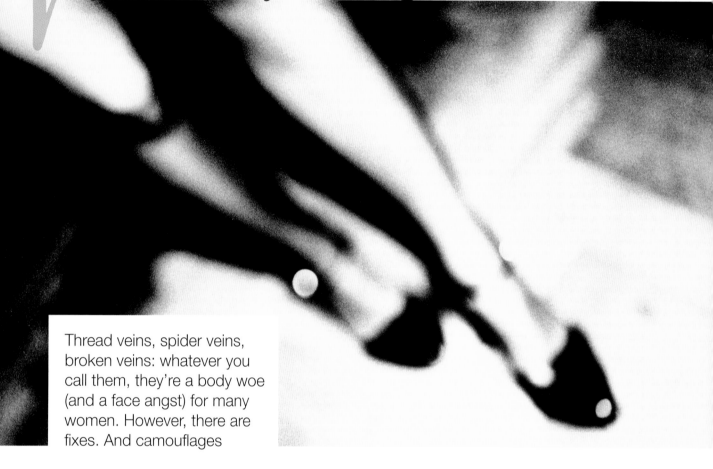

Thread veins, spider veins, broken veins: whatever you call them, they're a body woe (and a face angst) for many women. However, there are fixes. And camouflages

When a truly gorgeous-in-every-way friend in her early fifties was deserted by her (daft) husband, part of her fresh start was to tidy up the 'hated spider veins which creep in at various places up my legs and fan out over my thighs', as she put it. It isn't just legs that can be affected: many women are troubled by the appearance of thread veins on their face (cheeks, forehead, eyelids and around the nostrils), also neck and upper chest. They're particularly noticeable in people with pale thin skin. (And, says Jo, 'certainly the curse of my beauty life – the price for an English rose complexion'.)

The technical name for these clusters of tiny dilated blood vessels (capillaries), which appear just under the surface of the skin, is 'dermal flares'. They're incredibly common and while not serious, they are unsightly. On the legs, they can also lead to heavy aching legs and even pain. 'Little nerves in the veins can be painful if the veins get stretched,' explains consultant vascular surgeon Mr John Scurr of the Lister Hospital in London (our long-time 'veins' expert). They may be worsened by fluctuating levels of hormones, pre- and post-menopause, as well as standing up for long periods. (Men get them too.) Before treating leg veins, Mr Scurr explains that it's vital to have a scan first to check that there are no underlying problems, such as varicose veins (or, at the worst, deep vein thrombosis) – and be aware that varicose veins need to be treated before treating dermal flares. The following two treatment options are Mr Scurr's preferred choices.

For spider veins on legs, consider microsclerotherapy. Getting rid of these 'dermal flares' can be simple – but it's likely to be time-consuming. Mr Scurr recommends a process called microsclerotherapy, where each capillary is injected with a very fine needle containing a 'sclerosant' solution that expels blood from the vein, and leaves the walls of the vein stuck together so the blood can't return.

The sessions last about 20 minutes and are usually carried out by a nurse. Veins may sting a little but shouldn't be painful. A cylinder of tightly rolled cotton wool is stuck on each injection site immediately after to minimise bruising, and legs are wrapped in a light bandage before you leave. Both bandage and cotton wool can be taken off three hours later. Legs may ache slightly for a few days.

If you have a number of flares this process can take several weeks. And while microsclerotherapy is the most effective for legs, it's not appropriate for faces, where laser is the best and safest option.

Electrolysis is another option. In this treatment – suitable for faces as well as legs – an electrical current is passed through a fine needle to cauterise the vein so the blood is absorbed back into the body. (See right for more about facial thread veins.) Electrolysis is available at beauty salons, but you should always have potential 'deep veins' on legs checked out by a doctor first. Make sure you go to an experienced therapist who has the back-up to deal with potential problems, such as infection.

Schedule treatment for the tights season! Microsclerotherapy (and sclerotherapy which can be used for some varicose veins) can leave legs looking a bit battle-scarred so, if possible, time your treatment when you can cover up with black opaques. The process is definitely not a quick fix but, says our friend, it's worth it: 'Wonder of wonders, I now have unblemished thighs and legs. For the first time in years, I can leave the sarong behind when I walk to the pool.'

Remember dermal flares may stage a comeback. Mr Scurr warns that those pesky flares may return and need further treatment. Natural products, either to take internally or rub on, may help. Try Diosmin Complex by LifeTime Vitamins, a combination of natural compounds, or Zinopin Daily, a natural blend developed to prevent DVT for air travellers. Spider Veins Cream by Provenance features glycosaminoglycans (GAGs) that may help repair the damaged capillaries and possibly toughen the outer cell layers, minimising the appearance of spider veins. (Find a source for these in DIRECTORY.)

FACE YOUR THREAD VEINS

Cosmetic dermatologists treat unsightly thread veins on your cheeks and face with state-of-the-art lasers. Individual broken capillaries can be treated with walk-in-and-out lunchtime therapy which doesn't cause any bruising. (But you must, absolutely must, wear a sunblock for at least three months after.) Why not sclerotherapy? Experts including Dr Nick Lowe of the Cranley Clinic, London, and Dr Andrew Markey, say that while sclerotherapy is the gold standard for treating leg veins, they disapprove of using it on the face, because injecting the wrong vein may provoke an emergency and, in the worst-case scenario, lead to loss of vision. (Plus we've heard from a woman who had it done – unwisely – around her nose, that it's agony.) However, if you have developed thread veins during pregnancy, try waiting a few months after the birth because they may disappear on their own. And if you have acne rosacea with inflamed skin that looks like thread veins, you should probably be treated with antibiotics first. (For more on rosacea see page 168.)

In any case, please do make sure you consult a qualified and experienced dermatologist – it is your face after all! We recommend following Wendy Lewis's checklist of questions to ask, even before something which seems as minor as veins treatment (see page 46).

For us, a little bit of concealer (see camouflage suggestions right, and also top concealers on page 91) plus topical treatments minimise the problem very satisfactorily, without recourse to expensive treatments. Also see page 170 for products that have done well for facial redness. And do avoid scrubs or using anything scratchy on your face.

PS Sarah had more veins on her cheeks and round her nose in her twenties than she does now, and can only put that down to taking more care of her skin – with plenty of nourishing moisturiser in cold/windy weather and lots of anti-inflammatory foods and supplements, notably oily fish and omega-3 essential fatty acids (again!) – and leading a calmer life generally. Oh, and not drinking alcohol!

OUR TOP CAMOUFLAGERS

Products we know work include Estée Lauder Maximum Cover Camouflage Make-up for Face and Body and Vichy Dermablend Ultra-Corrective Foundation Cream Stick together with the same brand's Setting Powder. Laura Mercier Secret Camouflage can be very effective for faces, too.

TIP

Visible facial veins often come as a result of sun damage so – once again – please can we remind you to slap on the SPF! And avoid roasting and frying in the hottest parts of the day. And while we're at it, please avoid sunbeds too – they're a short cut to ageing and pose a significant risk of skin cancer. Remember: when it comes to tans, fake it to make it!

Take up yoga. Just do it, please

For us, this is almost the most important advice in this book. If you do it already, you will know the absolutely miraculous results of an hour or so's practise (sometimes just five minutes is enough to turn you round). Done regularly long-term, yoga can transform your life

We find yoga THE perfect exercise for a more mature body – and for ironing out any wrinkles in our minds. If you've never done it before, it can help enormously with flexibility – and bone strength, too. And there is nothing – repeat nothing – we've found that's better for stress, and for making us feel like we're on top of the mountain of different things we have to juggle. Plus it makes you look fabulous! At the end of a long day – or if you get up in the morning feeling and looking exhausted – the most effective way to go from tired and drab to glowing and gorgeous is to do some yoga. (Just try it.)

Take up yoga for your bones. As yoga teacher Jan Maddern, author of *Yoga Builds Bones*, observes, 'Yoga creates a balanced harmony between the ovaries, adrenal, parathyroid, pituitary and pineal glands, ensuring that the body receives a steady supply of the right hormones for maintaining bone strength and maximum health and wellbeing. The regular practise of weight-bearing hatha yoga postures offers women everywhere a safe way to build bone strength.' There is even some evidence that yoga can help people who have already developed symptoms of osteoporosis: according to Dr Andrew Weil, the world's leading expert in integrated medicine, two studies have shown that elderly women who took part in regular yoga classes, two to three times a week for between three and six months, saw a slight reduction in curvatures of the upper spine ('dowager's hump'). In one study the control group who didn't practise yoga actually saw an increase in upper spinal curvatures. In another study, older women who did a nine-week yoga programme gained a centimetre in height.

Take up yoga to balance your hormones. Consultant gynaecologist Michael Dooley recommends yoga to all his patients, particularly any going through the hormonal roller-coasters around menopause. Teachers have always held that certain postures can reduce hot flushes and night sweats as well as promote calm and restful sleep, and this was confirmed by researchers in India. (It also sharpened mental function – yippee!) During the long, slow asanas (postures), certain glands in the body are gently pressurised and depressurised, helping to stimulate and control the hormones produced by those glands. Yoga for menopause should place an emphasis on moving slowly and smoothly.

It is never too late to take up yoga, but

REACH A STATE OF UNITY

Yoga means 'union' in Sanskrit, the language of ancient India where the system originated more than 3,000 years ago. It unites body, mind and spirit through a combination of breathing, meditation, stretching and postures (asanas). There are different ways of practising yoga, varying from slow (eg, Hatha yoga) to dynamic (eg, Ashtanga) which suit different personalities. Iyengar yoga (a fairly recent development by BKS Iyengar) set out to be therapeutic and focuses on bodily alignment. Some people see yoga as a spiritual practice but it is certainly not a religion.

it's also never too early: as Suza Francina, a teacher who writes books about yoga for women (rather than babes) points out, 'If you practise yoga before the menopause, all the poses that are useful for coping with uncomfortable symptoms are familiar, and you can reach for them like an old friend. If you are familiar with restorative poses, then you have the best menopause medicine at your disposal.'

If you Google 'yoga for menopause' you may even be lucky eough to find a specific class in your area, as some teachers are starting to offer this type of yoga specifically (it's a baby-boom thing). Failing that, it's important to explain to your teacher if you have hot flushes, because they can guide you through the more restorative and cooling postures. The use of supportive props such as bolsters, blankets and blocks can help adapt postures so that you avoid gripping or straining, which can cause over-heating. Specific postures that are recommended during menopause include:

● Legs-up-the-wall pose (viparita karani), which is great for grounding.
● Head-to-knee forward bend (janu sirsasana) and seated forward bend (paschimottanasana) for irritability.
● Plough pose (halasana) and Shoulder Stand for hormonal balance.

The Shoulder Stand is known as 'the posture for eternal youth', but we would certainly recommend that shoulder stands are always done in a supervised class, unless you have been practising for some years.

LESS PAIN, MORE GAIN

Research by the US National Institute of Health revealed that taking regular yoga classes can reduce chronic back pain and enhance flexibility. In a 12-week study, volunteers who took 90-minute yoga classes twice a week showed 42 per cent reduction in pain and therefore reduced their dependency on pain medication. NB: it's vital to find qualified and experienced teachers who specialise in backs, however, as practising the wrong postures can make things worse.

OUR TOP YOGA PICKS

The accessories and websites we find helpful...

● **prAna Yoga Mats.** Nicely non-slip, with good 'give' (which helps wrists). If visiting a studio, we lay our mat on top of the mat provided, for extra support (whipping it away during balancing postures, when less 'squish' helps).

● **Gossypium yoga pants.** The Cropped Foldover Trouser is genius as the small amount of Lycra in the super-wide foldover waistband keeps the trousers (and your tummy) in place, without any restricting elastic. (As a close second, we also like prAna yoga gear.)

● **Beech sandals.** An important exercise in yoga is learning to stretch the toes so that the body is perfectly 'grounded'. These help: they contain built-in 'toe-separators', which help to train the toes to spread naturally, and help with balance and body alignment.

● **Yoga Journal iPractice App.** For iPhone users there is now no excuse not to practise when you're away from home: this app from the iTunes Store (put together by *Yoga Journal*, probably the best magazine about yoga published anywhere) features sequences put together by respected teachers – and you can set the speed at which you follow them.

● **www.lotusjourneys.com.** A holistic travel agency which arranges wellbeing holidays worldwide, including an excellent selection of yoga vacations and destinations.

● *Yoga for Beginners* **DVD with Patricia Walden.** A practical introduction which is precise and easy to follow if you can't get to a class.

Take up yoga for flexibility. There's a famous concept in yoga philosophy that a person's age is determined by the flexibility of his spine, not the number of years he has lived. (And recent research suggests that stretching the body may help prevent age-related stiffening of the arteries – we'd rather have ours flowing freely.) The improved balance and flexibility that come from regular yoga practise can also help prevent – or reduce the impact – of falls: a stiff body goes down like a ninepin, which is more likely to lead to bone breaks and fractures. And, of course, it's great to hang on to the ability to reach down to your shoelaces or up to a jar on the top shelf, because (even if this seems a long way off) it helps us remain as independent as possible for as long as possible. But we also very much like this quote, frequently repeated by one of Jo's yoga teachers: 'Flexible spine equals flexible mind'. The more we do yoga, the more we find we can roll with life's punches – going with the flow and adapting to change, as well as accepting that change is inevitable.

Take up yoga to tackle your wrinkles. Marie-Véronique Nadeau – who we met when she was visiting from Berkeley, California – is in her sixties, and she's her own best advertisement: almost line-free and with plumped-up, resilient skin. Marie-Véronique (who also has her own skincare line, Marie Veronique Organics) has put together a programme called The Yoga Facelift which we recommend if you feel you can make the commitment to facial exercises. As she says, 'The adage "If you don't use it, you lose it" really applies to the muscles of your face.' Women we know who practise yoga into their later years have sharper jaws and more defined facial contours, as well as glowing skin (it's the improved circulation). We also have a theory that the amount of time you spend 'inverted' helps hair growth, by boosting blood flow to the scalp. (Completely unsubstantiated, but we both have hair that grows like grass.)

Take up yoga for clarity, balance and to quieten 'monkey mind'. In the Yoga Sutras (sacred writings), there's a wonderful phrase: 'Yoga is the ending of disturbances of the mind'. We both find it gives us amazing focus, improves memory – and, when faced with a problem, shows us a clear way to deal with it for a positive outcome. We could cite endless scientific studies to back this up (and explain why), but we can also just tell you: it's true.

So we say, just take up yoga. Don't fret too much about which 'style' of yoga – but we would suggest that Hatha, Iyengar and Scaravelli yoga (which are more gentle) would be most appropriate. We recommend that peri- and menopausal women avoid Bikram (heated) or fast Ashtanga yoga, as these focus on creating heat within the body – and at this phase in life, that's something many of us are trying to avoid. The most important thing is to find a class/classes that fit with your schedule, as you're more likely to go, and the closer to home (or work) the better.

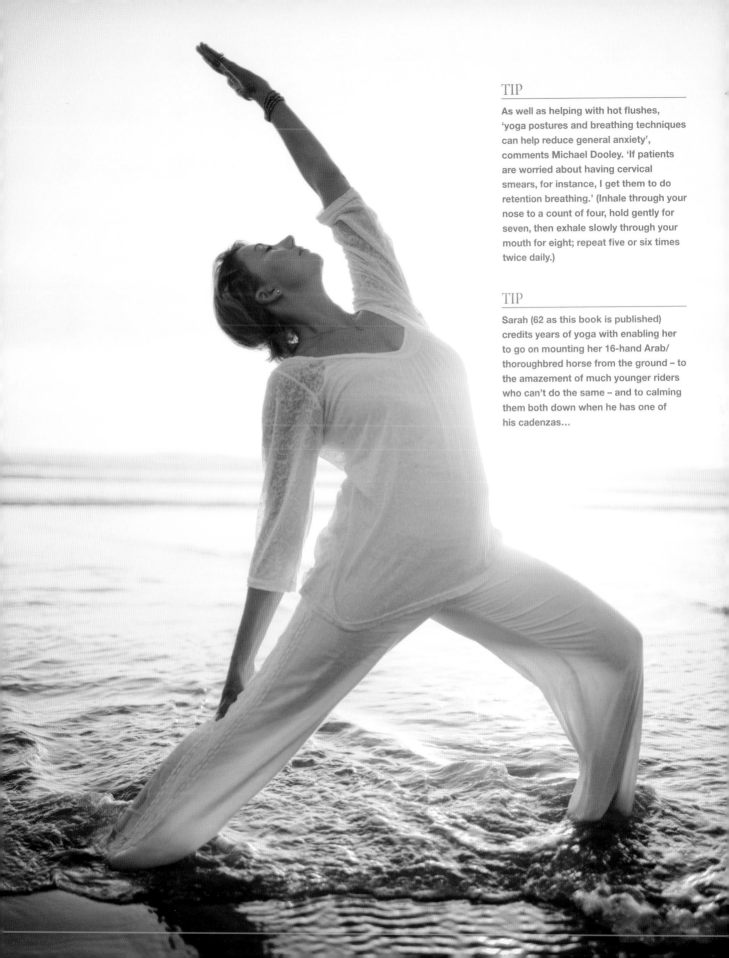

TIP

As well as helping with hot flushes, 'yoga postures and breathing techniques can help reduce general anxiety', comments Michael Dooley. 'If patients are worried about having cervical smears, for instance, I get them to do retention breathing.' (Inhale through your nose to a count of four, hold gently for seven, then exhale slowly through your mouth for eight; repeat five or six times twice daily.)

TIP

Sarah (62 as this book is published) credits years of yoga with enabling her to go on mounting her 16-hand Arab/ thoroughbred horse from the ground – to the amazement of much younger riders who can't do the same – and to calming them both down when he has one of his cadenzas…

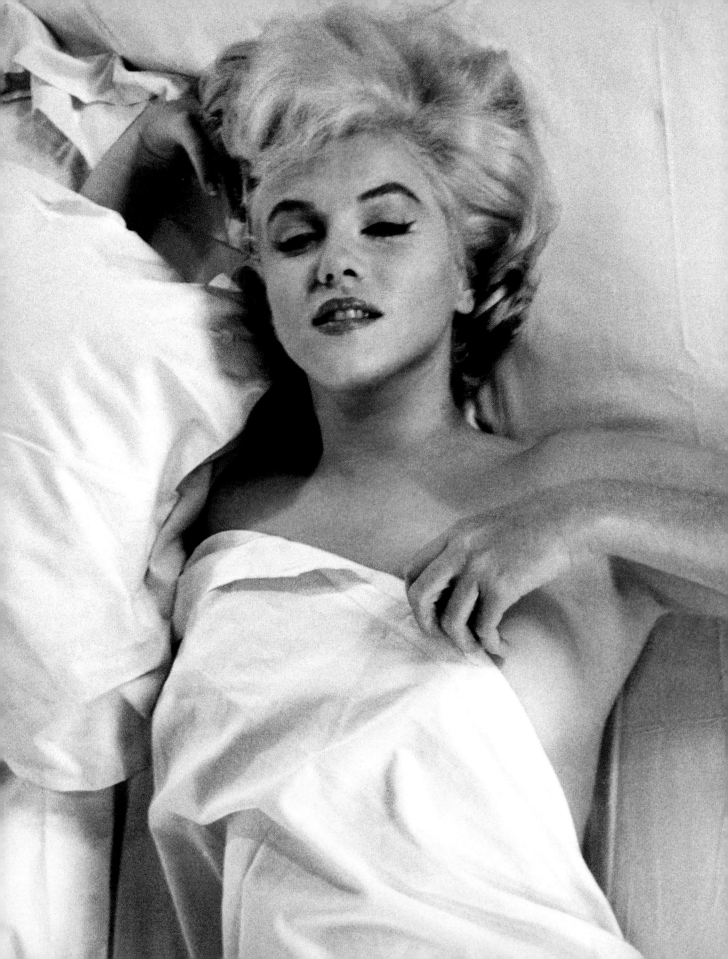

Get your Zzzzzs!
How to sleep better

No doubt about it, getting enough good sleep is beautifying. And de-stressing. And energising. All-round wonderful stuff. And every good woman deserves slumber!

Trouble is we don't all get enough sleep. Especially as the years roll by. While some lucky souls can slumber through anything – from thundering traffic and snoring partners, to super-stress – others wake as a feather drops or there's the slightest ripple of anxiety. So, if it's less than restorative, how can you improve your sleep pattern?

As the queens of 'sleep hygiene', doing all the right things to optimise a good night's sleep, we are keen to pass on the stuff we know works. We're both occasionally prone to sleeplessness (and both 'larks' with a tendency to wake up at 4am in summer – or when we're fretting about something, see page 211), so when it comes to sleep aids we've been there, done that, gone to bed in the T-shirt. In other words, we know what works. First of all, get the kit. These are the 'accessories' to good sleep, and the simple steps you can take right now, in your own bedroom, to help get the zzzzzs you need. (See DIRECTORY for sources.)

If you get too hot at night, check out linen. Linen is the most amazingly cooling fabric. On a hot day, you can touch a linen pillowcase on your bed and it will be cool, whereas a cotton pillowcase on the same bed can be room temperature. If you are menopausal or peri-menopausal and you suffer from night sweats or hot flushes, at the very least treat yourself to a couple of linen pillowcases. If you can indulge yourself with linen sheets, even better. A very simple trick to cool down in the night is to flip your pillow over. We thought we were the only people who knew this, but it turns out to be so popular that there is even – we kid you not – a Facebook group called, 'I flip my pillow over to get to the cold side', with nearly one million members when we last looked. (Jo also sleeps in a French linen nightshirt, which has an equally cooling effect.)

And/or buy a Chillow. Again, if you find that you can't sleep because you're too hot at night, the Chillow is an extraordinary innovation that we've heard very good things about. (The Chillow was first brought to our attention by consultant gynaecologist Michael Dooley whose patients were raving about it for hot flushes.) It's made of a patented substance which, when activated by water (you only need to do this once), creates a memory-foam-like layer that you put between you and your pillowcase. (If you don't like the flock-y surface, you can slip it under your pillowcase – ideally linen, see left.) There's a larger version (the Chillow PLUS), originally designed for reducing fevers, which some women prefer because they can wrap it around their pillow and slip a hand underneath while they rest, getting a double cooling whammy. If you're really having a problem with hot flushes, you'll want to know about the Petite Relief Chillow which you keep in the fridge to apply when you're feeling too hot to bear. Another excellent application, for anyone who uses a laptop on their – umm, lap: put the Petite Relief Chillow under your laptop and instead of getting very hot legs, you'll feel cucumber-cool.

'There is no pillow so soft as a clear conscience'
French proverb

(And lots of hospitals are now recommending Chillows for hot flushes associated with treatment for breast and prostate cancer.)

And get yourself a Bucky sleep mask. Jo has road-tested just about every sleep mask known to woman, and is convinced that this is the best, the most light-excluding and the most comfortable to wear of any sleep mask out there. It's super-soft and padded, cradling the eyes without pressure. It has soft padding over the nose and cheeks, which avoids even a molecule of light peeking in. The Bucky sleep mask also Velcros around the back (so is infinitely adjustable whatever your head size). There are several designs but the one you want is Eye Shades with Ear Plugs (these are stored in a little pouch on the front). Lots of

SLEEP REGIME

This natural regime is more effective than drugs at re-establishing a sound sleep structure, says psychiatrist Dr David Servan-Schreiber. Go to bed at the same time every night including weekends but get up two hours earlier than usual. Don't nap for more than 20 to 30 minutes during the day. If you wake, get up and read a book or magazine for an hour before going back to bed. Once sleep is continuous again – which may take a few weeks – increase the time you sleep by 15 minutes every three days until you're back to your normal length.

colours, all lined with black – but we think midnight or black are the most alluring.

Have an Aromatherapy Associates Deep Relax bath before bedtime. For many years we have been slavishly devoted to Aromatherapy Associates Deep Relax Shower & Bath Oil. It is knock-out drops for us. (After you've had a few baths with this there's probably a Pavlovian response, so you only have to smell the potent blend of vetiver, chamomile and sandalwood to start to feel sleepy.) Our one caveat: if you do get toasty at night, don't have the water too hot because the effect of heating the body will linger when you slip between the sheets. We love this oil so much we give it to friends for birthdays, then they start giving it to everyone they know, like an aromatherapy chain letter.

Or pour in the magnesium flakes. Magnesium is known as 'nature's tranquilliser' and as well as taking a supplement before bed (which helps with restless legs too), we pour Magnesium Flakes in the bath so this soothing mineral can cherish aches and pains and racing minds. (There's also an oil version.) PS Researcher Dr Paula Baillie-Hamilton tells us that putting magnesium in the bath is a wonderful treatment for over-excited/hyperactive children.

Spritz your pillow. We are both incredibly impressed by the Les Fleurs de Bach range, based on the principles of Bach Flower Remedies. Two products stand out in the quest for better sleep: the Anti-Stress Treating Fragrance is amazingly relaxing (and smells awfully nice, with its blend of sage, lavender, bergamot or eucalyptus). We recommend having two: one for the desk (for moments of stress), one for the night-stand; a few spritzes before bedtime – including on the pillow – help prepare the mind for sleep. (We love the whole Les Fleurs de Bach range, and also recommend the Les Fleurs de Bach Sleep Elixir, from the same range.)

Switch off the standby. There is now evidence that even the little standby light on your TV (if you have one in the bedroom) may affect your sleep pattern – not just preventing you from drifting off but interfering with the depth of your sleep. Only when the bedroom is totally dark will your body start to produce melatonin, which not only regulates sleep but also has an important role in reducing your risk of cancer. So: ditch the digital clock. Switch off any appliance that's on standby, and if you have a multi-gang plug with an orange light that tells you it's working, put gaffer tape over it.

Try a pelmet! Jo recently had a moment of absolute revelation, on a midsummer's morning when light was streaming into her bedroom before 4am: 'Ah – THAT's what a pelmet's for…' With the fashion for curtain poles rather than tracks, pelmets have very much fallen from favour – but perhaps our mothers (and grannies) knew a thing or two about keeping light out of a bedroom. If you really can't bear the look of a pelmet, try installing blackout blinds on the windows underneath, which can cover the top of the window but be half rolled up in the night, allowing air in. Meanwhile, if you have to sleep in a house where someone needs the landing light on, we suggest putting a rolled-up towel or a draught excluder at the bottom of the door, to prevent light seepage there.

Invest in a truly fabulous bed. Never, ever buy a new bed without trying it in a store. Or – better still – in a hotel: by popular request many hotels nowadays are offering for sale the actual beds that guests slumber peacefully in. (Jo is right now building up to buying one of the beds from her favourite London sleeping spot, The Langham hotel, where she gets a night's sleep like no other.) The beds with the best reputations are Hästens (made in Sweden out of bundles of horsehair, cotton, flax and pure new wool), and Hypnos (who make beds for the Queen, upholstered with cashmere, silk and lambswool). We are also impressed with the organic beds by Abaca. Some of these are very far from cheap. However, considering we spend one third of our lives in bed, we feel that investing in a great bed is probably as important as choosing a safe car as both are so essential to life.

Treat yourself to good pillows, too. It's up to you whether you like hard or soft, but make sure you replace them regularly. Do 'the pillow trick': hold out your arm, place the pillow over it – and if it flops down either side, it's definitely overdue for replacement. By reputation, the very best pillows are Hungarian or Siberian goose down, which are both very soft. Personally, we've always been impressed with Ikea pillows (they know a thing or two about sleep in a country with such long winter nights), although annoyingly they aren't quite the same size as standard UK pillows. Close enough to fudge it, though. When you want to treat yourself, try www.thebestbedlonenintheworld.com for pillows: Jo's came from Claridge's (a generous gift from Clarins – she didn't nick them!), and are – as she puts it – 'like a blissful firm cloud…'.

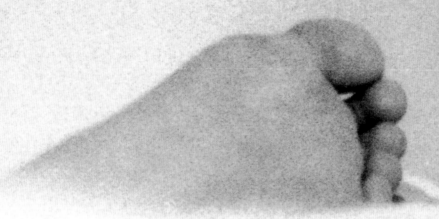

WHAT TO DO IF YOU WAKE UP IN THE WEE SMALL HOURS

Many older women get off to sleep fine but then wake between 3am and 5am. Often they can't get back to sleep; if they do, it's usually not restful slumber. Whatever the cause – and some swear it can be the phases of the moon – the result is a loss of energy and focus, and a feeling of having to drag yourself through the day until the next broken night. As well as the general advice on the previous pages, experts suggest the following ways to woo sleep; we've tried their advice and it works.

● Relax in the evening; don't drink coffee, tea or cola after 6pm and avoid fatty or sugary foods and excess alcohol which your body has to process during the night; cool your body by walking barefoot, opening a window, wearing light night clothes and having a warm bath.

● Dim lights through the evening: until electric lighting became commonplace, people naturally downshifted with the onset of dusk. Today, the light assault continues until we go to bed and we still expect to fall asleep immediately. Which is dotty since the sleep hormone melatonin needs darkness to switch it on. Last thing at night, spend a few moments gazing at the vast velvet darkness of the night sky.

● Try this delicious drink to calm the nervous system. Stir together over gentle heat: 250ml organic full-fat cow's milk or almond or rice milk, 2 teaspoons organic ground almonds, 2 cardamom pods, 5 strands saffron and a pinch of nutmeg. Strain and add one teaspoon honey, Manuka if possible.

● Take one to two capsules of Valerian and Ashwagandha Formula by Pukka Herbs before bed. Keep a capsule handy to take if you wake.

● And if you do wake up, refuse to fret about missed sleep: until recently, people took it for granted they'd wake in the long periods of natural darkness and talk, make love, tell stories or let their minds roam. Lie there and think of all the nice things you've done this year.

● Breathe: lie flat on your back, eyes closed, one hand on your chest. Inhale for a count of four, hold for seven, then exhale slowly to eight: visualise waves shimmying up a beach, hovering for a moment, then receding gently… slowly… into the sea.

● Low blood sugar may rouse you, so have a small banana and/or a small pot of organic natural yoghurt (plus teaspoon!) by your bed, also a glass of still water with a few drops of Bach Rescue Remedy in it (dehydration can lead to poor sleep and bad dreams).

● If anxieties beset you, remember that around 4am is the 'dark hour of the soul' when your brain can't process worries – thus the jangling cacophony in your head. Keep a pen and paper by your bed, and write them down.

● If you toss and turn for more than 15 minutes, turn on the radio (we love the BBC World Service), read a trashy novel (nothing stimulating), do the ironing or washing-up (nothing energetic).

Instant face revivers: our award winners

Sometimes, what you really want is to LOOK GOOD RIGHT NOW – the instant confidence-boost of a product that perks up your skin, makes you look radiant, peels back the years – especially after a short or disturbed night, before a Big Night Out, or if you've been poorly. Masks are pretty brilliant – see page 82 for our testers' reviews – but there are also serums, spritzes, gels (among other textures) which make you look as if you've had eight hours' peaceful and restorative slumber. We know some of them work (see our favourites in We Love…) and our testers do too now!

REVIEWS

Clarins Beauty Flash Balm

 8.56/10 Well, what do you know? Clarins invented this beauty category with the creation of Beauty Flash Balm over 30 years ago, winning countless awards before this one. According to our testers, it's still a wow, living up to its reputation as 'Cinderella in a tube'. With radiance-boosting ingredients, Beauty Flash Balm 'sets' to a comfy, firming film which makes skin look instantly fresh and gorgeously glowy.

Comments: '10/10! My skin felt lovely instantly, no tautness, make-up went on with no sliding or greasiness, there's nothing to compare to this' • 'skin looked brighter and plumper, fresher and more radiant, and it evened out skintone; fantastic product' • 'make-up looked smoother and lasted longer' • 'slight tingling sensation at first, which felt invigorating; very effective, quite a few people remarked on how bright and radiant my skin was' • 'skin looked dewy, glowy and radiant, lovely!'.

Liz Earle Superskin Concentrate

 8.39/10 We'll admit that we hadn't thought of using this facial oil as an instant face-saver until the brand put it forward for this category. But now we have, we're impressed at how this aromatic blend of vitamin E and plant oils (avocado, rosehip, argan) does speedily revive the skin. (The chamomile, neroli and lavender fragrance is especially lovely.) If you wanted to use this before

going out, we'd suggest applying, leaving to sink in, then blotting firmly with a tissue before applying make-up. Most testers loved it so much they chose to use it every night!

Comments: 'Top marks, made my skin really soft and plump, face uplifted and spirits too! I've been recovering from a hysterectomy and this has really balanced and evened out my skin, people say I look really well and healthy' • 'I was worried about using an oil on a spotty area, but it has really cleared my skin and sorted out the dry areas, it's done wonders' • 'skin felt gorgeous!' • 'made skintone perkier and more even, skin felt comfy but supported – like Spanx for the face…' • 'wore this just with some concealer and blush' • 'loved the smell of lavender which really helped to relax me at bedtime'.

Guerlain Issima Midnight Secret

 8.25/10 Another iconic beauty product: a super-silky emulsion which is best applied at bedtime, for skin that will look much better than you'll probably feel the morning after a late night or a smoky party. (The 'Hydronoctine' complex boosts microcirculation and helps cell oxygenation.) Gorgeous rose scent, and a little bit of real gold in there (which always helps with radiance!).

Comments: 'I'm convinced I look better as soon as I smooth it on! Glowy and relaxed…don't think my face was uplifted but my features did look smooth and comfy' • 'my skin is in a poor state and this improved it instantly, calming down the redness and

AT A GLANCE

Clarins Beauty Flash Balm

Liz Earle Superskin Concentrate

Guerlain Issima Midnight Secret

Elemis Visible Brilliance Instant Radiance Serum

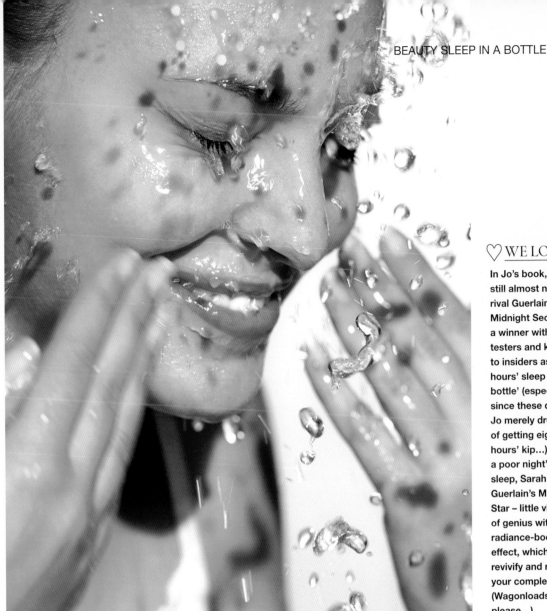

ANTI-AGEING
AWARD
WINNERS
BEAUTY BIBLE

♡ WE LOVE...

In Jo's book, there's still almost nothing to rival Guerlain Issima Midnight Secret, also a winner with our testers and known to insiders as 'eight hours' sleep in a bottle' (especially since these days, Jo merely dreams of getting eight hours' kip...). After a poor night's sleep, Sarah adores Guerlain's Midnight Star – little vials of genius with a radiance-boosting effect, which smooth, revivify and rejuvenate your complexion. (Wagonloads please...)

heat' • 'immediate improvement in my skin, it felt awake! Definitely beauty sleep in a bottle! I moisturise regularly and use this and my skin looks youthful and bright' • 'skin seemed firmer and more dewy-looking in the morning, nicely plumped-up and a good base for make-up: I absolutely loved everything about this product'.

Elemis Visible Brilliance Instant Radiance Serum

 A 'double action' serum, so we're told, from this global spa brand – with a multi-mineral complex (zinc, copper, magnesium), plus red seaweed, Swiss garden cress, 'dew bean' and a vitamin complex, for instant luminosity and a rested

appearance. We love the way the lid swivels up and the nozzle appears...!

Comments: 'Skin felt very smooth, looked brighter, more even and seemed less pink in red areas; make-up went on very smoothly and stayed put; held skin together really well' • 'I apply this serum at night if my skin is a bit blotchy or spotty, and definitely see an improvement in the morning, skin is clearer, smooth, silky and a bit brighter – I like the visible results' • 'made my rather sallow complexion brighter, wrinkles on brow definitely lessened and cheeks seemed a tad plumper and younger-looking; my beautician remarked how well I looked' • 'never known for the most wonderful complexion but suddenly people say how well I look and how good my make-up is...'.

TIP

'To brighten your skin, fill a basin with warm water and add several drops of lavender essential oil. Dip a face cloth in the water then lay over your face for a few moments. Repeat five times.'
– Ole Henriksen

Directory

The following includes stockist contacts for the brands featured in these books. But we also suggest that you first visit www.beautybible.com and have a look at the INSIDER DISCOUNTS section (it's one of the buttons along the top), as many of the brands featured in this book are available at very nice discounts from a handful of websites which we consider to be 'Beauty Bible-approved' sites (www.victoriahealth.com, www.lovelula.com, www.HQhair.com, www.beautyexpert.co.uk and www.lizearle.com which often put together special kits just for Beauty Bible) – all offering great, swift service and a terrific selection of ranges. A good place to start. (NB: all the brands in INSIDER DISCOUNTS are listed alphabetically.)

Beauty Bible Beauty Steals is available as an App for your iPhone – go to www.beautybible.com and click on the icon on the pink splash page for more info and to order.

All the supplements mentioned in this book, plus advice and information, are available from Victoria Health, tel: 0800 3898 195, www.victoriahealth.com

A

Abaca, tel: 01269 598491, www.abacaorganic.co.uk

AD Skin Synergy, from Victoria Health, tel: 0800 3898 195, www.victoriahealth.com

Adonia LegTone, www.adonialegtone.co.uk

Aerosoles, available via www.aerosoles.com and from stores in Paris

Alida, from Victoria Health, tel: 0800 3898 195, www.victoriahealth.com

AloeDent, from Victoria Health, tel: 0800 3898 195, www.victoriahealth.com

Alterna, tel: 01179 270435, www.alternauk.com

Amanda Lacey, www.amandalacey.com

Dr Andrew Markey, the Lister Hospital, tel: 020 7730 1219, www.thelisterhospital.com

Dr Andrew Weil, www.drweil.com

Anastasia Achilleos, at Urban Retreat, tel: 020 7893 8333, www.urbanretreat.co.uk

Andy Wadsworth, My Life Personal Training, tel: 07889 940888, www.mylifept.com

Annee de Mamiel, tel: 07516 099010, www.demamiel.com

Aquafresh, www.aquafresh.co.uk

Aromatherapy Associates, from Victoria Health, tel: 0800 3898 195, www.victoriahealth.com

Aveda, tel: 0800 054 2979, www.aveda.co.uk

B

Balance Me, www.balanceme.co.uk

Barbara Daly, www.barbaradalymake-up.co.uk

Bare Escentuals, tel: 0870 850 6655, www.bareescentuals.co.uk

Barefoot Botanicals, from Victoria Health, tel: 0800 3898 195, www.victoriahealth.com

BareMinerals, see Bare Escentuals above

Bastien Gonzalez, tel: 07766 663271, www.bastiengonzalez.com

Beech Sandals, from Victoria Health, tel: 0800 3898 195, www.victoriahealth.com

Benefit, tel: 0800 496 1084, www.benefitcosmetics.co.uk

Beverly Hills Formula, from Victoria Health, tel: 0800 3898 195, www.victoriahealth.com

Bliss, tel: 0808 100 4151, www.blissworld.co.uk

Blood test (at home): Ideal Omega 3 Test Kit from Victoria Health, tel: 0800 3898 195, www.victoriahealth.com

Bobbi Brown, tel: 0800 054 2988, www.bobbibrown.co.uk

The Body Shop, tel: 0800 092 9090, www.thebodyshop.co.uk

Botanicals, tel: 01664 464005, www.botanicals.co.uk

Bourjois, tel: 0800 269836, www.bourjois.co.uk

Bowen technique, tel: 01373 832340, www.thebowentechnique.com

Bremenn Research Labs, from Victoria Health, tel: 0800 3898 195, www.victoriahealth.com

Bucky, www.amazon.co.uk

Bumble & Bumble, tel: 0800 014 7424, www.bumbleandbumble.com

By Terry, www.byterry.com

C

CACI, tel: 020 8731 5678, www.caci-international.co.uk

Caudalie, tel: 00800 4429 2424, www.caudalie.com

Celgenics, tel: 01246 868808, www.celgenics.com

Cellulite Busting Kit, from Victoria Health, tel: 0800 3898 195, www.victoriahealth.com

Chanel, tel: 020 7493 3836, www.chanel.com

Professor Charles Clark, tel: 020 7935 0640, www.charlesvclark.com

Chie Mihara, tel: 0034 9669 80415 www.chiemihara.com

Chillow, tel: 08700 117174, www.chillow.co.uk

Chinese herbal medicine: Register of Chinese Herbal Medicine, tel: 01603 623994, www.rchm.co.uk

Christophe Robin, tel: 0033 14020 0283, www.christophe-robin.com

Clarins, tel: 0800 036 3558, www.clarins.co.uk

Clarks, tel: 08444 995544, www.clarks.co.uk

Clinique, tel: 0800 054 2666, www.clinique.co.uk

Cosmetic surgery: helpful organisations (see also Wendy Lewis, under 'W')

● British Academy of Cosmetic Dentistry, www.bacd.com

● The British Association of Aesthetic Plastic Surgeons, www.baaps.org.uk

● The British Association of Dermatologists (British Cosmetic Dermatology Group), www.bad.org.uk

● British Association of Oral and Maxillofacial Surgeons, www.baoms.org.uk

● The British Association of Otorhinolaryngologists, www.entuk.org

● British Association of Plastic, Reconstructive and Aesthetic Surgeons, www.bapras.org.uk

● British Oculoplastic Surgery Society, www.bopss.org

● The Care Quality Commission, www.cqc.org.uk

● The European Academy of Facial Plastic Surgery, www.eafps.org

● European Association of Plastic Surgeons, www.euraps.org

● European Society for Laser Dermatology, www.esld.org

● European Society of Plastic, Reconstructive and Aesthetic Surgery, www.espras.org

● General Medical Council, www.gmc-uk.org

● International Society of Aesthetic Plastic Surgery, www.isaps.org

● The Royal College of Anaesthetists, www.rcoa.ac.uk

Cosmetics à la Carte, tel: 020 7622 2318, www.cosmeticsalacarte.com

Cowshed, tel: 020 7534 0871, www.cowshedonline.con

Crème de la Mer, tel: 0800 054 2661, www.cremedelamer.co.uk

D

Daniel Galvin, tel: 020 7486 9661, www.danielgalvin.com

Darphin, tel: 0870 034 2318, www.darphin.co.uk

Dr David Cook, London Holistic Dental Centre, tel: 020 7323 1363, www.londonholisticdental.com

Davina Peace, tel: 020 7819 0262, www.davinapeace.com

Decléor, tel: 020 7313 8787, www.decleor.co.uk

Dental Miracle, from Victoria Health, tel: 0800 3898 195, www.victoriahealth.com

Dermalogica, tel: 0800 591818, www.dermalogica.com/uk

Dermol 500, from Victoria Health, tel: 0800 3898 195, www.victoriahealth.com

Dior, tel: 020 7216 0216, www.dior.com

Dr Brandt, from Space NK, tel: 020 8740 2085, www.spacenk.co.uk

Dr Hauschka, tel: 01386 791022, www.drhauschka.co.uk

E

Ecco, tel: 01590 679254, www.ecco-shoes-uk.co.uk

Electrolysis: British Institute & Association of Electrolysis, tel: 0844 544 1373, www.electrolysis.co.uk

Elemis, tel: 01278 727830, www.elemis.co.uk

Elizabeth Arden, www.elizabetharden.co.uk

Ellis Faas, www.ellisfaas.com

Emma Hardie, tel: 01923 839505, www.emmahardie.com

Erbaviva, from Love Lula, tel: 0870 242 6995, www.lovelula.com

Espa, tel: 01252 352231, www.espaonline.com

Essential Care, from Victoria Health, tel: 0800 3898 195, www.victoriahealth.com

Essie, tel: 0844 800 9396, www.nailsbymail.co.uk

Estée Lauder, tel: 0800 054 2444, www.esteelauder.co.uk

Eucerin, from Victoria Health, tel: 0800 3898 195, www.victoriahealth.com

Eve Lom, tel: 020 8740 2076, www.evelom.com

EyeSlices, from Victoria Health, tel: 0800 3898 195, www.victoriahealth.com

F

FitFlops, tel: 0845 359 9884, www.fitflop.com

G

Garnier, tel: 0800 085 4376, www.garnier.co.uk

Gillette Venus, www.gillettevenus.co.uk

Giorgio Armani, www.giorgioarmanibeauty.co.uk

Gossypium, tel: 0870 850 9953, www.gossypium.co.uk

Green Hands, from Victoria Health, tel: 0800 3898 195, www.victoriahealth.com

Green People, from Victoria Health, tel: 0800 3898 195, www.victoriahealth.com

Guerlain, www.guerlain.com

H

Hästens, www.hastens.com

Head & Shoulders, tel: 0800 731 2892, www.headandshoulders.co.uk

Heal Gel, from Victoria Health, tel: 0800 3898 195, www.victoriahealth.com

Huiles & Baumes, from House of Fraser, www.houseoffraser.co.uk

Hypnos, tel: 01844 348200, www.hypnosbeds.com

I

Ikea, tel: 0845 358 3363, www.ikea.com

Ila, tel: 01608 677676, www.ila-spa.com

Inika, tel: 020 7494 4571, www.inikacosmetics.co.uk

Inlight, from Victoria Health, tel: 0800 3898 195, www.victoriahealth.com

Institut Esthederm, from Space NK, tel: 020 8740 2085, www.spacenk.co.uk

J

Jane Scrivner, tel: 07899 906957, www.janescrivner.com

Jason, from Victoria Health, tel: 0800 3898 195, www.victoriahealth.com

Jemma Kidd, tel: 0844 800 2636, www.jemmakidd.com

Jenny Jordan Eyebrow and Make-up Clinic, tel: 020 7483 2222, www.jennyjordan.co.uk

Jessica Vartoughian, www.jessica-nails.co.uk

JetRest eye masks, from Victoria Health, tel: 0800 389 8195, www.victoriahealth.com

Jo Hansford, tel: 020 7409 7020, www.johansford.com

John Frieda, tel: 020 7491 0840, www.johnfrieda.com

John Scurr, tel: 020 7730 9563, www.thelisterhospital.com

Joico, available from salons nationwide, www.joico.com

Professor Jon Kabat-Zinn, Mindfulness-Based Cognitive Therapy, www.mbct.co.uk

Jurlique, tel: 020 3205 3845, www.jurlique.co.uk

K

Dr Karen Burke, tel: 00 1 212 754 1100, www.empowereddoctor.com

Kérastase, www.kerastase.co.uk

Kevin Murphy, tel: 01179 270434, www.kevinmurphystore.com

Kiehl's, tel: 020 7240 2411, www.kiehls.co.uk

Kimberly Sayer, from Love Lula, tel: 0870 242 6995, www.lovelula.com

Korres, from www.lookfantastic.com

L

La Clarée, tel: 0800 027 1102, www.laclaree.co.uk

Label.m, tel: 0870 770 8080, www.labelm.co.uk

Lancôme, www.lancome.co.uk

Lanolips, from Victoria Health, tel: 0800 3898 195, www.victoriahealth.com

La Prairie, www.laprairie.com

Laura Mercier, from Space NK, tel: 020 8740 2085, www.spacenk.co.uk

Lavera, tel: 01557 870266, www.lavera.co.uk

Lee Stafford, www.leestafford.com

Liz Earle Naturally Active Skincare, tel: 01983 813913, www.lizearle.com

L'Occitane, tel: 020 7907 0301, www.loccitane.com

L'Oréal, tel: 0800 030 4032, www.loreal-paris.co.uk

Lotus Journeys, www.lotusjourneys.com

Louise Galvin, tel: 0800 334 5933, www.louisegalvin.com

Lulu, tel: 0844 800 1694, www.lulusplace.co.uk

Lulu & Boo, tel: 029 2040 0036, www.luluandboo.com

Lumosity, www.lumosity.com

M

MAC, www.maccosmetics.co.uk

Mádara, tel: 01557 870266, www.madara-cosmetics.com

Margaret Dabbs, tel: 020 7487 5510, www.margaretdabbs.co.uk

Marie Veronique Organics, www.mvorganics.com

Marks & Spencer, tel: 0845 609 0200, www.marksandspencer.com

Mason Pearson, tel: 020 7491 2613, www.masonpearson.com

Matrix, tel: 0845 601 0122, www.matrixhaircare.co.uk

Maybelline, tel: 0845 399 0304, www.maybelline.co.uk

McTimoney Chiropractic, tel: 01491 829211, www.mctimoneychiropractic.org

Medik8, tel: 020 8997 8541, www.medik8.co.uk

Melvita, tel: 0800 138 7045, www.melvita.com

Michael Dooley, The Poundbury Clinic, tel: 01305 262626, www.thepoundburyclinic.co.uk

Monu, tel: 0870 220 9094, www.monushop.co.uk

Dr Mosaraf Ali, The Integrated Medical Centre, tel: 020 7224 5111, www.integratedmed.co.uk

Murad, from Victoria Health, tel: 0800 3898 195, www.victoriahealth.com

MV Organic Skincare, tel: 020 3075 1006, www.mvskincare.co.uk

MyFace Cosmetics, tel: 0844 335 6492, www.myfacecosmetics.co.uk

N

Nadia Brydon, practitioner of Western and Chinese herbal medicine, acupuncture and homeopathy, email: nadia@chanters.fsnet.co.uk

Nails Inc, tel: 020 7529 2340, www.nailsinc.com

Natio, from Debenhams, tel: 08445 616161, www.debenhams.com

Natura Bissé, www.naturabisse.es

Neal's Yard Remedies, from Victoria Health, tel: 0800 3898 195, www.victoriahealth.com

New CID Cosmetics, www.newcidcosmetics.com

Nia 24, from Space NK, tel: 020 8740 2085, www.spacenk.co.uk

Dr Nick Lowe, The Cranley Clinic, tel: 020 7499 3223, www.drnicklowe.com

Nivea, www.nivea.co.uk

No7, www.boots.com

Nude, tel: 0800 634 4366, www.nudeskincare.com

O

Ojon, tel: 0870 034 2454, www.ojon.co.uk

Ole Henriksen, www.olehenriksen.com

Origins, tel: 0800 054 2888, www.origins.co.uk

Orly, tel: 01827 280080, www.orlybeauty.co.uk

Oskia, tel: 01600 710710, www.oskiaskincare.com

P

Palmer's, from Victoria Health, tel: 0800 3898 195, www.victoriahealth.com

Paul Mitchell, tel: 0845 659 0012, www.paul-mitchell.co.uk

Per-fékt, www.perfektbeauty.com

Philip B, www.philipb.com

Phil Smith, www.philsmithhair.com

Philosophy, from www.HQhair.com

Pilates:
● **The Pilates Foundation**, tel: 020 7033 0078, www.pilatesfoundation.com

● **Body Control Pilates Association**, tel: 020 7636 8900, www.bodycontrol.co.uk

Pinks Boutique, tel: 01332 204804, www.pinksboutique.com

Pixi, www.pixibeauty.com

prAna Yoga Mats, from www.yogastudio.co.uk

Provenance, from Victoria Health, tel: 0800 3898 195, www.victoriahealth.com

Prtty Peaushun, www.prttypeaushun.com

Pureology, tel: 0800 783 3026, www.pureology-uk.com

Q

Qtica, tel: 01753 573423, www.nailcareclub.com

R

REN, tel: 020 7724 2900, www.renskincare.com

Renu, see Monu above

Repêchage, www.repechageuk.com

RéVive, www.reviveskincare.com

RevitaLash, tel: 01209 617146, www.skinbrands.co.uk

Revlon, tel: 0800 085 2716, www.revlon.com

Rigby & Peller, tel: 0845 076 5545, www.rigbyandpeller.com

Rimmel, www.rimmellondon.com

Rituals, tel: 0845 602 5446, www.rituals.com

Rodial, tel: 020 7351 1720, www.rodial.co.uk

Roja Dove, www.rojadove.com

S

Sarah Chapman, tel: 020 7589 9585, www.skinesis.com

Sebastian Professional, www.sebastianprofessional.co.uk

Sensodyne, www.sensodyne.co.uk

Serious Readers lamps, tel: 0800 028 1890, www.seriousreaders.com

Seven Wonders, from Victoria Health, tel: 0800 3898 195, www.victoriahealth.com

Shoe Therapy, www.shoetherapy.com

Shower water filters:
● Ethical Superstore, tel: 0845 009 9016, www.ethicalsuperstore.com
● Pure Showers, tel: 0800 612 7174, www.pureshowers.co.uk

Shu Uemura, tel: 020 7240 7635, www.shuuemura.co.uk

Sisley, tel: 020 7591 6380, www.sisley-cosmetics.co.uk

Soap & Glory, www.soapandglory.com

Space NK, tel: 020 8740 2085, www.spacenk.co.uk

St Tropez, tel: 0115 983 6363, www.st-tropez.com

Steve Mason, tel: 01273 771441, www.brightonacupuncture andmassage.co.uk

Sue Devitt, from Harvey Nichols, tel: 020 7235 5000, www.harveynichols.com

Susan Posnick, www.susanposnick.com

Suzie Mitchell, tel: 01424 430389, www.spaghetti-tree.com

T

T'ai chi: The UK T'ai Chi Association, tel: 020 7407 4775, www.taichiuk.co.uk

Taryn Rose, from Footwise, tel: 01483 455586, www.footwiseuk.com

Temple Spa, from Victoria Health, tel: 0800 3898 195, www.victoriahealth.com

Terra Plana, tel: 01458 449081, www.terraplana.com

Thalgo, www.thalgo.com

This Works, tel: 020 8543 3544, www.thisworks.com

Tim Hutchful, The British Chiropractic Association, tel: 0118 950 5950, www.chiropractic-uk.co.uk

Tom's of Maine, www.tomsofmaine.co.uk

TRI-AKTILINE, from www.boots.com

Trilogy, from Victoria Health, tel: 0800 3898 195, www.victoriahealth.com

Trish McEvoy, www.trishmcevoy.com

Tweezerman, www.tweezerman.co.uk

U

Ugg, tel: 01475 746000, www.uggaustralia.com/gb

Une, www.unebeauty.com

Upper Canada Soap, tel: 01277 220842, www.uppercanadasoap.com

Urban Retreat, tel: 020 7893 8333, www.urbanretreat.co.uk

V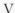

Vaishaly Patel, tel: 020 7486 7705 (products); tel: 020 7224 6088 (clinic), www.vaishaly.com

Valerie Beverly Hills, from Victoria Health, tel: 0800 3898 195, www.victoriahealth.com

Vaseline Intensive Care, www.vaseline.co.uk

Vichy, tel: 0800 169 6193, www.vichyconsult.co.uk

Viscotears, widely available at chemists

W

Weleda, from Victoria Health, tel: 0800 3898 195, www.victoriahealth.com

Wendy Lewis, tel: 00 1 212 861 6148, www.wlbeauty.com email: wl@wlbeauty.com Wendy Lewis Beauty Forum: www.beautyinthebag.com facebook.com/beautyinthebag twitter.com/beautyinthebag

Wild Organics, tel: 01955 609064, www.wildorganicsbeauty.com

X

Xyliwhite, from Victoria Health, tel: 0800 3898 195, www.victoriahealth.com

Y

Yes to Carrots, from Victoria Health, tel: 0800 3898 195, www.victoriahealth.com

Yes to Tomatoes, from Victoria Health, tel: 0800 389 8195, www.victoriahealth.com

Yoga: British Wheel of Yoga, tel: 01529 306851, www.bwy.org.uk

Youngblood, tel: 0845 246 4666, www.ybskin.co.uk

YSL, www.ysl.com

ANTI-AGEING BOOKSHELF

Food Rules by Michael Pollan (Penguin)

Healing Without Freud or Prozac by Dr David Servan-Schreiber (Rodale International)

I Feel Bad about My Neck by Nora Ephron (Black Swan)

The Lowdown on Facelifts and Other Wrinkle Remedies by Wendy Lewis (Quadrille)

Plastic Makes Perfect by Wendy Lewis (Orion)

The New Yoga for People Over 50 by Suza Francina (Health Communications)

Yoga and the Wisdom of Menopause by Suza Francina (Health Communications)

Yoga Builds Bones by Jan Maddern (Element)

The Yoga Facelift by Marie-Véronique Nadeau (Conari Press)

The Ultimate Natural Beauty Book by Josephine Fairley (Kyle Cathie)

DVD:
Yoga for Beginners by Patricia Walden (from www.yogastudio.co.uk)

Index

Acknowledgements

This book is the result of decades of research. We would like to thank all the friends, colleagues and experts worldwide who have helped us so generously over the years. Also our doughty and dedicated teams of testers, without whose commitment to trialling products and writing up their findings, Beauty Bible wouldn't be here.

A vast vote of thanks to our illustrator David Downton (who's also included in the dedication), who has surpassed himself – and made us laugh a lot too: our Beauty Bible publications would not be so stylish and beautiful without his support and super-talented input.

Particular thanks to:

Maggie Alderson
Bobbi Brown
Nadia Brydon
Dr Karen Burke
Sarah Chapman
Professor Charles
  Clark
Dr David Cook
Margaret Dabbs
Barbara Daly OBE
Shabir Daya
Carmen dell'Orefice
Michael Dooley
Roja Dove
Liz Earle MBE
Mary Greenwell
Terry de Gunzburg
Newby Hands
Tim Hutchful
Eve Lom
Dr Nick Lowe
Lulu
Trish McEvoy
Lorna McKnight
Annee de Mamiel
Dr Andrew Markey
Laura Mercier
Suzie Mitchell
Marie-Véronique
  Nadeau
Tim Petersen
Philip B
Kathy Phillips
John Scurr
Gill Sinclair
Dr Andrew Weil
Andreas Wild

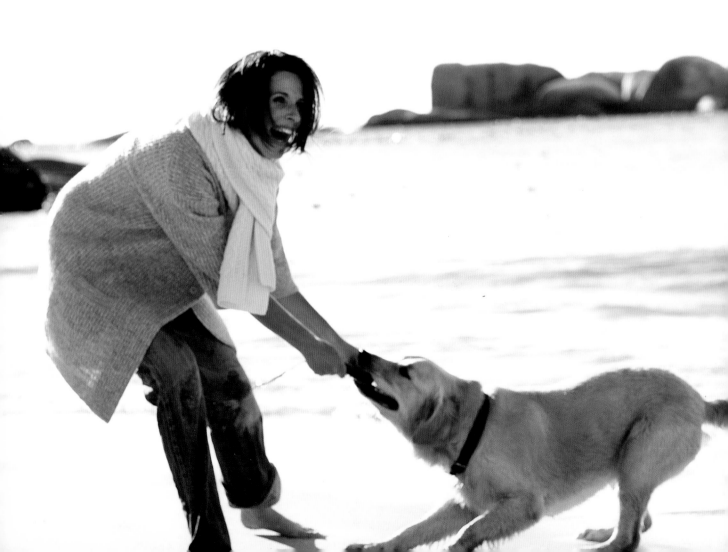

Photo acknowledgements

We would also like to thank a raft of beauty PRs who supported us so efficiently with our project but would need an extra book to include them all. But special thanks go to Emma Dawson and her team at L'Oréal; Sarah Griffiths and her team at Estée Lauder Companies; Julietta Longcroft and Tom Konig Oppenheimer at TCS (who went so far as to appoint a special 'Beauty Bible Liaison Officer', Ellie Howden, who we also thank); Nancy Brady and all at NBPR; Jenny Halpern and her crew at Halpern PR; Jo Fox Tutchener and Michelle Boon at Beautyseen; Rick Havemann at www.avea.co.uk; Fiona Dowal, Owen Walker, Max Flower and the team at Modus Dowal Walker; Phily Keeling at Chanel; Lesley Chilvers at Bourjois; Kate Hudson and Helen Mitchell at Guerlain; Jazz Kaur at Benefit (who helped us with this book wearing her former Guerlain chapeau); Aude Chatelin at Dior; Carri Kilpatrick and the Kilpatrick PR team; Kelly Marks and all at Pure PR – plus everyone at Liz Earle (especially Kim Buckland, who set up Liz Earle Naturally Active Skincare with Liz herself).

Thanks to our publisher Kyle Cathie, as ever, and to our colleagues at YOU magazine, Sue Peart, Catherine Fenton and Rosalind Lowe.

And, of course, to our wonderful Beauty Bible team (see dedication).

Title page Plainpicture/beyond
p7 Adrian Peacock, Charlotte Murphy
p9 Icon Photo/C.Watts
p10-11 Kellie Hindmarch
p14-15 Photolibrary/D&L Jacobs
p20 www.urbanlip.com
p22 Photolibrary
p26 Rex Features/T.Logan
p32 Getty/E.Estabrook
p35 Camera Press London/Brigitte
p36 Plainpicture/Ableimages
p39 www.urbanlip.com
p40 www.urbanlip.com
p45 Camera Press London/B.Coster
p46-47 www.urbanlip.com
p50-51 Photolibrary/Photoalto
p52-53 Photolibrary/B.Lark
p54 Photolibrary/Superstock Inc
p57 www.urbanlip.com
p58 Corbis/S.Prezant
p61 Trunk Archive.com/A.Bettles
p63 Getty/Superstudio
p65 Photolibrary/Imagesource
p66 Getty/J.Tisne
p67 Getty/B.Yee
p69 Photolibrary/M.Constantini
p71 Photolibrary/Photoalto
p75 Photolibrary/S.Zulawinski
p79 www.urbanlip.com
p81 Photolibrary/J.Feingersh
p83 Photolibrary/B.Vogel;
p86 Camera Press London/*Journal für die Frau*
p92 Getty/P.de Villiers
p94 Photolibrary/C.Sharp
p97 Photolibrary/T.Kruesselmann
p98 Plainpicture/applypictures
p106 Trunk Archive.com/H.Salinas
p106 Camera Press London/J.Veysey
p106 Corbis
p106 Photolibrary/Z.Smith
p106 Getty/A.Mo
p107 Rex Features/Col Pics/Everett
p107 Camera Press London/J.Veysey
p107 Camera Press London/C.Djanogly

p108 Getty/Tedfoo
p115 Trunk Archive.com/Pamela Hanson/ Hair: Julien d'Ys/Make-up: Stephane Marais
p122 Photolibrary/It Stock RF
p125 Photolibrary/F.Wirth
p129 Photolibrary/B.Erlinger
p132 Photolibrary/A.Oliel
p133 www.urbanlip.com
p139 Photolibrary/Photoalto
p140 Photolibrary/B.Lark
p143 Getty/Dorling Kindersley
p144 Photolibrary/R. Kaufma/L. Hirshowitz
p146 Photolibrary/Radius Images
p151 www.urbanlip.com
p153 Photolibrary/M.Burkhart/Corbis
p154 Photolibrary/Stockbrokerxtra images
p158-159 Photolibrary/Fancy
p161 Photolibrary/Fotosearch
p165 Getty/B.Fraker
p166 Tim Petersen
p168-169 Photolibrary/Pixtal Images
p171 Photolibrary/Corbis
p173 Photolibrary/F.Cirou
p177 Camera Press London/Titti Fabi
p178 www.urbanlip.com
p179 Photolibrary/J.Klee
p181 Getty/A.Rohmer
p182-183 Photolibrary/Tetra Images
p185 Photolibrary/C.Chiossone/Photex
p186 Magnum Photos/Robert Capa/International Centre of Photography
p189 Getty/T.Barwick
p191 www.urbanlip.com
p193 Photolibrary RF
p194 Photolibrary/Uppercut Images
p196 Photolibrary/M.Anderson
p201 Photolibrary/Emotive Image
p202 Photolibrary/P.Leonard;
p204-205 Photolibrary/Innerhofer Photodesign
p207 Getty/LaCoppola-Meier
p208-209 Magnum Photos/Eve Arnold
p210-211 Arcangel/R.Musyhiar
p213 www.urbanlip.com
Acknowledgements page www.urbanlip.com

We would like to dedicate this book to the Beauty Bible 'team' who worked so hard to help us make it happen: Sally Cole, David Downton, Amy Eason, David Edmunds, Jessie Lawrence, Ben Lovegrove, Liz Murray, Jenny Semple, and also to our divine agent Kay McCauley, who we want to be like – and look as good as – when we grow up...

This edition published in Great Britain in 2011 by
Kyle Books,
23 Howland Street,
London W1T 4AY
email: general.enquiries@kylebooks.com
website: www.kylebooks.com

First published in Great Britain in 2011 by Kyle Cathie Ltd

ISBN: 978 1 85626 945 2

Design: Jenny Semple
Illustrations: David Downton
Copy editor: Liz Murray
Picture researcher: Sally Cole, Perseverance Works Ltd
Production: Gemma John, Sheila Smith and Nic Jones

Colour reproduction by Scanhouse in Malaysia
Printed and bound in Slovenia by DZS